Manual of Outpatient Gynecology
Fourth Edition

Manual of Outpatient Gynecology
Fourth Edition

Editors

Carol S. Havens, M.D.
Associate Clinical Professor of Family Practice
University of California, Davis, School of Medicine
Staff Physician, Chemical Dependency Clinic
Kaiser Permanente Medical Center, Sacramento
Director, Clinical Education
Northern California Region
Kaiser Permanente, Oakland, California

Nancy D. Sullivan, M.S., F.N.P.
Staff Nurse Practitioner, Department of Medicine
Kaiser Permanente Medical Clinic
Vacaville, California
Clinical Instructor
Holy Names College
Oakland, California

LIPPINCOTT WILLIAMS & WILKINS
A **Wolters Kluwer** Company
Philadelphia · Baltimore · New York · London
Buenos Aires · Hong Kong · Sydney · Tokyo

Acquisitions Editor: Richard Winters
Developmental Editor: Jenny Kim
Production Editor: Thomas Boyce
Manufacturing Manager: Colin J. Warnock
Cover Designer: Jeane Norton
Compositor: Circle Graphics
Printer: Vicks Litho

Printed in the USA

Library of Congress Cataloging-in-Publication Data

ISBN 0-7817-3278-6

Care has been taken to confirm the accuracy of the information presented and to describe generally accepted practices. However, the authors, editors, and publisher are not responsible for errors or omissions or for any consequences from application of the information in this book and make no warranty, expressed or implied, with respect to the currency, completeness, or accuracy of the contents of the publication. Application of this information in a particular situation remains the professional responsibility of the practitioner.

The authors, editors, and publisher have exerted every effort to ensure that drug selection and dosage set forth in this text are in accordance with current recommendations and practice at the time of publication. However, in view of ongoing research, changes in government regulations, and the constant flow of information relating to drug therapy and drug reactions, the reader is urged to check the package insert for each drug for any change in indications and dosage and for added warnings and precautions. This is particularly important when the recommended agent is a new or infrequently employed drug.

Some drugs and medical devices presented in this publication have Food and Drug Administration (FDA) clearance for limited use in restricted research settings. It is the responsibility of the health care provider to ascertain the FDA status of each drug or device planned for use in their clinical practice.

10 9 8 7 6 5 4 3 2 1

To our mothers,
who had the stamina and courage
to raise us to be the best that we can be

CONTENTS

CONTRIBUTING AUTHORS

Victor Chan, M.D.
Department of Obstetrics and Gynecology, University of California, Davis, Medical Center, Sacramento, California

Victor P. Chin, M.D., M.P.A.
Chief, Department of Obstetrics and Gynecology, Kaiser Permanente Medical Center, Oakland, California

Mary Ciotti, M.D.
Department of Obstetrics and Gynecology, University of California, Davis, Medical Center, Sacramento, California

Jeanne A. Conry, M.D., PH.D.
Staff Physician, Obstetrics and Gynecology, Kaiser Permanente Medical Center, Roseville, California

Condessa M. Curley, M.D., M.P.H.
Clinical Instructor, Maternal Child Health Fellow, Family Health Center, Los Angeles, California

Raymond Frink, M.D., PH.D.
Staff Physician, Obstetrics and Gynecology, Kaiser Permanente Medical Center, Roseville, California

Harley Goldberg, D.O.
Director of Complementary and Alternative Medicine, Oakland, California

William M. Green, M.D.
Clinical Professor, Emergency Medicine, University of California, Davis, School of Medicine, Sacramento, California

Kenneth Griffis, M.D.
Department of Obstetrics and Gynecology, University of Mississippi Medical Center, Jackson, Mississippi

Carol S. Havens, M.D.
Associate Clinical Professor of Family Practice, University of California, Davis, School of Medicine; Staff Physician, Chemical Dependency Clinic, Kaiser Permanente Medical Center, Sacramento; Director, Clinical Education, Northern California Region, Kaiser Permanente, Oakland, California

Rebecca King, M.D.
Department of Obstetrics and Gynecology, University of California, Davis, Medical Center, Sacramento, California

Cheryl L. Lambing, M.D.
Medical Education Office, Ventura County Medical Center, Family Practice Residency, Ventura, California

Gary S. Leiserowitz, M.D.
Associate Professor, Department of Obstetrics and Gynecology, Division of Gynecologic Oncology, University of California, Davis, School of Medicine, Sacramento, California

Arthur F. Levit, M.D.
Assistant Chief and Residency Program Director, Department of Obstetrics and Gynecology, Kaiser Permanente Medical Center, Oakland, California

Mary K. Miller, PHARM.D., M.D.
Associate Clinical Professor, University of California, Davis, Clinical Medical Director, Department of Obstetrics and Gynecology, HIV Gynecology, CARES— Sacramento (Center for AIDS Research, Education, and Services), Department of Obstetrics and Gynecology, University of California, Davis, Medical Center, Sacramento, California

Michael J. Murray, M.D.
Clinical Assistant Professor, Department of Obstetrics and Gynecology, University of California, Davis, School of Medicine, Sacramento; Director, Division of Reproductive Endocrinology and Infertility, Kaiser Permanente Medical Center, Sacramento, California

Richard H. Oi, M.D.
Professor Emeritus, Clinical Obstetrics and Gynecology and Pathology, Department of Obstetrics and Gynecology, University of California, Davis, Medical Center, Sacramento, California

Clara K. Paik, M.D.
Associate Professor, Division of Gynecology, University of California, Davis, Medical Center, Sacramento, California

Maureen Park, M.D.
Department of Obstetrics and Gynecology, University of California, Davis, Medical Center, Sacramento, California

Kara Riley-Paull, M.D.
Department of Surgery, Kaiser Permanente Medical Center, Walnut Creek, California

Michel E. Rivlin, M.D.
Associate Professor, Department of Obstetrics and Gynecology, University of Mississippi Medical Center, Jackson, Mississippi

Patricia A. Robertson, M.D.
Associate Professor, Director, Medical Student Education in the Department of Obstetrics, Gynecology, and Reproductive Sciences, University of California, San Francisco, San Francisco, California

Caryn Rybczynski, M.D.
Department of Obstetrics and Gynecology, Kaiser Permanente Medical Center, Hayward, California

Patricia R. Salber, M.D.
Medical Director, Managed Care, General Motors Corporation in conjunction with the Permanente Company, Co-founder and Co-President, Physicians for a Violence-free Society, Larkspur, California

Nancy D. Sullivan, M.S., F.N.P.
Staff Nurse Practitioner, Department of Medicine, Kaiser Permanente Medical Clinic, Vacaville; Clinical Instructor, Holy Names College, Nurse Practitioner Program, Oakland, California

Kathleen E. Taylor, M.D., F.A.C.O.G.
Department of Obstetrics and Gynecology, Kaiser Permanente Medical Center, Hayward, California

Stephen E. Thorn, M.D., F.A.C.O.G.
Staff Physician, Obstetrics and Gynecology, Alberta Lea Medical Center, Mayo Health Care System, Albert Lea, Minnesota

Patti Tilton, M.D.
Staff Physician, Department of Obstetrics and Gynecology, Kaiser Permanente South Sacramento Medical Center, Sacramento, California

Gerald W. Upcraft, M.D.
Department of Obstetrics and Gynecology, Kaiser Permanente Medical Center, Sacramento, California

Janet M. Walker, M.D.
Department of Obstetrics and Gynecology, Kaiser Permanente Medical Center, Roseville, California

Ty Yarnel, L.C.S.W.
Auburn, California

PREFACE

Manual of Outpatient Gynecology, Fourth Edition, is a practical text designed to aid in the treatment of outpatient gynecologic problems. It is meant to emphasize office diagnosis and treatment for the most frequently encountered problems and various sensitive subjects encountered in office medicine.

Women are often the health care monitors for family members and frequently ask questions regarding different age groups. Since there is a heightened interest in herbal and vitamin remedies, various "natural" treatments have been added to several chapters throughout the manual, and a chapter has been devoted to complimentary and alternative medicine. The health care maintenance chapter includes updated recommendations for health care maintenance for all age groups. Discussions of inpatient management and of most surgical therapies are beyond the scope of this book.

The *Manual* is intended for anyone treating gynecologic problems, including gynecologists, family physicians, internists, house officers, medical students, nurse practitioners, and physician assistants.

We have kept the format practical and simple. Each chapter covers a specific issue and is written in an outline format with headings that include, but are not limited to, history, physical examination, investigative procedures, and management. Some chapters have tables that can also be used for patient handouts. Each chapter also includes references for the reader who desires more comprehensive information.

C.S.H.
N.D.S.

ACKNOWLEDGMENTS

Our heartfelt gratitude is extended to all who have contributed their expertise and time to this edition. The contributors and editors from the third edition are indeed included in our thanks, for without them there would never have been a fourth one. We also acknowledge Jenny Kim of Lippincott Williams & Wilkins for her assistance and gentle prodding.

We personally thank Kyra and Jessica for their support and patience during this edition.

Notice: The indications and dosages of all drugs in this book have been recommended in the medical literature and conform to the practices of the general medical community. The medications described do not necessarily have specific approval by the Food and Drug Administration for use in the diseases and dosages for which they are recommended. The package insert for each drug should be consulted for use and dosage as approved by the FDA. Because standards for usage change, it is advisable to keep abreast of revised recommendations, particularly those concerning new drugs.

1. VULVOVAGINITIS

Nancy D. Sullivan and Caryn Rybczynski

Vulvovaginitis is the most common of all outpatient gynecologic problems and accounts for 10% of office visits annually for the primary care provider (35). The diagnostic accuracy with patients complaining of vaginal irritation, odor, and discharge has been enhanced over the past several years by a greater understanding of bacterial vaginosis (BV). By using current knowledge and simple office laboratory methods, a precise etiologic diagnosis can be made in more than 95% of patients. These patients can be divided into five diagnostic categories, each with different management strategies. In a study of vaginal infections or discharges in 20,000 consecutive patients, BV was the most common diagnosis (33%), followed by cervicitis (20%–25%); monilial infection (20.5%); excessive, but otherwise normal, secretions (10%); *Trichomonas* (9.8%); and diagnosis undetermined (2%–5%) (10).

The approach to diagnosing the patient with vulvovaginitis consists of a careful history, pelvic examination, and microscopic examination of the vaginal fluid as well as assessment of vaginal pH and amine tests. All of these parts of the evaluation contribute to, and are essential for, a precise diagnosis.

A normal physiologic vaginal discharge consists of cervical and vaginal secretions, epithelial cells, and bacterial flora. The normal vaginal pH is 3.8 to 4.2. A physiologic vaginal discharge is usually white and odorless, and does not cause itching, burning, or other discomfort. The amount of discharge varies with the day of the menstrual cycle. The normal vaginal flora consists of primarily Lactobacillus as well as streptococci, staphylococci, diphtheroids, *Gardnerella vaginalis, E. coli,* and several anaerobic organisms. *Candida* and *Mycoplasma* species are also commonly found.

This chapter describes the evaluation and treatment of the common causes of vulvovaginitis. These are candidiasis; BV *(Gardnerella), Trichomonas,* cervicitis; chemical or irritative causes; and atrophic vulvovaginitis. Sexually transmitted diseases (STDs) such as herpes genitalis, chlamydia, and gonorrhea, are discussed in Chapter 3.

I. **History.** The classic presentation of vaginitis is found in fewer than 33% of cases. The discharge color, presence of pruritus, and the color of the cervix may lead to inappropriate diagnosis and therapy. **Treatment based on symptoms alone has been clearly shown to be inaccurate and should be avoided.**

The following questions should be asked of all women presenting with any vulvovaginitis complaint:

A. **Current symptoms**
  1. Focus on changes from her personal norm.
  2. **Discharge.** Most women have some degree of leukorrhea. "How is the current discharge different?"
  3. **Odor**
    a. Is there **any** odor?
    b. Is the odor **constant**?
    c. Does the odor occur **after coitus**?
  4. **Pruritus**
    a. Is there a **pattern** to the itching?
    b. Does the itching seem to be **internal, external,** or **both**?
  5. **Burning**
    a. Is there burning **with urination**?
    b. Does the burning occur **while urinating**?
    c. Does the burning occur as the **urine touches the skin**?
  6. **How long have the symptoms been occurring?**
    a. What makes them better?
    b. What makes them worse?

This chapter is a revision of the third edition chapter by Nancy D. Sullivan.

1

7. Skin irritation or lesions
   a. Is the skin irritated?
      (1) What areas are involved?
         (a) Vulva
         (b) Vagina
         (c) Rectum
   b. Is there a history of **sensitive** skin?
   c. Is there a history of **dry** skin?
   d. Is there any rash or sore on any part of the body?
8. Sexual activity
   a. Are the sexual partners male, female, or both?
   b. Are the **symptoms increased** with sexual activity?
   c. In the past year, has there been **more than one coitus** partner?
   d. Is the **sexual partner** in a **monogamous relationship** with the patient?
   e. Is there a **need** for **contraception**?
9. Medication and **contraceptives.** Medications, contraceptives, and barrier methods have **all been contributory causes** for vulvovaginitis, consequently, they all need to be identified.
10. Menses history
   a. Date of last menstrual period (LMP).
   b. Do the **symptoms** occur in any **relationship** to the menstrual cycle?
   c. Is the patient **pregnant**?
11. Feminine hygiene products. Some women use over-the-counter (OTC) sprays, perfume, or douches, or a combination thereof, regularly. If this practice is identified, it should be discouraged. These **products can be the cause of vulvovaginitis.**
12. Recurring vulvovaginitis symptoms need to include the following questions:
   a. Have any medications **caused itching**?
   b. Have any medications **caused burning**?
   c. What **medications have been used** for this problem? It's important to recognize that many women will have tried OTC therapies or will have been prescribed a medication after a telephone consultation only.
      (1) Miconazole (Monistat)
      (2) Terconazole (Terazol)
      (3) Ketoconazole
      (4) Clotrimazole (Gyne-Lotrimin)
      (5) Metronidazole (Flagyl)
      (6) Antibiotics
      (7) Hydrocortisone
      (8) Estrogen cream
      (9) Acyclovir (Zovirax)
      (10) Fluorouracil (5-FU) cream
      (11) Others including OTCs
   d. Systemic diseases. Some systemic diseases **can cause vulvovaginitis** symptoms leading the provider to potentially conclude an inaccurate diagnosis. A few of these include:
      (1) Diabetes mellitus
      (2) Acquired immunodeficiency syndrome (AIDS)
      (3) Rheumatoid arthritis
      (4) Lupus
      (5) Hodgkin's disease
      (6) Leukemia
      (7) Skin diseases such as **psoriasis** and **eczema**
II. Physical examination (PE). The PE must include the vulva, vagina, and cervix. On occasion, the uterus, ovaries, and rectum also need to be evaluated. When **managing difficult or recurring cases** of vulvovaginitis, the **goal of the PE shifts to identifying cutaneous lesions** (which may need biopsy); **obtaining**

vaginal secretions for further evaluation; and **investigating the possibility of obscure diagnoses,** such as rectovaginal fistula, vesicovaginal fistula, bladder leakage, and urethral diverticulum.

III. **Laboratory procedures**

    A. **Saline and potassium hydroxide (KOH) preparations** generally take less than 3 minutes yet are **invaluable** in identifying what is or is not causing the vulvovaginitis complaint. If there is an excess of white blood cells (WBCs), a mixed infection must be considered.

    B. **Cultures** of the vaginal fluids or cervix **may be necessary** to clarify the diagnosis.

    C. **The pH** of the normal vaginal discharge is 3.8 to 4.2. An alkaline pH suggests BV or *T. vaginalis.*

IV. **Vulvovaginal candidiasis** (VVC), **formerly called monilia or candidiasis,** is a common fungal infection of the vulva and vagina caused by *Candida albicans, Candida tropicalis, Candida glabrata* (formerly *Torulopsis glabrata*), and *Candida parapsilosis.* Since the 1980s, the incidence of non-*C. albicans* infection has more than doubled and now accounts for more than 21% of cases.

It has been estimated that 75% of all women will have an episode of candida vaginitis at least once and as many as 40% to 50% will have recurrent infections. A small subpopulation, **approximately 5%, will have several recurrent, often intractable episodes of VVC.**

Sexual intercourse is not the means of transmission because these organisms are part of the endogenous flora in up to 50% of asymptomatic women. Environmental changes in the vagina, including the vaginal flora, result in the infection. Predisposing factors for VVC include diabetes, systemic antibiotics, pregnancy, use of oral contraceptives or corticosteroids, tight clothing, obesity, warm weather, and a decreased host immunity to *Candida* species.

    A. **History.** The symptoms of VVC depend on the degree and location of tissue inflammation.

        1. In mild cases, the most common complaint is **pruritus.**

        2. As the disease progresses, **burning, soreness,** and **dyspareunia** occur.

        3. **Dysuria** is a common symptom of VVC in the urethra and must be distinguished from infection of the urinary tract to avoid the inappropriate use of antibiotics.

        4. **Vaginal discharge may not be present;** however, some patients describe a characteristic white curd drainage.

    B. **Physical examination**

        1. Monilial infection of the vulva and vagina may cause **erythema.**

        2. **Occasionally,** excoriation from scratching and small red satellite lesions are present on the vulva.

        3. If present, the curdlike discharge may be localized or may coat the entire vagina.

        4. **In severe cases,** vulvar edema and tissue fissuring may occur.

    C. **Investigative procedures**

        1. A **wet-mount preparation** with saline or 10% KOH demonstrates pseudohyphae and spores in most patients (Fig. 1.1). When these are present, the diagnosis is confirmed. They may be absent, however, in a significant number of cases because non-*Albicans* species may not be readily identifiable on KOH.

        2. When pseudohyphae and spores are not seen, the clinician must decide whether to treat on the basis of signs and/or symptoms or to obtain a culture.

            a. A **gonorrhea culture** can also be used as a yeast culture since *Candida* grows on Thayer-Martin medium despite the presence of nystatin.

            b. **Culture media,** such as Sabouraud's or Nickerson's, should be used. Growth is evident within 1 to 3 days.

            c. The **presence of** *C. albicans* in the **absence of clinical disease** is not diagnostic of candidal vaginitis.

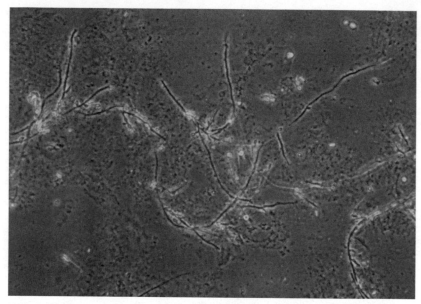

FIG. 1.1. Pseudohyphae and spores of *Candida* on wet smear. (Reproduced with permission from Fleury FJ. Adult vaginitis. *Clin Obstet Gynecol* 1981;24:407.)

    D. Management. It is often helpful to classify candidiasis as uncomplicated or complicated to facilitate the selection and duration of therapy.

        Uncomplicated *Candida vaginitis* is infection that occurs in a normal, healthy woman and involves symptoms that are sporadic and infrequent and not chronic or recurrent. Most often the symptoms have been present for 48 to 72 hours. In this setting, most patients do very well with a short course of therapy, regardless of whether it is topical or oral.

        Complicated candidiasis represents approximately 10% of all cases and includes:
- Severe infection with severe vulvovaginal signs and symptoms including severe erythema, edema, severity pruritus, and dyspareunia.
- Recurrent disease, that is four or more episodes in the last 12 months.
- Evidence, on wet-mount KOH, of budding yeast but not hyphal elements, which increases the likelihood of *C. glabrata* or *Saccharomyces cerevisiae*, species that are less likely to respond to traditional therapy.
- An abnormal host. Most of these patients require a minimum of 7 days of therapy but may need more prolonged treatment, up to 14 days, to achieve complete resolution of symptoms.

        1. Pharmacologic treatment. Creams have the advantage over suppositories in that they may be directly applied to the vulva. Oral medications are easy to use but can have substantial side effects and can be costly.

            a. Miconazole (Monistat) and **clotrimazole** (Gyne-Lotrimin) creams or suppositories are rapidly effective for monilial vulvovaginitis, when used intravaginally at bedtime. These products are now available OTC.

                (1) In mild cases, 3 days of treatment may be sufficient, with 7 days adequate for most cases.

                (2) Severe cases may require 10 to 14 days.

    (3) Suppositories are given as 100 mg qhs for 7 nights, 200 mg qhs for 3 nights, or 500 mg qhs for 1 night only.

    (4) Monistat 5 vaginal tampons contain 100 mg of miconazole nitrate. For 5 consecutive nights, the medicated tampon is inserted Hs and removed in the morning. There does not appear to be any difference in efficacy when compared to other methods of administration. The tampons may not be available in all states.

  b. Terconazole (Terazol) is more effective against *C. tropicalis* and *C. glabrata* strains. Both a 3-day suppository and 7-day cream are available.

  c. Fluconazole (Diflucan) is available in a 150-mg tablet taken once PO. This treatment has been compared with 7-day topical treatments. It offers essentially 100% compliance but is expensive and requires a prescription. It is the only Food and Drug Administration (FDA) approved oral agent for VVC.

  d. Boric acid suppositories as well as **gentian violet topically** are alternatives to the standard antifungal creams or pills. These are static agents that suppress the growth of organisms and to some extent eradicate them. However, they will not sterilize the genital tract.

  2. Nonpharmacologic methods have been proposed for VVC. It is likely that the following methods simply assist in restoring acid pH to the environment so that other host factors can contribute to eradicating the infection.

    a. Vinegar-in-water douching has been considered effective if used very early in mild cases. The recommended dose is 1 to 2 tablespoons of vinegar per quart of water qd or bid for no more than 5 days.

    b. Unprocessed yogurt douching daily for 5 days has also been proposed, with only anecdotal reports of its effectiveness.

    c. Recurrent VVC infections may benefit from **alternative strategies** including prophylactic fluconazole 100 mg PO q week or clotrimazole 500 mg suppository q week or biweekly administration of 600 mg of boric acid or nystatin powder. Nearly all of these prophylactic regimens should be used for 3 to 6 months to be effective. For recurrent yeast infections, consider testing for HIV and diabetes mellitus. See Table 1.1 for a list of alternative strategies for treating recurrent yeast infections.

  3. Patient education. The predisposing factors for VVC should be controlled, if possible, to prevent recurrent infections.

    a. Excessive moisture to the vulva can be avoided by wearing loose clothing and cotton underwear, which is more absorbent than nylon.

    b. Wiping the buttocks from front to back after bowel movements decreases the exposure of the vulva and vagina to candidal organisms.

    c. Diabetes should be tightly controlled.

    d. At the **first sign of symptoms,** vinegar-in-water or antifungal cream may be the only treatment needed to control the infection.

    e. In most cases, general antibiotic use does not result in candidal infection with enough frequency to warrant the prophylactic use of vaginal creams. However, **prophylactic treatment should be considered** for those patients with a history of candidal infection from antibiotics.

V. Bacterial vaginosis (gardnerella vaginitis). This common, clinically distinct, and readily recognizable form of vaginitis was first described by Gardner and Dukes in 1955. It was not until 1978, however, when a group of researchers in Seattle reported that this infection was responsible for virtually all cases of what was being called **nonspecific vaginitis,** that widespread understanding of this form of vaginitis and the current therapy began to emerge. The organism identified with this infection has been reclassified from *Corynebacterium vaginale* to *Haemophilus vaginalis,* and currently, to *G. vaginalis*. BV consists of the presence of *G. vaginalis* as well as an increase in anaerobic bacteria, especially

Table 1.1. Alternative strategies used for treating recurrent yeast infection

---

Increase rest, and reduce stress exposure

Four to six acidophilus capsules a day (especially 2–3 days before menses)

A daily drink of a mixture of 1 tablespoon honey to 1 cup apple cider vinegar

Boric acid capsules (600 mg intravaginally each night for 2 wk) or 1 Tbsp boric acid powder in 1 qt warm water. It is toxic systemically and potentially poisonous and should not be used until its safety has been established

Topical application of fluorouracil; may cause severe genital ulceration

Vitamin C 500 mg bid–qid to increase acidity of vaginal secretions

Lubricated condoms to decrease vaginal irritation

Douches of goldenseal-myrrh (1 Tbsp to 3 cups of water, cooled and strained)

Gentian violet 1% painted on the vagina once a week for 4 wk or monthly after menses for 4 mo; rare risk of severe irritant reaction (epithelial exfoliation)

Daily topical application of nonirritating moisturing preparations such as petrolatum, vegetable shortening, or mineral oil

Douching with potassium sorbate 3% (a commercial preparation to retard mold on cheese) used as a douche in a quart of warm water

Routine use of antifungal a few days before and after menses

Vinegar and water douche each month following menses

From Carcio HA, Clark-Secor RM. Vulvovaginal candidiasis: a current update. *Nurse Pract. Forum* 1992;3(3):135, with permission.

bacteroides, peptococci, and mobiluncus. *G. vaginalis* may be present in 30% to 70% of asymptomatic women without the abnormal proliferation of anaerobes and is only one component of BV. The presence of *G. vaginalis* in asymptomatic women need not be treated.

The significance of *G. vaginalis* found in the vaginal discharge of **prepubertal girls** remains controversial. However, one published study found prepubertal girls with a **history** of **sexual abuse** were **more likely to have** *G. vaginalis* on vaginal culture (14.6%) than control patients (4.2%) or girls with genitourinary complaints (4.2%). No association between vaginal erythema or discharge and the presence of the organism was found (3). Consequently, **prepubertal girls with** *G. vaginalis* **should be considered as possibly having been sexually abused and should be evaluated appropriately.**

A. **History.** The **characteristic symptoms** of BV (gardnerella vaginitis) are discharge and odor.
   1. The **discharge** is described as grayish or white.
   2. The **odor,** which is the most diagnostic symptom of BV (gardnerella vaginitis) is described as fishy and increases in intensity after sexual intercourse.
   3. Since there is often little tissue inflammation with this infection, **irritative symptoms** such as itching, burning, or soreness **may be absent.**

B. **Physical examination.** The pelvic examination is unremarkable except for the presence of the odorous homogenous gray-white discharge that coats the vaginal walls and has a pH greater than 4.5.

C. **Investigative procedures**
   1. The vaginal fluid pH is almost always greater than 4.5.
   2. The **saline wet-mount preparation** in BV shows 20% of epithelial cells stippled with coccobacilli, giving them a granular appearance with indistinct cell margins (clue cells, Fig. 1.2). There is often a paucity of leukocytes and a virtual absence of the normally appearing lactobacilli.

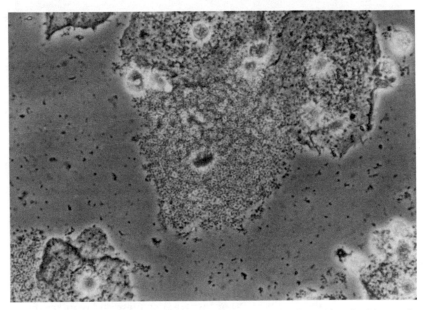

FIG. 1.2. Clue cells on wet smear in gardnerella vaginitis. (Reproduced with permission from Fleury FJ. Adult vaginitis. *Clin Obstet Gynecol* 1981;24:407.)

     3. The fishy **odor** becomes much worse when a smear of the discharge is mixed with a drop of 10% KOH (whiff test).

     4. A culture medium for *G. vaginalis* is now readily available and can be used when the clinical and microscopic findings are equivocal.

  D. Management. Controversy exists concerning the treatment of sexual partners. Both men and women may carry the organisms asymptomatically (see section **D.1.f.**).

     1. Pharmacologic treatment

        a. The current drug of choice is **metronidazole** 250 mg PO tid or 500 mg PO bid for 7 days.

           (1) The 2-g single dose of metronidazole given PO and repeated on day 3 has been effective. **However,** the 7-day regimen cures between 5% and 20% more patients than does this two-dose regimen.

           (2) Metronidazole 0.75% gel intravaginally bid for 5 days has also been effective.

           (3) Patients taking this drug orally should be instructed to **avoid alcoholic beverages** during the course of treatment since there may be a disulfiram-like (Antabuse-like) reaction.

        b. Clindamycin (Cleocin) 300 mg bid PO for 7 days, or clindamycin 2% cream intravaginally qhs for 7 nights, is equally effective.

           (1) This oral preparation is safer for pregnant women than is metronidazole.

           (2) Currently, this medication is more expensive than metronidazole.

        c. Ampicillin, 500 mg PO qid for 7 days, or a cephalosporin (e.g., cephalexin [Keflex], 500 mg PO qid for 7 days), is an alternative to metronidazole but is much less effective.

        d. Topical sulfonamide creams are not effective.

       e. BV can cause serious upper genitourinary tract infections and should be treated. Studies have shown the following:
         (1) Women undergoing a **cesarean section** have a sixfold **increased rate of postpartum endometritis.**
         (2) A threefold **increased rate** of **postabdominal hysterectomy cuff cellulitis** has been found.
         (3) An **increased premature birth rate** has been associated with BV and several studies have shown that treatment with metronidazole reduces prematurity. However, the screening and treatment of BV in pregnancy is controversial because some studies have failed to demonstrate any benefit to these protocols. The Centers for Disease Control and Prevention (CDC) currently recommends screening for BV early in the second trimester in women with a history of preterm delivery, followed by treatment with oral metronidazole, if appropriate.
         (4) There is a **linkage between BV and chorioamnionitis.**
      f. BV recurrence treatment
         (1) Women who **fail oral therapy can be switched to topical treatment.**
         (2) Studies show that **oral metronidazole given to male partners does not influence recurrence rates.** However, other antimicrobial agents have not yet been studied.
         (3) Women whose **male partners** use **condoms** have a much **lower recurrence rate.**
         (4) **A one-time PO or intravaginal metronidazole treatment at time of coitus may prevent recurrence** for those women who have intercourse-related infections.
         (5) When recurrences do not have an identifiable relation to coitus, **suppression of microorganisms** associated with BV **while allowing lactobacilli to reestablish is** the goal.
           (a) Initial metronidazole treatment for a 7-day course is recommended.
           (b) Then treat with either an oral or intravaginal medication every third or fourth day for an additional month.
    2. Patient education. BV is the least serious of the common forms of vulvovaginitis in a non-pregnant woman because of the relative absence of tissue inflammation. Patients can harbor this infection for years and may consider the odorous discharge normal.
      a. The **possible sexual transmission** of the infection must be explained to all patients.
      b. Douching with acidic solutions may decrease the discharge and odor temporarily but will rarely eradicate the infection.
VI. Trichomonas vaginitis. *Trichomonas vaginalis* is a flagellated protozoan for which human reservoirs are the vagina and urethra. It can be carried asymptomatically in both men and women, particularly in the postmenopausal period. The mode of transmission is almost always sexual intercourse.
    The infection caused by *T. vaginalis* in women is more variable than the other common forms of vulvovaginitis and may involve the cervix, vagina, and vulva.
    A. History. Patients with trichomonas vaginitis vary in their symptoms depending on the severity of the inflammatory response. The history is less specific than for candidal vaginitis or BV (gardnerella vaginitis).
      1. A vaginal discharge may be the only symptom.
      2. As the inflammatory response progresses, the discharge increases, and **vaginal soreness, itching, dyspareunia, postcoital spotting,** or a combination of these, can occur. The abnormal bleeding comes from the inflamed endocervical cells, which bleed from direct contact.
      3. Some patients with *Trichomonas* infection complain of pelvic or lower abdominal pain. Whether this represents inflammatory involvement of the upper genital tract or referred pain from the cervix is uncertain.

B. Physical examination. The appearance of the discharge in trichomonas vaginitis also varies with the inflammatory response.

1. Although the discharge may be minimal, most patients have a **gray-white secretion.** The commonly described frothy green discharge is seen in only about 10% of patients.
2. The vulva, vagina, and cervix can become **swollen and red,** depending on the severity of the infection.
3. **Bleeding** from the endocervix is common when touched with a cotton-tipped applicator or spatula.
4. **A nonspecific discomfort** with bimanual palpation of the uterus and adnexa is present in some patients.

C. Investigative procedures

1. The **diagnosis** is usually made by observation of the motile flagellate on a **saline smear.** Although this microscopic examination has been considered highly sensitive for detecting *Trichomonas* infection, studies have shown that the organisms may not be visible in many patients with a symptomatic infection. Patience and diligence at the microscope are often necessary.
2. *Trichomonas* **cultures** are available at some laboratories and can be used when the infection is suspected but not seen under the microscope, especially in the setting of a high pH.
3. **Polymerase chain reaction** (PCR) is being investigated as a diagnostic method. However, it is too expensive to be practical except for patients who have a persistent purulent discharge despite treatment.

D. Management. The asymptomatic patient in whom *T. vaginalis* is discovered does not require treatment unless there is a concern for sexual transmission. Sometimes the presence of this organism is suggested on a Papanicolaou (Pap) smear or urinalysis report. Many cytotechnicians cannot reliably detect this infection and confirmation should be obtained by a wet smear or culture if treatment is considered (Fig. 1.3) (10).

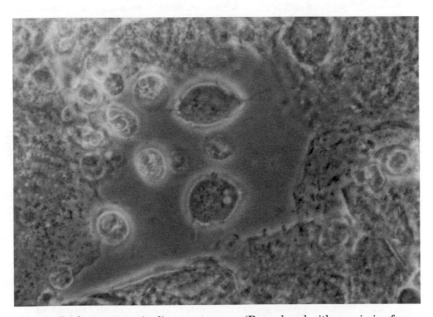

FIG. 1.3. *Trichomonas vaginalis* on wet smear. (Reproduced with permission from Fleury FJ. Adult vaginitis. *Clin Obstet Gynecol* 1981;24:407.)

1. **Metronidazole,** as a 2-g single dose, or 250 mg PO tid for 7 days, is the treatment of choice. Both regimens are 90% to 95% effective.
   a. The sexual partner should also be treated.
   b. Those being treated should be instructed to **avoid alcohol** during treatment.
   c. *T. vaginalis* has become **slightly more resistant to metronidazole** in recent years. When a patient has a treatment failure, **not reinfection,** the following regimens have been tried with varying results:
      (1) Metronidazole 1 g PO bid, and metronidazole intravaginally (cream base) bid for 7 to 10 days. In general, this is poorly tolerated owing to gastrointestinal upset.
      (2) Metronidazole 500 mg PO tid for 7 days.
      (3) Metronidazole 2 g PO qd for 3 to 5 days (1998 CDC STD Treatment Guidelines).
2. **Nonoxynol-9,** 100-mg spermicidal suppositories qhs for 2 nights serendipitously cured a woman with trichomoniasis infection that had resisted treatment for 3 years. Another provider tried this intravaginal suppository qhs, for 1 week on two different patients; one was cured. There is no prescribed regimen for nonoxynol-9.
3. **Tinidazole** 2 g PO, one-time dose, has been as effective as metronidazole. This drug is not yet available in the United States but formulating pharmacies can make it up.
4. In a symptomatic **breast-feeding patient,** metronidazole can be used in a single-dose treatment. The woman is then instructed to pump her breasts, as necessary, for 24 hours before resuming breast-feeding.
5. **In pregnancy,** trichomoniasis causes a dilemma since metronidazole should be avoided, especially in the first trimester. Some concern exists about the role *T. vaginalis* may play in either causing premature rupture of membranes or predisposing to an ascending infection if rupture occurs.
   a. There has not yet been a birth defect in humans or animals associated with the use of metronidazole. The package insert sanctions its use in the second or third trimester if local measures fail to relieve symptoms.
   b. Vagisec cream has been used in pregnancy for vaginal discomfort. This cream is OTC and can be used bid up to q6h.
6. **Local measures** that may be tried in trichomonas vaginitis are acidic vaginal cleansing (this infection, like others, makes the vagina more alkaline) and povidone-iodine (Betadine) vaginal washing. In Europe and Canada, clotrimazole is approved for topical therapy against *Trichomonas* infection, but is limited in its effectiveness.

VII. **Cervicitis** is really an **endocervicitis,** which is an inflammation of the **endocervical mucosa, rather than the squamous epithelium** of the cervix. **Approximately one third** of all women **with vaginal discharge** have **endocervicitis** and **not** a **vaginal infection.**

Endocervicitis is generally overlooked as a cause of vaginal discharge. Consequently, women are treated with topical creams that fail. Topical therapy does not reach the infected cervix since the inflammation extends into the underlying stroma.

The **cause of endocervicitis is infection with <u>Chlamydia</u>, gonorrhea, <u>Trichomonas</u>, or herpes simplex virus. Other causes have yet to be identified.**

A. **History**
   1. The woman generally presents with a nonirritating, nonodorous, mucoid **discharge** that may be yellow.
   2. Intermenstrual or postcoital **spotting** or both may be noted.
   3. **Dyspareunia** or **pelvic discomfort** or both may also be present.

B. **Physical examination**
   1. The cervical mucosa appears **inflamed** with focal hemorrhages.

   2. The cervix is **friable** and bleeds easily when touched with the speculum or when doing a Pap smear or culture.
   3. The **discharge** tends to be cloudy yellow or tan tenacious mucus from the endocervical glands.
   4. If herpes simplex virus is the etiologic agent, **lesions** will be seen on the vulva, vagina, or cervix.
   C. Investigative procedures
   1. Wet-mount preparations usually show multiple WBCs and no particular pathogen unless *Trichomonas* is the etiologic agent.
   2. A recent study found that patients in whom a **Gram's stain** of a vaginal discharge showed no gram-negative intracellular diplococci and fewer than ten WBCs per oil-immersion field had a high incidence of chlamydial infections.
   3. A culture for gonorrhea and chlamydiae should be obtained routinely, and one for herpes simplex virus should be obtained if indicated.
   4. A Pap smear should **not** be **done prior** to treatment since abnormal results may be obtained during the infection.
   D. Management is dependent on the etiology (see Chapter 3 for treatment).
VIII. Chemical vulvovaginitis. The etiologies of chemical vulvovaginitis are **different for children and adults. In children,** the offending agents tend to be **bubble baths, harsh soaps, and body lotions that often contain strong perfumes.** In adolescents and adults, the involved agents tend to be any chemically harsh substance that comes into direct contact with the vulvovaginal area, such as soaps, perfumed toilet paper or pads, powders, contraceptive agents, or feminine hygiene products. Strong vinegar douches are frequent offenders. A detailed history is very important.
   A. History may include persistent vulvar burning, itching, dysuria, dyspareunia, or a combination of these.
   B. Physical examination. Inspection reveals an inflamed or edematous (or both) vulva and vagina.
   C. Investigative procedures
   1. The only necessary investigative procedure is the pelvic examination.
   2. Wet-mount preparations are necessary, however, to rule out causes such as monilia.
   3. Cultures for gonorrhea and chlamydia as indicated by history.
   D. Management is dependent on the severity of the vulvovaginitis.
   1. Pharmacologic treatment
      a. For mild or moderate cases, the treatment is nonfluorinated topical corticosteroids, such as 1% hydrocortisone cream, applied twice daily for 7 to 10 days to the involved perineal area.
      b. In the more **severe cases,** hospitalization may be necessary for pain management and bladder catheterization.
   2. Patient education
      a. Regardless of the severity, the woman must be instructed to discontinue all current and future use of the offending agent.
      b. Douching can cause chemical vulvovaginitis as well as alter the pH balance of the vagina, which predisposes it to a candidal infection. Consequently, the primary care provider should instruct women to **discontinue the routine use of douching.** Douching should be done as a treatment for an infection only, and when used, the appropriate quantity is 1 to 2 tablespoons of vinegar per quart of water, twice daily.
IX. Irritative causes of vulvovaginitis. As is true for chemical vulvovaginitis, the **etiology** for irritative causes is different for children, adolescents, and adults.
   Infants and children have an innate curiosity that leads to exploration and insertion of objects into various body orifices, and the vagina is no exception. Foreign bodies must be considered as a cause of vaginal discharge and bleeding in this age group. Other causes include local trauma from play and irritation from

clothing. **Molestation or abuse must be suspected in infants younger than 10 to 12 months who present with a foreign body in or trauma to the genital area.** In general, this age group is not coordinated enough to insert a foreign body into the vagina.

The most common foreign body in the **adolescent and adult** groups is the tampon. Tampons may have strings that have broken off or are difficult to reach, or they may have been forgotten until the symptoms of infection have manifested.

A. History

1. The **presenting complaint** is vaginal discharge, persistent foul-smelling odor, or both.
2. The history of a foreign body is often unknown or not remembered.

B. Physical examination. Purulent discharge surrounding the foreign object is present. The examination techniques vary for the different age groups.

1. **At younger than 2 years of age,** the child should be placed in the supine position, and either an otoscope or nasal speculum can be used for vaginal inspection. The perineal area should be examined for contusions or abrasions. If present, abuse must be suspected.
2. **At 2 years or older,** the girl should be placed in the knee-chest position. With deep breaths, the spine and abdomen relax, which in turn allows the vaginal wall to open and relax. Frequently, no instrument is needed for visualization. If one is needed, the nasal speculum or otoscope may be used.
3. **Adolescents and adults** are placed in the lithotomy position, and the appropriate-sized vaginal speculum is used.

C. Investigative procedures

1. The PE is the only procedure necessary for foreign bodies.
2. Wet-mount preparations and cultures are not necessary unless abuse is suspected.

D. Management

1. Management consists of removing the object.
2. Antibiotic therapy is usually unnecessary.

X. Atrophic vaginitis is defined as inflammation of the vaginal epithelium that is due wholly or in part to a lack of estrogen. It is important for the clinician to distinguish between the symptomatic woman with an inflamed atrophic vagina and the woman who has vaginal atrophy, which is considered generally asymptomatic and is not inflamed. The importance of this distinction lies in the fact that atrophic vaginitis is uncommon, whereas atrophic vaginas are common.

There are **three stages during life when the vagina is atrophic.** These times are before menarche, during breast-feeding, and postmenopausally. The physiology of the vagina during these stages is similar. The epithelium is thin and lacks glycogen owing to a decrease in the endogenous estrogen. The pH increases to 6.5 to 7.0, which can support smoldering bacterial infections. However, this pH environment usually does not support candidal, trichomonal, or gonorrheal infections.

A. History

1. Atrophic vaginitis is very rare in **children.** However, if present, the signs tend to be discharge or spotting (or both), which occurs from the development of a chronic vaginitis.
2. If atrophic vaginitis occurs during **breast feeding,** the complaint is of vaginal dryness or dyspareunia.
3. **Postmenopausal** women are the ones most commonly affected with atrophic vaginitis. The presenting signs and symptoms are localized burning, dryness, soreness, dyspareunia, vulvar and vaginal irritation, occasional spotting, or a combination of these symptoms.

B. Physical examination. The vaginal walls appear thin, dry and smooth with little or no rugations. Inflammation, petechial hemorrhages, or exudate may be present.

C. Investigative procedures

1. The **wet-mount preparation** shows multiple WBCs with many bacteria present.

2. **Vaginal and cervical cultures are not recommended** since the microorganisms present are secondary invaders and not the cause of the vaginitis.
D. **Management** is dependent on the etiology and age group.
  1. **Children.** Trauma, foreign bodies, and neoplasms must be ruled out first. When the diagnosis of atrophic vaginitis has been established, the following treatments are recommended:
     a. **Nonpharmacologic** methods of treatment include sitz baths every day, improved local hygiene, white cotton underwear, Tucks to the perineal area, and avoidance of harsh soaps. If vulvitis is present, calamine lotion applied to the affected area provides some relief.
     b. **Pharmacologic** methods should be used only if the girl is unresponsive to the nonpharmacologic treatments. Topical estrogen (e.g., Premarin or Delestrogen) can be applied to the introitus twice daily for 2 to 4 weeks.
  2. **Breast-feeding women.** Atrophic vaginitis is not uncommon; however, women should be evaluated for lesions other than atrophic changes. Topical estrogens as described previously can alleviate symptoms readily.
  3. **Postmenopausal women**
     a. If there is **no history of bleeding,** the **topical treatment** is 0.5 to 1.0 applicator full of estrogen cream applied intravaginally at bedtime for 1 to 2 weeks, then reduced to every other night for 1 to 2 weeks, and then continued every week as needed. Alternatively, Estring, a vaginal silicone ring impregnated with estradiol and time released over 3 months, is very well tolerated by most women and may have less systemic absorption than vaginal creams.
        (1) Vaginal estrogen creams are absorbed systemically. When used for extended periods, the risk of endometrial hyperplasia or carcinoma must be considered. One should consider the intermittent use of progesterone to counteract the effects of estrogen on the endometrium.
        (2) For long-term therapy, the use of an oral or transdermal estrogen and oral progesterone combination may be preferable.
     b. If there is a **history of bleeding or spotting,** despite the apparent bleeding from the atrophic wall, dilation and curettage (D & C) or endometrial biopsy is recommended since there is no guarantee that the bleeding is not from the endometrial cavity.
        (1) A Pap smear is also recommended.
        (2) **No** treatment should be instituted until after the D & C or an adequate workup has been done.

References
1. Alderete JF, et al. Vaginal antibody of patients with trichomoniasis is to a prominent surface immunogen of *Trichomonas vaginalis*. *Genitourin Med* 1991;67:220.
2. Burns FM, et al. Diagnosis of bacterial vaginosis in a routine diagnostic laboratory. *Med Lab Sci* 1992;49:8.
3. Carcio HA, Clark-Secor RM. Vulvovaginal candidiasis: a current update. *Nurse Pract Forum* 1992;3(3):135.
4. Centers for Disease Control and Prevention. 1998 guidelines for treatment of sexually transmitted diseases. *MMWR* 1998;47(RR-1):1–118.
5. Colli E, Landoni M, Parazzini F. Treatment of male partners and recurrence of bacterial vaginosis: a randomized trial. *Genitourin Med* 1997;73(4):267–270.
6. Egan ME, Lipsky MS. Diagnosis of vaginitis. *Am Fam Physician* 2000;62(5):1095–1104.
7. Emans SJ. Significance of *Gardnerella vaginalis* in a prepubertal female. *Pediatr Infect Dis J* 1991;10:709.
8. Ferris DG, Dedle C, Litaker MS. Women's use of over-the-counter antifungal pharmaceutical products for gynecologic symptoms. *J Fam Pract* 1996;42:595–600.

9. Fidel PL, et al. Systemic cell-mediated immune reactivity in women with recurrent vulvovaginal candidiasis *J Infect Dis* 1993;168:1458.
10. Fleury FJ. Adult vaginitis. *Clin Obstet Gynecol* 1981;24:407.
11. Grinbaum A, et al. Transient myopia following metronidazole treatment for *Trichomonas vaginalis* [letter]. *JAMA* 1992;267:511.
12. Haefner HK. Current evaluation and management of vulvovaginitis. *Clin Obstet Gynecol* 1999;42(2):184–195.
13. Hamed KA, Studemeister AE. Successful response of metronidazole-resistant trichomonal vaginitis to tinidazole: a case report. *Sex Transm Dis* 1992;19:339.
14. Hauth JC, Goldenberg RL, Andrews WW, et al. Reduced incidence of preterm delivery with metronidazole and erythromycin in women with bacterial vaginosis. *N Engl J Med* 1995;333:1732–1735.
15. Holst E. Reservoir of four organisms associated with bacterial vaginosis suggests lack of sexual transmission. *J Clin Microbiol* 1990;28(9):2035–2039.
16. Hoosen AA, et al. Vaginal infections in diabetic women: is empiric antifungal therapy appropriate? *Sex Transm Dis* 1993;20:265.
17. Ingram DL, et al. *Gardnerella vaginalis* infection and sexual contact in female children. *Child Abuse Negl* 1992;16:847.
18. Klebanott M, Carey JC. Metronidazole did not prevent preterm birth in asymptomatic women with bacterial vaginosis. *Am J Obstet Gynecol* 1999;180:S2.
19. Livengood CH, Lossick JG. Resolution of resistant vaginal trichomoniasis associated with the use of intravaginal nonoxynol-9. *Obstet Gynecol* 1991;78:954.
20. McDonald HM, et al. Bacterial vaginosis in pregnancy and efficacy of short course oral metronidazole treatment: a randomized controlled trial. *Obstet Gynecol* 1994; 84:343.
21. Morales WJ, Schorr S, Albritton J. Effect of metronidazole in patients with preterm birth preceding pregnancy and bacterial vaginosis: a placebo-controlled double-blind study. *Am J Obstet Gynecol* 1994;171:345–347; discussion 348–349.
22. Patel HS, et al. Is there a role for fluconazole in the treatment of vulvovaginal candidiasis? *Ann Pharmacother* 1992;26:350.
22a. Paterson BA, Garland SM, Bowden FJ, et al. The diagnosis of *Trichomonas vaginalis*: new advances. *Int J STD AIDS* 1999;10:68–69.
23. O-Prasertsawat P, Jetsawangsri T. Split-dose metronidazole or single-dose tinidazole for the treatment of vaginal trichomoniasis. *Sex Transm Dis* 1992;19:295.
24. Pearlman MD, Yashar C, Ernst S, et al. An incremental dosing protocol for women with severe vaginal trichomoniasis and adverse reaction to metronidazole. *Am J Obstet Gynecol* 1996;174:934–936.
25. Rosenfeld WD, Clark J. Vulvovaginitis and cervicitis. *Pediatr Clin North Am* 1989;36:3.
26. Ryu JS, Chung HL, Min DY, et al. Diagnosis of trichomoniasis by polymerase chain reaction. *Yonsei Med J* 1999;40:56–60.
27. Smith SM, et al. Involvement of *Gardnerella vaginalis* in urinary tract infections in men. *J Clin Microbiol* 1992;30:1575.
28. Sobel JD, Chaim W. Treatment of *Torulopsis glabrata* vaginitis: retrospective review of boric acid therapy. *Clin Infect Dis* 1997;24:649–652.
29. Sobel JD, Faro S, Force RW, et al. Vulvovaginal candidiasis: epidemiologic, diagnostic, and therapeutic considerations. *Am J Obstet Gynecol* 1998;178:203–211.
30. Sobel JD, Nagappan V, Nyirjesy P. Metronidazole-resistant vaginal trichomoniasis: an emerging problem. *N Engl J Med* 1999;341:292–293.
31. Sobel JD. Vaginitis. *N Engl J Med* 1997;337(26):1896–1903.
32. Sobel JD. Vulvovaginitis in healthy women. *Compr Ther* 1999;25(6–7):335–346.
33. Stein GE, et al. Comparative study of fluconazole and clotrimazole in the treatment of vulvovaginal candidiasis. *Ann Pharmacother* 1991;25:582.
34. Summers PR, Sharp HT. The management of obscure or difficult cases of vulvovaginitis. *Clin Obstet Gynecol* 1993;36:206.
35. Willard, M. Vulvovaginitis. A concise guide to office diagnosis and treatment. *Female Patient* 1994;19:52.
36. Vejtorp M, Bollerup AC, Vejtorp L, et al. Bacterial vaginosis: a double-blinded randomized trial of the effect of treatment of sexual partners. *Br J Obstet Gynecol* 1988;95:920–926.

2. DISEASES OF THE VULVA

Patti Tilton

By definition, the vulva includes the mons veneris, the labia minora and majora, the fourchette, the upper vestibule, the orifices of the urethra and the vagina, and ducts of Skene's and Bartholin's glands.

I. **Bartholin's glands** are bilateral structures located between the superficial and deep perineal compartments. The glands are lined by tall, mucous-secreting cells that empty their contents into ducts. The ducts are lined by transitional epithelium, are about an inch long, and open in the vestibule on the lateral external portion of the hymenal ring. **The exact function of the glands is not known.** At one time, it was postulated that the function of Bartholin's glands was to lubricate the vagina during intercourse. This theory has been disputed by others, who claim that these glands secrete very little during erotic stimulation. It has been suggested that the glands may lubricate the vestibular surface, because women who have had unilateral excision of the gland experience dryness and scaliness on the affected side. Bartholin's glands **do not function prior to puberty.**

A. **Bartholin's cysts are one of the most common vulvar disorders.** They arise from the duct system when there is occlusion and continued secretory activity of the gland.

1. **Etiology. Causes of obstruction** include infection; congenital stenosis or atresia; thickened or inspissated mucus near the ductal opening; and mechanical trauma, such as a laceration or episiotomy.

2. **The differential diagnosis** of swelling in the posterior third of the vulva should include carcinoma, abscess and cyst of the Bartholin's gland, enterocele, perineal hernia, ischiorectal abscess, large sebaceous cyst, hydrocele of the canal of Nuck, fibroma of the diverticular apparatus, pudendal hematoma, and metastatic carcinoma.

3. **History.** Most **women** who **have small Bartholin's cysts** are asymptomatic. However, some women may experience dyspareunia or inadequate genital lubrication or report the presence of a mass. **Extremely large cysts** may cause difficulty in walking or constant localized pain. The patient should be questioned about infection or trauma to the area.

4. **Physical examination**
   a. Physical examination reveals a **cystic, unilateral** (usually), **nontender, tense mass** measuring 1 to 10 cm in diameter.
   b. The **location** is in the posterior third of the labia majora just external to the hymenal ring, immediately beneath the skin and vestibular mucosa.
   c. The **contents of the cyst** vary depending on the cause of the obstruction and may appear sanguineous, cloudy, or brown.

5. **Investigative procedures**
   a. **Specimens for cultures** (anaerobic and aerobic organisms, gonorrhea, and chlamydia) and sensitivity testing should be obtained from all draining cysts so that appropriate antibiotic therapy can be instituted, if necessary.
   b. In patients **older than 40, cytologic studies** should be done on cyst fluid to investigate the possibility of cancer.

6. **Management**
   a. If the **cyst is asymptomatic and small, no treatment** is necessary.
   b. Cysts that are subject to recurrent abscess formation, are symptomatic, or both require **surgical treatment.** Simple incision and drainage may provide temporary relief. However, the opening tends

to become obstructed, and recurrent cystic dilation, infection, or both may result. Thus, a permanent opening for drainage should be established, or total excision of the gland and duct should be done.

c. **Marsupialization** may be performed under local, regional (pudendal), or general anesthesia, the last rarely being necessary.

   (1) After appropriate preparation, a longitudinal or elliptic **incision** approximately 1.5 cm long is made in the mucosa over the cyst parallel to and outside the hymenal ring.

   (2) The cyst is then entered, and the contents sent for **culture** (see section I.A. 5.a), **sensitivity testing,** and **cytologic studies** if indicated.

   (3) A **portion of the cyst wall is excised** so that the resulting stoma is at least 1 cm in diameter.

   (4) **Exploration of the cavity** to ensure that all loculations are broken is **followed by a thorough rinsing with saline.**

   (5) The **edges of the cyst lining are then everted and fixed** to the surrounding skin and mucous membrane using 2-0 chromic interrupted sutures.

   (6) **Drains or packs are not needed** after surgery.

   (7) **Postoperative discomfort** can be treated with simple analgesics and sitz baths (on the third postoperative day).

   (8) **Appropriate antibiotics** should be given if considerable inflammation develops (see section I.B.5.b).

   (9) **Within 2 to 3 weeks,** the opening shrinks to a fraction of a centimeter and functions as an outlet for secretions. **Six weeks later,** the stoma will have contracted to a few millimeters in diameter and the gland will be functioning normally.

   (10) **Marsupialization eliminates** many of the complications resulting from total excision of the cyst.

d. **The Word catheter** is a bulb-tipped inflatable catheter that is inserted into the cyst through a stab wound.

   (1) The **mucosal surface over the cyst is washed** with an antiseptic solution and is anesthetized with 1% lidocaine with epinephrine.

   (2) The vulva is spread apart, and a **0.5-cm stab wound** is made in the area of the original duct opening immediately adjacent to the hymenal ring.

   (3) **Penetration of the cyst wall** is evidenced by the outflow of its contents.

   (4) The **bulb tip of the catheter is then inserted into the stab wound** and injected with 2 to 4 mL of water through the sealed stopper end. The inflated catheter occupies only a portion of the cyst cavity.

   (5) The **plugged end** of the catheter is then **placed in the vagina.**

   (6) **Adequate and continuous drainage** is provided through the stab wound around the catheter stem.

   (7) **Continuous pain 24 hours following insertion indicates** that the bulb is too large, and fluid should be withdrawn from it. Overinflation of the bulb can result in pressure necrosis of the cyst wall, and an extensive defect may ensue.

   (8) **Sexual intercourse is permitted** as soon as tenderness subsides.

   (9) The **catheter should remain in place for at least 4 weeks or longer** (6–8 weeks) if possible, until the orifice is epithelialized. At that time, the bulb is deflated and the device removed. Some women cannot tolerate the catheter for the entire 4 weeks, so removal can be done sooner.

   (10) After the new "accessory" duct has been established, the **recurrence of a Bartholin's cyst is greatly minimized.**

e. **Total excision** should be done **if cancer is suspected,** or if there are **repeated recurrences** following treatment.

B. **Bartholin's abscess**

1. **Etiology.** A Bartholin's abscess is formed when a Bartholin's cyst becomes secondarily infected. A **primary abscess** develops when virulent bacteria enter the duct, creating an edematous response that closes the orifice. Such an abscess is usually more acute and more extensive than one that occurs in a previously existing cyst. The infectious process can be acute or chronic. **Organisms that have been implicated** in causing infection include *Neisseria gonorrhoeae, Escherichia coli, Staphylococcus aureus, Trichomonas vaginalis, Mycoplasma hominis, Chlamydia trachomatis,* and species of *Streptococcus* and *Bacteroides.*

2. **History**
   a. Most **abscesses develop over** a period of 2 to 3 days.
   b. The patient may complain of a low-grade **fever,** perineal **discomfort,** labial **swelling, dyspareunia,** inguinal **adenopathy,** purulent **discharge, difficulty in sitting or walking,** or any combination of these symptoms.

3. **Physical examination**
   a. The abscess is an **extremely tender, fluctuant mass** lateral to and near the posterior fourchette.
   b. There may be **local swelling, erythema, labial edema, painful inguinal adenopathy, and a low-grade fever.**
   c. Sometimes a **purulent exudate** can be expressed from the duct by gentle pressure.
   d. **Spontaneous rupture** usually occurs within 72 hours.

4. **Investigative procedures.** It is important to obtain cultures of the exudate (see section I.A.5.a). Cervical and urethral cultures may also be indicated.

5. **Management**
   a. **Treatment in the acute phase** should consist of bedrest; administration of analgesics; and local application of heat by hot, wet dressings or sitz baths four times daily.
   b. **Broad-spectrum antibiotics** should be given if *C. trachomatis* and *N. gonorrhoeae* are potential causative organisms (see Chapter 3).
   c. When abscess formation is evident, **incision and drainage** can be performed to provide temporary relief.
      (1) The **incision** is made through a topically anesthetized site on the distended mucosa in the vestibule as close to the hymenal ring as possible or through the skin if an area of impending rupture can be identified. If the abscess has begun to drain spontaneously, the opening can merely be enlarged.
      (2) The **cavity is then packed** with iodoform gauze for 24 hours, or a Word catheter is inserted.
      (3) **Once the infection has entered the quiescent phase** (e.g., decreased edema, erythema), the abscess wall is better identified, and marsupialization can be done if necessary (see section I.A.6.c).
   d. **Total excision may be indicated** for prolonged or repeated incidents of infection with abscess formation (chronic bartholinitis) or in women older than 40 when cancer is suspected.

C. **Carcinoma of Bartholin's gland. Any enlargement** of the gland occurring in a postmenopausal woman should be **considered a malignancy until proved otherwise.** The age of peak incidence is in the mid 60s. Uncomplicated inflammatory disease of the gland is uncommon after the fourth decade.

   Primary carcinoma of Bartholin's gland is uncommon and accounts for only 0.001% of female genital tract malignancies.

1. **History.** Women may present with complaints of **dyspareunia or a mass.**
2. **Physical examination.** Bartholin's tumors may appear **similar to cysts or present as a hard mass.** Inguinal nodes may be unusually enlarged if metastasis has occurred.
3. **Investigative procedures.** Diagnosis is confirmed by **biopsy.**
4. **Management.** The patient should be **referred to a gynecologic oncologist** for management.

II. **Inflammations**
  A. **Contact dermatitis** is probably the **most common benign disorder** of the external genitalia. It is sometimes **divided** into **two categories: irritant** (a nonimmunologic response) and **allergic** (a true immunologic response).
    1. **History**
      a. **Pruritus, rash,** or both are common presenting complaints.
      b. Since most cases are caused by local irritants, the patient **should be questioned** about tight-fitting clothes, synthetic underwear, aerosol sprays, bubble bath or oils, colored toilet paper, detergents, fabric softeners, perfumed soaps and powders, condoms, diaphragms, spermicides, and anything else that may have come in contact with the vulva.
    2. **Physical examination**
      a. The **skin may appear red, inflamed, eczematous, or edematous.**
      b. **Vesicles or bullae** may be present in severe cases.
      c. **Weeping, scaling, and crusting** are often followed by dryness, fissuring, and lichenification.
      d. **Excoriations and secondary infection can occur.**
    3. **Investigative procedures**
      a. Determining the causative agent is best accomplished through a **thorough history.** Once a suspected agent has been identified, the patient is instructed to **discontinue the use of that product.** If the trial of removal does not improve the patient's condition, **patch testing** can be done, or another diagnosis should be considered.
      b. Tissue scrapings should be examined microscopically with potassium hydroxide (KOH) to rule out fungal infections.
      c. A wet mount should be done to rule out causes of vulvovaginitis such as *Trichomonas* and bacterial vaginosis.
      d. Biopsy is indicated when simple measures fail to relieve symptoms.
    4. **Management**
      a. Most importantly, the **causative agent should be removed.**
      b. When vesicles or bullae are present, **compresses** soaked in Burow's solution at a 1:20 dilution should be used four times daily as needed.
      c. For symptomatic relief following the treatment in b, or initially in milder cases, **1% hydrocortisone cream** can be applied sparingly three times daily.
      d. Cases **unresponsive** to 1% hydrocortisone cream after 1 to 2 weeks can be treated with a **fluorinated hydrocortisone cream** twice daily for several weeks. Caution should be used since prolonged use produces systemic reaction, local fibrosis, or atrophy.
      e. Antihistamines or sedatives may relieve nighttime itching.
      f. Hygienic measures, such as wearing loose-fitting clothing and cotton underwear, using mild soaps, and drying the vulva thoroughly with a hair dryer twice daily, should be encouraged.
  B. **Intertrigo** is an inflammatory reaction involving the genitocrural folds or the skin under the abdominal panniculus. It is **more commonly seen in obese or diabetic patients** in areas where there is persistent moisture on skin surfaces. Superinfection by bacteria or fungi may occur.
    1. **History. Chafing, itching, and burning** are the chief symptoms.
    2. **Physical examination**

  a. In the **early stages,** the skin may appear erythematous or white from maceration.
  b. **Later, linear fissuring** may be present, followed by cracking, thickening, and hyperkeratosis.
  c. Eventually, **hyperpigmentation** may occur.
3. **Investigative procedures**
  a. A **KOH preparation** should be done to rule out fungal infection, and the **lesions can be cultured.**
  b. A **fasting blood sugar should be done,** if indicated, since this disease is more common in diabetics.
4. **Management**
  a. A **dry environment** should be maintained by wearing cotton underwear and loose-fitting clothing.
  b. **Weight loss** should be encouraged if the patient is obese.
  c. **Diabetes** should be managed appropriately.
  d. To control pruritus, **1% hydrocortisone cream** can be used (see section II.A.4.c).
  e. **Occasionally,** topical antibiotics or antifungal agents may prove beneficial if secondary infection has occurred.
  f. Some dermatologists recommend 1% hydrocortisone cream with nystatin in Schomberg's lotion bid, or miconazole (Zeasorb AF). Both preparations can be used topically bid.
C. **Other inflammatory conditions.** Seborrheic dermatitis, psoriasis, neurodermatitis, and lichen planus are other inflammatory conditions that may affect the vulva. They usually present in the same manner as elsewhere on the body and are discussed in most textbooks of dermatology.
III. **Bacterial infections** of the vulva are usually the result of injury to the skin or altered resistance of the host. The categories of **reaction patterns** to bacterial infection include erythema, pustules, ulcers, and abscesses.
  A. **Erythrasma** is a mild, chronic, superficial bacterial infection.
    1. **History.** Patients are usually **asymptomatic.** However, they may complain of a rash.
    2. **Physical examination.** Lesions are characterized by inflamed, dry, slow-spreading, slightly scaly, circumscribed **macular patches** that may occupy the genitocrural, pubic, axillary, and inframammary areas. **Smaller plaques** may be formed outside the border of the larger ones.
    3. **Investigative procedures**
      a. Uncleansed affected areas show a **coral-red fluorescence under a Wood's lamp.**
      b. Gram-stained scrapings examined under oil immersion reveals gram-positive rodlike, filamentous bacteria called **<u>Corynebacterium minutissimum.</u>**
    4. **Management**
      a. Erythrasma can be treated with **erythromycin,** 250 mg PO qid for 2 weeks. However, **recurrences are common.**
      b. An **alternative method** employs a **keratolytic agent,** such as salicylic acid (Keralyt Gel), applied qhs and left on overnight, or resorcinol.
      c. The affected areas should be scrubbed with an **antibacterial soap** twice daily.
  B. **Hidradenitis suppurativa** is a **resistant infection of the apocrine sweat glands,** usually caused by staphylococci or streptococci. Most frequently, it occurs after puberty.
    1. **History.** The patient complains of **pain and pruritus.**
    2. **Physical examination.** Initially, **multiple pruritic subcutaneous nodules** appear that eventually **develop into abscesses and rupture.** Physical examination may reveal suppurative lesions, draining sinuses, lymphedema, widespread scarring, pitting, and induration. The axillae can also be involved.

3. **Investigative procedures.** Purulent drainage should be **gram-stained** and sent for **culture and sensitivity testing.**
4. **Management**
   a. **Warm, moist compresses** should be applied for 20 minutes four times daily.
   b. **Broad-spectrum antibiotics,** such as tetracycline, 250 mg PO qid or amoxicillin-clavulanate (Augmentin), 250 mg PO q8h, until resolution occurs, can be administered while culture results are pending.
   c. **Oral contraceptives** may improve the situation by reducing secretions from the glands.
   d. **Extensive disease may necessitate a partial or complete vulvectomy** followed by skin grafting.
C. **Other infections** that may occur on the vulva include chancroid, condylomata lata, lymphogranuloma venereum, granuloma inguinale, impetigo, cellulitis, erysipelas, furunculosis, herpes simplex and zoster viruses, and condylomata acuminata. Some of these are discussed elsewhere in this book, whereas others are covered in most infectious disease textbooks.

IV. **Viral infections. Molluscum contagiosum** is a viral infection characterized by **mild local irritation.** It is caused by a mildly contagious virus that is transmissible by **direct and indirect contact.** Autoinoculation is also common.
A. **History.** The patient usually presents with the complaint of **small bumps.**
B. **Physical examination**
   1. **Lesions** are usually multiple, dome-shaped, pedunculated or sessile, and vary from 0.1 to 1.0 cm in diameter.
   2. **Necrosis and infarction** of the overlying skin may produce umbilication through which a gritlike, milky material can be expressed.
   3. The lesions **grow slowly** for weeks or months **or can remain dormant for years.**
C. **Investigative procedures.** Diagnosis is made by the appearance of the lesion.
D. **Management.** Treatment varies, and any of the following will suffice:
   1. **Manual expression of material** from the lesions, followed by application of carbolic acid or silver nitrate to the cavity (one treatment is usually sufficient).
   2. **Cryotherapy** with liquid nitrogen or carbon dioxide.
   3. **Curettage** of the lesion, with or without electrodesiccation or painting with Monsel's solution.
   4. Application of **bichloroacetic acid** to the lesions.

V. **Mycotic infections. Tinea cruris** is a fungal infection of the genitocrural area caused by *Epidermophyton floccosum, Trichophyton mentagrophytes,* or *Trichophyton rubrum.* Transmission is possible during coitus or by contaminated clothing. Tinea cruris is **frequently accompanied by fungal infection of the hands or feet** (tinea pedis).
A. **History.** Mild to intense pruritus is the chief symptom.
B. **Physical examination**
   1. The infection starts as a **small erythematous patch.** Vesiculation and crusting or scab formation may occur.
   2. The lesions **spread peripherally** and coalesce as they enlarge, sometimes healing in the center. They are usually well circumscribed and have erythematous margins that are slightly elevated and vesiculated.
   3. **Maceration and weeping** may result from scratching, which eventually leads to lichenification.
   4. **Distribution** can be unilateral or bilateral, most often in the upper inner thighs, groin, perineum, and buttocks.
C. **Investigative procedures**
   1. **Skin scrapings** in 20% KOH **reveal hyphae** under the microscope.
   2. The fungi can also be **cultured on Sabouraud's medium** if scrapings are negative (rarely done).
D. **Management**

1. The **acute inflammatory stage** should be treated with calamine lotion and frequent applications of Burow's solution, 1:20 dilution for itching, or 1% hydrocortisone cream tid.
2. **After the acute inflammatory stage** has been controlled, a **topical antifungal agent** (clotrimazole or miconazole) should be applied tid for 1 to 3 weeks.
3. **Griseofulvin,** 250 mg PO qid for 3 to 4 weeks, can be used for **extremely obstinate cases** insensitive to topical agents. However, this drug has **many side effects** and should be used with caution. Ketoconazole, 200 mg PO once daily for 4 weeks, can be used as an alternative.
4. The **patient should be instructed to avoid** friction, sweating, heat, tight clothing, and obesity.

VI. **Autoimmune diseases. Behçet's syndrome** (triple-symptom complex) is rarely seen in the United States and is found mainly in the Mediterranean area. It is **characterized by genital and oral ulcerations and ocular inflammation.** Occasionally, other manifestations occur, such as disorders of the skin resembling erythema nodosum and erythema multiforme, CNS disturbances, arthritic disease, and thrombophlebitis. Ocular lesions may lead to iridocyclitis and blindness. The **etiology is probably viral.**

A. **History.** Pain, dyspareunia, fever, and malaise can precede the lesions and persist afterward. The lesions can occur cyclically.

B. **Physical examination**
  1. Lesions appear as **small vesicles or papules that ulcerate** and are usually covered with a gray material.
  2. The **vulva, vagina, and cervix** may be involved.
  3. **Healing** can be followed by fibrosis, scarring, and labial perforation.
  4. The **buccal mucosa should be inspected for lesions, and the eyes** for iritis or iridocyclitis.

C. **Investigative procedures. Punch biopsy** of the lesions show an inflammatory infiltrate associated with vasculitis.

D. **Management.** Lesions often **regress spontaneously,** making the efficacy of any treatment questionable.
  1. Patients should be **referred to the appropriate specialist** (rheumatologist, dermatologist, or ophthalmologist) for treatment.
  2. **Systemic corticosteroids** such as prednisone, 40 to 60 mg PO once daily for 2 to 4 weeks, can be given, then tapered slowly.
  3. **Oral contraceptives** and pregnancy apparently cause regression of lesions.
  4. **Analgesics** are indicated for **pain relief.**
  5. Topical antibiotics can be used as needed **for secondary infection.**
  6. **Excision** of the lesion(s) preceded and followed by administration of prednisone is **occasionally beneficial.**

VII. **Disorders of pigmentation**
A. **Leukoderma** results from a **congenital lack of pigmentation** in the vulva or other areas of the body that often appears at puberty.
  1. **History.** Patients are usually **asymptomatic,** and lesions may be incidental findings.
  2. **Physical examination. Areas of hypopigmentation** are visible on the vulva or other areas of the body.
  3. **Investigative procedures.** None are indicated.
  4. **Management.** The treatment is an explanation of the lesion with reassurances that this is a **benign lesion.**

B. **Vitiligo** is hypopigmentation secondary to acquired causes such as trauma, chronic infection, and radiation scarring. It is **often transitory or migratory.**
  1. **History.** Patients are usually **asymptomatic,** and lesions may be incidental findings.
  2. **Physical examination.** Lesions are **well-demarcated areas of hypopigmentation** without evidence of atrophy or hypertrophy.

      3. Investigative procedures. None are indicated.

      4. Management consists of reassurance that this is a benign lesion.

  C. Melanosis consists of irregular, deeply pigmented macules and patches on vulvar mucosal surfaces.

    1. History. Patients are asymptomatic.

    2. Physical examination. Areas of hyperpigmentation with irregular borders are visible. They lack ulcerations and palpability seen with melanomas.

    3. Investigative procedures. Biopsy is indicated only if melanoma is suspected.

    4. Management consists of reassurance that this is a benign lesion. It has not been reported as a melanoma precursor.

VIII. Vulvar nonneoplastic epithelial disorders. The nomenclature and definitions of vulvovaginal disease have been evolving. In 1987, the Instructional Society for the Study of Vulvovaginal Disease (ISSVD), in collaboration with the International Society of Gynecological Pathologists, proposed the following classification of vulvar nonneoplastic epithelial disorders (previously called vulvar dystrophies):

- Lichen sclerosis.
- Squamous cell hyperplasia.
- Other dermatoses.

  A. Lichen sclerosis may affect women at any age, but usually it occurs in **postmenopausal women.** It has been postulated that malignancy develops in 2% to 3% if the symptoms are not relieved.

    1. History. In the initial phases, women are **asymptomatic. Later,** they may complain of **intense pruritus and dyspareunia.**

    2. Physical examination

      a. Areas involved can include the labia, perineum, and perianal regions (hourglass configuration).

      b. In premenarchal girls, the skin may appear patchy and white.

      c. In older women, lesions begin as small bluish-white papules that have comedo-like plugs and depressions. Eventually, these form white plaques.

        (1) Skin may appear atrophic or parchmentlike (cigarette paper).

        (2) Scratching can result in **ecchymoses beneath the skin.**

        (3) Adhesions may form between the labia minora and majora, and these may eventually dissolve into one another.

        (4) The **prepuce** can appear agglutinated and scarred and may be associated with clitoral swelling and phimosis. If the introitus becomes stenotic, this will lead to dyspareunia.

    3. Investigative procedures

      a. Punch biopsy is done to establish the diagnosis.

      b. Staining with 1% toluidine blue may reveal areas of atypia. However, false-positive and false-negative results do occur.

      c. Use of colposcopy may aid in directing biopsies.

    4. Management. If the patient is **asymptomatic, no treatment** is necessary. If the patient is **symptomatic,** the **following** should be **done.**

      a. In the prepubertal patient, mild cases may respond to topical emollients such as A and D ointment or 1% hydrocortisone cream. For **severe cases,** a potent corticosteroid such as clobetasol propionate 0.05% is used bid until symptoms improve, usually 2 to 12 weeks. With symptomatic improvement, a less potent steroid is started, such as triamcinolone or 1% to 2% hydrocortisone cream, which may be tapered over the course of several weeks.

      b. In the postpubertal patient, the current treatment includes very high potency topical corticosteroids such as 0.05% clobetasol propionate applied bid for 2 to 3 weeks and then decreased to once daily, usually at night, until symptoms and findings begin to subside. The dosage thereafter can be decreased to one or three times per week depending on response.

    c. Topical progesterone and 2% testosterone propionate in a petrolatum base (bid to tid for 3–6 months or until pruritus is relieved, followed by applications once or twice weekly) have been used with varying results. Testosterone is systemically absorbed and should not be used in children. Women may develop side effects such as acne, hair growth, and oily skin.

    d. Topical estrogens have been attempted as therapy for lichen sclerosis but have **no proven efficacy.**

    e. Nonmedical treatment includes maintaining good personal hygiene, keeping the vulva dry, avoiding irritants, and using simple emollients such as lanolin or hydrogenated vegetable oil.

    f. Careful follow-up is indicated as the **malignant** potential is still **unknown.**

B. Squamous cell hyperplasia is an **epithelial reaction caused by external irritants** such as synthetic underwear, laundry detergents, feminine hygiene sprays, perfumed douches, tight clothing, vinyl seats, and excessive sweat. It is more common than lichen sclerosus in younger women and usually occurs before age 50.

    1. History. Intense **pruritus** may be present.

    2. Physical examination

       a. Lesions are **pink, white,** or both, **usually raised,** and **well delineated.**

       b. Thick, white plaques or lichenification is frequently seen.

       c. Fissures and excoriations caused by chronic scratching may be present.

       d. The vulva can appear **dusky red.**

    3. Investigative procedures

       a. Before treatment is started, **multiple punch biopsies** should be taken from suspicious areas.

       b. Toluidine blue is a nuclear stain that can help detect abnormal areas when used in the following manner:

          (1) A 1% **aqueous solution** is applied to the vulva with a cotton-tipped applicator.

          (2) The area is **allowed to dry** for several minutes; then a 1% **acetic acid solution** is applied to the same area.

          (3) Suspicious areas appear dark blue or at least darker than the surrounding areas of normal skin.

       c. Use of the colposcope may aid in directing biopsies.

       d. Aggravating factors such as fungal infections and vaginitis should be ruled out (see Chapter 1).

    4. Management

       a. Potential aggravating factors should be eliminated first.

       b. A 1% hydrocortisone cream can be used topically three times daily until the skin appears normal.

       c. If 1% hydrocortisone fails, 0.1% triamcinolone or 0.025% or 0.01% fluocinolone acetonide bid **or** tid, or 7:3 betamethasone valerate plus 0.1% crotamiton (Eurax) bid for 4 weeks can be used.

       d. If a fungal infection is also present, then a combination of 3% iodochlorhydroxyquin (Vioform) with 1% hydrocortisone, or nystatin with 0.01% triamcinolone, should be used.

       e. Antihistamines or sedatives may relieve nighttime itching. Hydroxyzine HCl (Atarax), 25 to 50 mg q6–8h PRN, has been very effective for skin pruritus.

C. Other dermatoses

    1. Lichen simplex chronicus. Lichen simplex chronicus is a dermatosis that can occur on the vulva. In some clinics, it may be the most commonly encountered dermatosis.

       a. History. Vulvar pruritus.

       b. Physical examination reveals thickened white epithelium, which is often unilateral and localized.

        c. Investigative procedures. Diagnosis is made by punch biopsy.

        d. Management

           (1) Topical, medium-strength corticosteroids bid for 2 to 3 weeks (triamcinolone acetonide 0.1%).

           (2) Removal of irritating agents.

IX. Vulvar neoplasms. This topic is beyond the scope of this book and will be mentioned only briefly here. **Vulvar anaplasia** constitutes 3% to 4% of all primary malignancies of the genital tract. Wide local invasion or extension often precedes lymphatic or hematogenous dissemination. The average age of onset is 60 to 65 years.

    A. History. The initial symptom of carcinoma is usually pruritus. However, the lesion may present as a lump or be relatively asymptomatic.

    B. Physical examination. Cancerous lesions may present as **scaly red plaques.** Others are **entirely white, red, or a combination of the two.** Inguinal lymph nodes should be examined.

    C. Investigative procedures. Toluidine blue directed or colposcopic directed biopsies should be taken.

    D. Management. The patient should be **referred to a gynecologic oncologist** for treatment.

X. Vulvodynia is **chronic vulvar discomfort,** especially characterized by complaints of burning, stinging, irritation, or rawness. Several sign-symptom complexes have been identified including vulvar dermatoses, cyclic vulvitis, vulvar papillomatosis, essential vulvodynia, and vulvar vestibulitis. Vulvar vestibulitis is the only problem addressed since it is the most frequently encountered condition of these relatively rare disorders.

    A. Vulvar vestibulitis is a **chronic, persistent clinical syndrome** characterized by severe pain on vestibular touch or attempted vaginal entry, tenderness to pressure localized within the vulvar vestibule, **and physical findings confined to vestibular erythema of various degrees.**

        1. Etiology. The endodermally derived vestibule may be intrinsically more sensitive than other areas of the vaginal mucosa. Vulvar vestibulitis may be caused by hypersensitivity to an as yet undetermined agent or agents such as urinary oxalate.

        2. History. Complaints may include vulvar irritation or burning precipitated by intercourse, tampons, touching, bicycle riding, or wearing tight clothing.

        3. Physical examination. Erythematous foci that are extremely **tender** when touched are located **in or around Bartholin's glands or between them posteriorly.** In some cases, erythema and tenderness may be more diffuse, but still limited to the vulvar vestibule. A cotton-tipped applicator is useful in establishing the diagnosis and in mapping out the affected areas.

        4. Investigative procedures

           a. Vaginitis should be **ruled out.**

           b. Colposcopy and **biopsies** can be done to **rule out HPV** and **vulvar dermatoses.**

           c. Measuring urinary calcium oxalate levels is under investigation.

        5. Management

           a. 5% lidocaine (Xylocaine) ointment topically PRN for pain or prior to intercourse.

           b. Estrogen cream may be helpful in atrophic patients.

           c. All potential irritants should be removed including harsh soaps, scented toilet paper, detergents, douches, and feminine deodorant sprays.

           d. Cotton underwear should be worn and pantyhose, tights, or close-fitting clothing avoided. Cotton menstrual pads can be used.

           e. Antidepressants, such as amitriptyline, 25 to 50 mg PO qhs, may be helpful.

           f. Surgical resection of the painful areas of the vestibule is successful in 60% to 70% of patients.

g. A low-oxalate diet may be helpful.

h. Other treatment modalities have included topical steroids, topical capsaicin cream, interferon alfa injections, calcium citrate, lactobacillus capsules (vaginal), comfrey leaves, tea sitz baths, and aloe vera.

i. Women may want to contact
The Vulvar Pain Foundation, 433 Ward Street, Graham, NC 27253.

References

1. American College of Obstetrics and Gynecology. ACOG technical bulletin no. 139. *Vulvar dystrophies.* Chicago: Author; January 1990.
2. American College of Obstetrics and Gynecology. Precis V. *An update in obstetrics and gynecology.* 1994.
3. Egart ML. Sexually transmitted diseases of the vulva. *Dermatol Clin* 1992;10:2.
4. Friedrich EG. Benign vulvar dystrophy: how to diagnose and treat it. *Contemp Obstet Gynecol* 1982;20:197.
5. Hill AD, Lensi JJ. Office management of Bartholin gland cysts and abscesses. *Am Fam Physician* 1988;57(7).
6. ACOG educational bulletin. Vulvar neoplastic epithelial disorders. *Int J Gynecol Obstet* 1997;241:181–188.
7. Jones HW, Jones GS. Diseases of the vulva. In: Jones HW, Jones GS, eds. *Novak's textbook of gynecology.* Baltimore: William & Wilkins, 1981.
8. Kaufman RH. Vulvovaginal disease. *Clin Obstet Gynecol* 1991;54(3).
9. Lynch PJ. Vulvar dystrophies and intraepithelial neoplasias. *Dermatol Clin* 1987;5(4).
10. Rock B. Pigmented lesions of the vulva. *Dermatol Clin* 1992;10:2.
11. Savage EW. Bartholin's cysts and abscesses. *Current concepts in ob/gyn.* Quilligan, 1980.
12. Schroeder B. Vulvar disorders in adolescents. *Obstet Gynecol Clin North Am* 2000; 27:1.
13. Tovell HM, Young AW. Classification of vulvar diseases. *Clin Obstet Gynecol* 1978; 3:955.
14. Zellis S, Pincus SH. Treatment of vulvar dermatoses. *Semin Dermatol* 1996; 15:71–76.

3. SEXUALLY TRANSMITTED DISEASES AND OTHER CONTAGIOUS DISEASES

Michel E. Rivlin

Twenty or more infectious diseases may be transmitted by sexual contact. This chapter reviews those associated with cervicitis, gonorrhea and chlamydia, and those characterized by genital ulcers, syphilis, herpes, chancroid, lymphogranuloma venereum, and granuloma inguinale as well as the parasitic skin infestations, pediculosis pubis and scabies. Sexually transmitted diseases (STDs) often coexist. It is strongly recommended that whenever serologic testing is done, screening for syphilis (rapid plasma reagin test [RPR]), HIV, hepatitis B surface antigen (HBsAg) and hepatitis C titer should be included routinely.

I. **Gonorrhea.** Urogenital purulent inflammation is the most common form of infection with the gram-negative, intracellular diplococcus *Neisseria gonorrhoeae,* which has an avidity for columnar and transitional epithelium. Transmission is almost always by sexual contact, with a usual incubation period of 2 to 8 days. In the United States, an estimated 600,000 new infections are reported annually.

  A. **History.** The acute attack usually follows sexual exposure or a menstrual period. Symptoms include vaginal discharge, urinary frequency and dysuria, menstrual irregularity, and bilateral lower abdominal pain. An **asymptomatic carrier state** is common in both sexes. The incidence of asymptomatic gonorrhea in men has been estimated to be as low as 12% and as high as 50%. The estimated incidence for asymptomatic women ranges from 50% to 80%. **Infections in other mucosal sites,** such as the oropharynx and anorectal area, are usually asymptomatic, but may lead to complaints of pain and discharge. **Hematogenous spread** may occur, causing manifestations such as septic arthritis and skin lesions. The most common dissemination, however, is by mucosal passage to the fallopian tubes and ovaries, resulting in pelvic inflammatory disease (PID), occurring in 10% to 15% of infected women (see Chapter 5).

  B. **Physical examination.** In the asymptomatic case, the physical examination may be entirely normal. There may be a purulent discharge, or Skene's or Bartholin's glands may be inflamed. However, these are nonspecific signs, and the diagnosis is dependent on **bacteriologic investigations.** The classic presentation of acute gonococcal PID, with fever, abdominal and adnexal tenderness, and a purulent discharge, is often absent.

  C. **Investigative procedures**

    1. **A Gram stain** of urethral or cervical secretions is unreliable since there is a 60% to 70% false-negative rate in female patients.

    2. **Gonorrhea culture,** on Thayer-Martin or equivalent medium. The culture should be placed in a candle jar since the organism is fastidious, requiring aerobic conditions with an increased carbon dioxide atmosphere to grow. Incubation should begin as early as possible. Depending on the history, cultures may also be required from the pharynx and rectum.

    3. **Enzyme immunoassay (ELISA),** polymerase chain reaction (PCR), and ligase chain reaction (LCR) assays on endocervical or urine samples have largely replaced culture methods of diagnosis and are at least as accurate.

    4. **Serologic testing** for syphilis should be done on all patients. HIV testing and screening for HBsAg and hepatitis C are strongly recommended.

    5. **Chlamydia** testing should be done at the same time the gonorrhea culture is obtained.

  D. **Management.** Therapy is based on antibiotic sensitivity, site of infection, and concurrent STDs. Antibiotic resistance is mediated through two genetic mechanisms: chromosomal-mediated resistant *N. gonorrhoeae* and plasmid-mediated resistance. Two types of plasmids are important: one for penicillinase and one for high-level tetracycline resistance. Rectal infections are relatively refractory to amoxicillin and tetracycline, and pharyngeal infections to amoxicillin and spectinomycin. *Chlamydia trachomatis* is a common coinfective agent and should be covered with empiric therapy. A summary of the guidelines for treatment recommended by the Centers for Disease Control and Prevention (CDC), **Atlanta,** in 1998 follows.

1. Treatment of adults

  a. Uncomplicated gonococcal infections are treated with empiric single-dose therapy consisting of ceftriaxone, 125 mg IM once. Mixing 1% lidocaine reduces the discomfort of the injection. Other recommended **single-dose regimens include** cefixime, 400 mg PO; or ciprofloxacin, 500 mg PO; or ofloxacin, 400 mg PO. **Alternative regimens include** spectinomycin, 2.0 g IM for patients who cannot tolerate cephalosporins or quinolones. **Injectable cephalosporins** that are **also effective** include ceftizoxime, 500 mg IM; cefotaxime, 500 mg IM; cefotetan, 1 g IM; and cefoxitin, 2 g IM. Oral cephalosporin regimens include cefuroxime axetil, 1 g PO; and cefpodoxime proxetil, 200 mg PO. These two regimens are **less effective against pharyngeal infections.** Other quinolone regimens include enoxacin, 400 mg PO; lomefloxacin, 400 mg PO; and norfloxacin, 800 mg PO. Many other antibiotics are effective, and this does not represent a comprehensive list of all suitable treatments.

   (1) All treatment regimens should include a single dose of azithromycin 1 g PO or a **7-day course** of **oral tetracycline** or **doxycycline** to eradicate concurrent chlamydial infection, which has been documented in up to 45% of gonorrheal cases in some populations. These drugs are **not** considered adequate therapy for gonorrhea. Generic doxycycline costs a little more than tetracycline but provides the advantage of a 100-mg bid dosage unrelated to meals, compared with a 500-mg qid dosage between meals with tetracycline. The **alternative regimen** is erythromycin stearate, 500 mg; erythromycin ethylsuccinate, 800 mg; or erythromycin base, 500 mg PO qid for 7 days (see section III.D.1.).

   (2) All patients should have a serologic test for syphilis and should be offered counseling and testing for HIV infection. Most patients with incubating syphilis (in who there is no clinical evidence and who are seronegative) may be cured by any of the foregoing regimens, with the exception of spectinomycin and the quinolones. Patients treated with these drugs should have a syphilis serologic workup in 1 month.

  b. Pharyngeal infections should be treated with ceftriaxone, 125 mg IM. Those who cannot receive this drug should be treated with ciprofloxacin, 500 mg PO, as a single dose; and these patients **require repeat culture** 5 to 7 days later. Trimethoprim, 720 mg; sulfamethoxazole, 3600 mg (Septra 9 tablets) PO once daily for 5 days may be an effective alternative therapy.

  c. Sexual partners should be identified, examined, cultured, and treated presumptively.

  d. Follow-up culture (so-called test of cure) following combined ceftriaxone-azithromycin or doxycycline therapy is not essential since treatment failure is rare. Reculture 1 to 2 months later **(rescreening)** detects both treatment failures and reinfections. Patients treated with other regimens and those with persistent symptoms should have cultures 4 to 7 days after completion of therapy.

  e. Treatment failures after one of the recommended regimens are usually due to reinfection, indicating a need for improved contact tracing and patient education. Nevertheless, antibiotic sensitivities and chlamydial cultures are indicated. Additional treatment with ceftriaxone and azithromycin or doxycycline should be given.

2. **Pregnant women** should be treated with ceftriaxone, 125 mg IM, plus azithromycin 1 g PO or erythromycin base, 500 mg PO qid for 7 days. (Erythromycin stearate, 500 mg; erythromycin ethylsuccinate, 800 mg; or an equivalent may be substituted for erythromycin base). **Tetracyclines** (including doxycycline) and the **quinolones** are **contraindicated in pregnancy** because of possible adverse fetal effects. Pregnant women allergic to beta-lactams should be treated with spectinomycin, 2 g IM, followed by erythromycin. **Test of cure is required for these cases.**

3. **Gonococcal PID** (see Chapter 5)

4. **Disseminated gonococcal infection (arthritis-dermatitis syndrome).** The condition may be monoarticular or polyarticular. Skin lesions are commonly present with the arthritis. They begin as small red papules, evolving through vesicular and pustular stages to lesions with a necrotic center superimposed on a hemorrhagic base. Healing is usually spontaneous. Hospitalization is usually indicated, especially for those who cannot reliably comply with therapy or who have an uncertain diagnosis, purulent joint effusions, or other complications. Treatment schedules for this syndrome are included in the CDC guidelines but are outside the scope of this chapter.

5. **Miscellaneous.** The CDC guidelines also recommend schedules of therapy for infants born to mothers with gonococcal infections, for gonococcal ophthalmia in adults, and for neonatal infections. These are problems seldom encountered in a medical or gynecologic outpatient department. However, adolescents may be seen and should receive similar regimens. Children weighing more than 100 lb (45 kg) receive adult dosage while those weighing less receive dosages adjusted to weight. **In all pediatric cases, the possibility of sexual abuse must be considered.**

E. **Sequelae.** The short-term and long-term complications and sequelae of gonococcal infections are mainly related to gonococcal PID (see Chapter 5).

II. **Syphilis.** The infectious agent is a spirochete, *Treponema pallidum*. Spread is by sexual intercourse or by intrauterine transmission (congenital syphilis). The **incubation period** is usually 2 to 6 weeks, with a primary sore (chancre) appearing at the site of infection and remaining for 1 to 6 weeks. Manifestations of the secondary stage may appear 2 to 12 weeks later. During **early latency** (1–4 years), relapses with mucocutaneous lesions may occur. Thereafter, there are no relapses and the syphilis is noninfectious, except transplacentally. **Late symptomatic syphilis** is generally characterized by cardiovascular or neurologic disease, although any tissue can be involved.

The incidence of syphilis in the United States in 1995 was 9 cases per 100,000 population.

A. **Early (primary, secondary, latent less than 1 year)**

1. **History.** The **primary chancre** usually appears on the genitalia, mouth, or anus and is painless. The secondary stage may present with **ulcerations** of mucous membranes or **skin eruptions.** Frequently there is only a flulike syndrome with a fever, sore throat, and muscle pain. During the latent phase, the patient is generally asymptomatic. Nearly two thirds of patients pass through the primary and secondary stages without realizing it. The clinical spectrum of syphilis acquired in utero includes stillbirth, neonatal death, neonatal illness, and development of the stigmata of congenital syphilis in later life.

2. **Physical examination. Chancres** vary in appearance but the usual feature is that of a nontender clean-cut ulcer with an indurated base and an associated regional adenopathy. The **secondary-stage skin lesions** tend to be widespread and symmetric, with 60% to 80% of patients having lesions on their palms and soles. Cutaneous lesions tend to be maculopapular. Condylomata latum are intertriginous papules

formed at areas of friction and moisture, such as the vulva. Mucosal or mucocutaneous lesions appear in 21% to 58% and include pharyngitis, tonsillitis, and the "mucous patch" (a papule with a central erosion found on the oral and genital mucosa). Lymphadenopathy is a very common finding in the secondary stage.

3. **Investigative procedures. Dark-field microscopy** of fluid expressed from lesions may demonstrate the organism. In practice, **serologic tests** are of major importance in diagnosis. **Nontreponemal tests** (Veneral Disease Research Laboratories test [VDRL] and RPR) are used for screening and may be repeated quantitatively as a guide to therapeutic response. The tests become positive 1 or 2 weeks after the appearance of the chancre. They are positive in approximately 66% of primary cases, in 99% of secondary cases, and in about 70% of late cases. These tests are nonspecific, with biologic false-positive results occurring in association with other infections and diseases (e.g., infectious mononucleosis, collagen vascular diseases). The titer is usually low (no more than 1:8), with a false-positive test. **Treponemal tests** (fluorescent treponemal antibody absorption test [FTA-ABS], *Treponema pallidum* immobilization test [TPI]) are specific, but are not quantitative, and remain positive even after adequate therapy. The treponemal tests, therefore, are used to confirm the diagnosis. The FTA-ABS test is positive in 85% of primary and 100% of secondary cases and may be the only positive test in tertiary cases. Positive serologic studies in the newborn may be passively acquired, but most physicians treat all VDRL-positive neonates. All patients with evidence of latent syphilis should have a **lumbar puncture** with a cerebrospinal fluid (CSF) VDRL to rule out neurosyphilis (7).

4. **Management.** The **CDC recommendations** (1998) are summarized as follows:

   a. **Drug therapy** for early syphilis is benzathine penicillin G, 2.4 million units IM in a single dose. Penicillin-allergic patients should receive doxycycline, 100 mg PO bid; or tetracycline hydrochloride, 500 mg PO qid for 14 days. An alternative regimen is erythromycin, 500 mg PO qid for 14 days. Various ceftriaxone regimens may also be considered. **Pregnant patients** are treated similarly, but **tetracyclines are contraindicated.** Penicillin is the only acceptable therapy for the pregnant patient. Following documentation of penicillin allergy by skin testing, reactive patients should be desensitized and treated with penicillin. Desensitization should be performed in consultation with an expert and only where adequate emergency facilities are available.

   b. **Quantitative nontreponemal tests** should be repeated at 3, 6, and 12 months after treatment. Pregnant women who are treated should have monthly tests until delivery.

   c. **Retreatment** may be indicated if there is a fourfold increase in titer, an initial high titer fails to show a fourfold decrease within a year, or clinical signs persist or recur. Retreatment should consist of schedules recommended for late syphilis (see section II.B.4.). **Pregnant women who are treated and who do not show a fourfold decrease in titer in a 3-month period should be retreated.**

   d. **Miscellaneous.** Cases of syphilis should be reported within 48 hours of diagnosis to a local or state health department, which usually offers referral and follow-up services. Sexual partners are notified without identification of the index case.

5. **Sequelae.** One third of all untreated patients develop sequelae that are generally confined to the CNS and cardiovascular system.

B. **Late (neurosyphilis, latent more than 1 year)**

1. **History, antecedent treatment, and previous serologic tests** are important in establishing the diagnosis. Patients with latent symptomatic

syphilis present with complaints relevant to the particular organs involved (see section II.B.2). The latent stage prior to clinical presentation ranges from 3 to 20 years.

2. **Physical examination.** The typical lesion of late syphilis is the **gumma.** These nodular ulcerative lesions can involve skin, mucous membranes, skeletal system, and viscera. Cardiovascular syphilis manifests with aortitis, aneurysm, or aortic regurgitation. Neurosyphilis may be asymptomatic or symptomatic, presenting as tabes dorsalis, meningovascular syphilis, or general paralysis of the insane. Iritis, choroidoretinitis, and leukoplakia may occur.

3. **Investigative procedures.** CSF VDRL should be done for clinical signs and symptoms consistent with a CNS lesion and for patients with syphilis of more than 1-year duration to exclude asymptomatic disease.

4. **Management**
   a. **Recommendations for therapy** of cardiovascular, late benign syphilis, and syphilis of more than 1-year duration are as follows: benzathine penicillin G, 2.4 million units IM weekly for 3 weeks; or if penicillin-allergic, doxycycline, 100 mg PO bid, or tetracycline hydrochloride, 500 mg PO qid, for 30 days. Alternatively, if the patient is pregnant or unable to tolerate tetracyclines, desensitization in consultation with an expert may be indicated.
   b. **Neurosyphilis** may be treated with aqueous crystalline penicillin G, 12 to 24 million units, administered as 2 to 4 million units q4h IV for 10 to 14 days. An alternative regimen is procaine penicillin, 2 to 4 million units IM daily, **with** probenecid, 500 mg PO qid, both for 10 to 14 days. After completion of these regimens, many authorities recommend the addition of benzathine penicillin G, 2.4 million units IM. Patients allergic to penicillin should be skin-tested and desensitized in consultation with an expert.
   c. Up to 80% of patients treated during the late stages of syphilis **remain seropositive indefinitely,** although their titers should decrease over time.
   d. The provider should keep in mind that the **Jarisch–Herxheimer reaction can occur,** producing fever, myalgia, tachycardia, and hypotension within 24 hours of treatment. Some authors recommend hospitalization of pregnant patients since this reaction places mother and fetus at increased risk.

III. **C. trachomatis** is a bacterial intracellular parasite that causes a wide range of infections. In women, these include cervicitis, salpingitis, perihepatitis, and urethritis. There are 15 serotypes, and those associated with genital infection are D to K, whereas the L strains are associated with lymphogranuloma venereum. In the United States, approximately 4% to 5% of sexually active women carry *Chlamydia* in their cervix; and this site appears to play a central role in transmission, with the horizontal spread to male partners and the vertical spread to neonates. There are an estimated 4 million cases annually in the United States. Chlamydial PID is discussed in Chapter 5.

A. **History.** Chlamydial cervicitis is frequently asymptomatic. However, a purulent discharge may be found. Dysuria and frequency (urethral syndrome) may be present. A history of nongonococcal urethritis in the male partner is associated with a 50% isolation of *Chlamydia* from the female partner. Neonates born to infected mothers have a 60% to 70% risk of infection, including a 10% to 20% risk of pneumonia and a 25% to 55% risk of conjunctivitis.

B. **Physical examination.** Although the cervix may appear normal, there is often a significant increase in the incidence of cervical ectopy, erythema, and friability, as well as the presence of mucopus readily seen on a cotton-tipped swab. Mucopurulent cervicitis is caused by chlamydial infection in approximately 50% of cases.

C. **Investigative procedures. Culture** is the only reliable way to establish the diagnosis. Endocervical samples are required and should be frozen if not cultured immediately. The organism must be grown in cell culture, and characteristic intracytoplasmic inclusions are identified after staining. If chlamydial cultures are not available, treatment should be given if the diagnosis is strongly suggested on clinical grounds. Direct tests for chlamydial antigen utilizing monoclonal antibodies, enzyme immunoassay, or a DNA probe are useful for screening high-prevalence populations. In low-prevalence groups, there are a significant number of false-positive results. Serologic testing is of little value.

D. Management. Tetracycline, erythromycin, and azithromycin are highly effective, with cure rates approaching 95%. Additional drugs that have demonstrated activity against *Chlamydia* include sulfamethoxazole-trimethoprim, rifampin, clindamycin, ofloxacin, and amoxicillin.

1. **The CDC-recommended regimens** are azithromycin 1 g PO in a single dose or doxycycline, 100 mg PO bid for 7 days. Alternative regimens are ofloxacin, 300 mg PO bid for 7 days; erythromycin base, 500 mg PO qid for 7 days; erythromycin ethylsuccinate, 800 mg PO qid for 7 days; or sulfisoxazole, 500 mg PO qid for 10 days (this has inferior efficacy to other regimens) (3).

2. The CDC-recommended regimen for **pregnant women** azithromycin, 1 g PO or erythromycin base, 500 mg PO qid for 7 days. Alternative regimens include erythromycin base, 250 mg PO qid for 14 days or erythromycin ethylsuccinate, 800 mg PO qid for 7 days or 400 mg PO qid for 14 days. If erythromycin cannot be tolerated, amoxicillin, 500 mg PO tid for 7 to 10 days or clindamycin, 300 mg PO tid for 7 days, are recommended. Limited data exist on these regimens.

3. **Sexual partners** should be **evaluated** and **treated.**

4. Follow-up testing is unnecessary unless symptoms persist or reinfection is suspected. **Pregnant patients,** however, **should be retested.** At least 3 weeks must elapse after completion of therapy before retesting.

E. Sequelae. The major serious complications are associated with PID and these are described in Chapter 5.

IV. Genital herpes simplex virus. Venereal transmission through intercourse or orogenital contact is common for herpesvirus, a DNA virus. After the genital skin is inoculated, the virus infects peripheral nerve endings and travels to the lumbosacral dorsal root ganglia. A persistent, but subclinical, infection is established in the ganglion cells. Periodically, the virus becomes active and travels by peripheral nerves to the skin, inducing the characteristic focal recurrent lesion. Infections with herpesvirus type I or II are the most common cause of vesiculoulcerative lesions of the female genital tract. Type I generally causes oral lesions (fever blisters), and 75% to 80% of genital lesions are type II. However, these percentages vary with the population screened. About 50% to 70% of patients with primary infection experience recurrence. The attack rate (percentage of those who contract herpes simplex virus after exposure) for susceptible individuals is believed to be about 75%. There are an estimated 500,000 new cases in the United States annually, with more than 20 million episodes of recurrence.

A. History. Incubation periods range from 1 to 30 days (median, 6–8 days). Generally, the **presenting complaint** is of blisters or ulcers on the vulva or severe vulvar pain. Much less often, severe dysuria, general malaise, fever, and enlarged inguinal nodes are the presenting features. The lesions typically evolve from vesicles to pustules to ulcers to crusts, with healing occurring over 14 to 21 days. They may be preceded by pruritus, burning, or hyperesthesia of the skin. **Some patients may have no symptoms;** thus it is not uncommon to miss the first infection. **Recurrent infections** are generally less severe than the primary infection and may be triggered by emotional stress, menses, intercourse, or may be totally unpredictable. Systemic symptoms rarely occur, and lesions last from 7 to 10 days. Recurrent lesions represent a reactivation of latent virus, not reinfection.

B. Physical examination. Exquisitely sensitive vesicles and erosions of the labia, vaginal canal, perineum, and oropharynx may be found. Intense edema of the labia and urethra, as well as inguinal adenopathy may be present. Recurrent disease follows essentially the same course except that it is less debilitating, there are few ulcers, and adenopathy is seldom present. It is generally believed that there is no clinical difference between the lesions caused by the two virus types.

C. **Investigative procedures.** The vesicles and ulcers characteristic of the disease are easily recognized, especially if there is a positive history. Cervical herpes virus is less obvious clinically. A Papanicolaou (Pap) smear of cervical herpes virus contains characteristic multinucleate giant cells in about 30% to 50% of patients. Definitive diagnosis can be confirmed by **viral culture.** Specimens should be taken using cotton-tipped or Dacron-tipped swabs placed in viral transport medium and held at 4°C until cultured. Direct detection of viral antigens using immunodiagnostic methods is available and provides sensitivities of 85% to 90%. These methods are much less sensitive in detecting asymptomatic viral shedding. Herpes virus antibodies appear within 4 days of primary infection and are present thereafter; therefore, they are not helpful in recurrent infection unless a change in titer is documented. Since herpesvirus is an STD, **culture for gonorrhea and chlamydia** infections and **a serologic workup for syphilis, HIV,** and **hepatitis B and C** should be obtained.

D. **Management**

1. **General measures include** keeping the **vulva** and **perineum** as **dry** as possible, wearing **cotton underwear**, and exposing the vulva to a **heat lamp** or a **hair dryer**, which may be soothing. Analgesics may be required because of pain and hypnotics may be required if there is interference with sleep. Occasionally, urinary retention may necessitate the use of an indwelling catheter. Sitz baths and local anesthetic creams may be helpful.

2. **Specific measures.** Oral acyclovir, valacyclovir, and famciclovir provide partial control of the symptoms and signs of herpes episodes but do not eradicate latent virus. Topical therapy is less effective and its use is discouraged. The CDC guidelines are as follows:

   a. For **first clinical episodes of genital herpes,** the recommended regimen is acyclovir, 200 mg PO 5 times a day for 7 to 10 days or until clinical resolution. Alternatives are famciclovir 250 mg PO 3 times a day for 7 to 10 days or valacyclovir 1 g PO twice a day for 10 days. The dose of acyclovir is doubled for **herpes proctitis** and treatment is for 10 days, experience with famciclovir or valacyclovir in proctitis is lacking.

   b. When treatment for **recurrent episodes** starts during the prodrome or within 2 days of lesion onset, limited benefit may result. The recommended regimen is acyclovir, 200 mg PO 5 times a day for 5 days or 400 mg PO tid for 5 days or 800 mg PO bid for 5 days. Drug therapy begun more than 2 days **after** onset of lesions has not been proven to be of benefit. Alternatives are famciclovir 125 mg PO twice a day for 5 days or valacyclovir 500 mg PO twice a day for 5 days.

   c. **Daily suppressive therapy** reduces recurrences by at least 75% in patients having six or more episodes per year. Safety and efficacy have been reported for as long as 6 years. Asymptomatic viral shedding and the potential for transmission are not totally eliminated. After 1 year, therapy should be discontinued to reassess the rate of recurrence. The recommended regimen is acyclovir, 400 mg PO bid or famciclovir 250 mg PO bid or valacyclovir 500 mg PO bid or valacyclovir 1000 mg PO once a day.

   d. For patients who have **severe symptoms** or **complications** that necessitate hospitalization, intravenous acyclovir shortens the median course of first episodes by approximately 7 days.

   e. Acyclovir has **not been adequately tested** in **pregnant** or **lactating women.** Use in pregnancy is recommended **only** in the presence of life-threatening maternal infection. However, evidence of adverse effects has not been shown in ongoing registries, and therefore first clinical episodes in pregnancy **may** also be treated with acyclovir.

3. Patients should be **counseled** about the disease and advised to abstain from sexual intercourse while lesions are present. The risk of transmitting herpes simplex virus during asymptomatic periods is unknown. The use of condoms should be encouraged during all sexual exposures. Women also need to be instructed to inform their clinicians of their history of genital herpes early in pregnancy since serious neonatal infection may occur during parturition.

E. **Sequelae.** In addition to a **possible link** with **cervical neoplasia** and **neonatal infections,** patients with the disease also have a **high incidence of depression and sexual dysfunction.** Much of the burden of this disease is of an emotional and social nature. Self-help groups, such as the American Social Health Association, may be of great assistance in helping herpes simplex virus patients cope with their problems.

V. **Chancroid** is an ulcerating disease of the genital region caused by *Haemophilus ducreyi.* Its exact incidence is unknown, although clinical infection is rare in women. The **incubation period** is generally 4 to 7 days, the male to female ratio is 10:1.

A. **CDC guidelines.** Chancroid is probably underreported because of the difficulty in proving the diagnosis. In an attempt to obtain more accurate incidence figures, the CDC has changed its reporting guidelines. The new case classification is:

1. **Probable: a clinically compatible case with one or more painful genital ulcers and both**
   a. No evidence of *T. pallidum* by dark-field examination of ulcer exudate or by a serologic test for syphilis performed at least 7 days after the onset of ulcers.
   AND
   b. **Clinical presentation of the ulcer is not typical of a disease caused by herpes simplex virus, or an HSV culture is negative.**
2. **Confirmed:** A case that is laboratory confirmed. Recently there has been a documented association of chancroid and HIV. The presence of HIV infection predisposes women to chancroid and increases the possibility of treatment failure.

B. **History.** The patient usually presents with the complaint of a painful lesion.

C. **Physical examination.** The initial lesion in women occurs on the fourchette, labia minora, urethra, cervix, or anus. Extragenital lesions may occur but are uncommon. Chancroid begins as an inflammatory pustule or papule that quickly ruptures to form a **painful, nonindurated, shallow ulceration.** Women tend to have multiple ulcers, with an average of four. The ulcer is 1 to 2 cm in diameter with ragged undermined edges, and the base is often covered with a purulent exudate. Approximately 1 week after the initial ulcer, lymphadenopathy, which is usually unilateral, develops in 50% of patients. This subsides without suppuration in more than half of the patients; however, if left untreated, the lymphadenitis may undergo unilocular suppuration. The involved nodes are inflamed and tender, and the overlying skin is erythematous. These nodes then break down, forming a single drainage sinus and/or fever may occur.

D. **Investigative procedures**
1. **A presumptive diagnosis of chancroid** may be made in the presence of a genital ulcer(s) with a negative examination for syphilis (dark-field examination, serologic tests, or both) and no evidence of herpesvirus during follow-up visits.
2. **A definitive diagnosis** is made by isolation of the organism from ulcers of lymph nodes on an appropriate selective medium, but the organism is difficult to culture.
3. DNA probes and the use of PCR may make diagnosis easier in the future.

E. Management

1. **Drug therapy.** Recommended regimens include azithromycin, 1 g orally; or ceftriaxone, 250 mg IM or ciprofloxacin, 500 mg PO bid for 3 days; or erythromycin, 500 mg PO qid for 7 days.
2. **Fluctuant nodes** should be aspirated through healthy adjacent skin as often as necessary to prevent the formation of a draining sinus. Incision and drainage of buboes may be necessary.
3. **All sexual partners** should be treated.
4. As with all STDs, examination should be undertaken for the presence of other STDs, HIV, and hepatitis B and C.
5. All patients should be counseled about the risk of transmitting chancroid **and** the risk of either transmitting or acquiring HIV and hepatitis B and C through sexual intercourse. Patients should be encouraged to abstain from intercourse until all lesions have healed. Condoms have also been shown to prevent the transmission of chancroid.

VI. Lymphogranuloma venereum (LGV) is a granulomatous disease of the genital region that is primarily sexually transmitted. The causative organism is *C. trachomatis,* and the serotype is different from that which causes cervicitis. The incubation period is unknown. It is more common in men than women. LGV is rare in the United States, however, the actual prevalence is unknown.

A. History. The **presenting complaints** may include a painless lesion, lymphadenopathy, lower abdominal pain, rectal bleeding, rectal purulent discharge, and proctitis with tenesmus, depending on the stage of development.

B. Physical examination

1. **The initial lesion** is a painless vesicopapule that appears on the external genitalia, vaginal walls, or cervix in women. It appears a few days to a few weeks after exposure. This quickly breaks down to form a small erosion that heals rapidly in men, but more slowly in women. As many as 50% of these lesions are asymptomatic and heal without scarring.
2. **The secondary stage** is characterized by **lymphadenopathy,** which is usually unilateral, but involves multiple nodes. This results in the formation of a large nodal mass with inflamed overlying skin. The involvement of inguinal and femoral nodes with a depressed area over the inguinal ligament **(groove sign)** is almost pathognomonic for LGV. These nodes then develop multiple foci of suppuration, followed by skin breakdown and formation of multiple draining sinuses (as opposed to chancroid, which has a single area of suppuration and one draining site). **Genital mutilation** often develops.
3. The inguinal adenopathy typically resolves after 2 to 3 months if untreated. However, in the **tertiary stage** involvement of internal nodes (perirectal and perivaginal) leads to an **anorectal syndrome** with lower abdominal complaints and proctitis with tenesmus, rectal bleeding, and a purulent discharge. This may lead to rectal strictures, elephantiasis of the labia, and rectovaginal fistulae. Although extragenital lesions are rare, LGV is associated with significant systemic signs such as fever, malaise, myalgias, and arthritis.

C. Investigative procedures

The diagnosis of LGV is best made by **complement fixation titers,** which are available through most laboratories. However, there is cross-reaction with other chlamydial serotypes. A fourfold increase in titer or a titer of greater than 1:64 should be considered diagnostic. A titer of 1:16 to 1:64 is suggestive, but can occur in individuals with other chlamydial infections. The organism can be recovered from nodal aspirations, but culture is technically difficult, expensive, and rarely available.

D. Management

1. **Drug therapy.** The recommended regimen is doxycycline 100 mg PO bid for 21 days. An alternative regimen is erythromycin 500 mg PO qid for 21 days.

2. As with chancroid, **involved lymph nodes (buboes) should be aspirated** through adjacent normal skin, and incision and drainage may be indicated.
3. **Sexual contacts** should be examined and treated.
4. Investigation for the presence of other STDs, including HIV and hepatitis B and C, should be undertaken.

VII. **Granuloma inguinale** is generally considered a disease of tropical and subtropical regions. It is rare in the United States. The causative organism is an intracellular gram-negative bacterium, *Calymmatobacterium granulomatis*.

   A. **History.** The presenting complaint is usually of an **enlarging painless ulcer.**

   B. **Physical examination.** The initial lesion is a painless ulcer that has little undermining and is usually located on the labia or fourchette. There is no lymphadenopathy unless the lesion is secondarily infected. Occasionally, a deep granuloma may appear to be a fluctuant node. These "pseudobuboes" may erode through skin and slowly extend by local enlargement. Constitutional symptoms are absent. **If left untreated,** these lesions progress insidiously, often along skin folds, and take on a granulomatous appearance. The central portions of the ulcer may heal spontaneously, leaving gray, fibrous scars with active advancing borders. These scars can produce deformities and strictures. Long-standing lesions often produce elephantiasis-like enlargement of the labia and extensive ulceration of the perineum. Extragenital lesions can occur almost anywhere by direct spread, and systemic dissemination (presumably blood-borne) has been described. In advanced cases, general debilitation may lead to death. The incidence of squamous cell carcinoma is increased within the chronic ulcers.

   C. **Investigative procedures.** The diagnosis of granuloma inguinale should be considered in any genital ulcer lasting more than several weeks, especially in the absence of lymphadenopathy. The diagnosis is best made by finding the typical organisms **(Donovan bodies)** with histiocytes on stained smears or tissue sections from the edge of lesions. The tissue should be crushed and spread between two glass slides and stained with Wright's or Giemsa stain. The Donovan bodies exhibit bipolar staining and are commonly described as having a "safety pin" appearance.

   D. **Management**
   1. **Drug therapy.** The recommended regimens include doxycycline, 100 mg bid for 3 weeks or until all lesions have healed (from 2–12 weeks); trimethoprim-sulfamethoxazole DS (160/800) bid for at least 3 weeks; erythromycin, 500 mg qid for 2 to 3 weeks; or ciprofloxacin 750 mg PO bid for at least 3 weeks.
   2. **Sexual partners** should be examined and treated.
   3. Patients should also be examined for the presence of other STDs.

VIII. **Pediculosis pubis.** The causative organism for pubic lice is *Phthirus pubis* (crab louse), which is different from body or head lice. Its life cycle is approximately 25 days and can be completed entirely on the human host. Soon after reaching maturity, impregnated females begin laying eggs (nits) that hatch in 7 to 8 days. Each egg is cemented to a single hair shaft.

   Transmission is generally by **direct body contact,** usually sexual. The risk of transmission from fomites is negligible. Pubic lice are the most contagious STD known, and the risk of acquiring the infestation is approximately 95% after a single exposure. The incidence is higher in young women from 15 to 19 years of age and is higher in men older than 20 years. There is no racial difference. Although pubic lice can be transmitted without sexual contact, abuse should be considered in any infection in a child.

   A. **History.** The chief complaint of infested persons is **pruritus** and, because of autosensitization, it is not always localized to the affected sites. Patients may report seeing organisms move in their pubic hair.

   B. **Physical examination.** The louse is usually found in the **pubic area, eyebrows, and eyelashes.** Nits may be seen at the base of the hair shafts in these areas. Scratching may lead to secondary excoriations, which may predispose to lymphadenitis or pyoderma. The infested patient may also present with a symptomatic, bluish, nonblanching, nodular **rash** on the lower trunk and upper thighs, known as **maculae ceruleae.** This rash is believed to be either secondary to altered blood pigments in the patient or an excretory substance from the louse's salivary glands.

C. **Investigative procedures.** A magnifying glass may be helpful in visualizing the lice or nits. They may also be placed on a slide with a drop of mineral oil and examined under the microscope. The lice look like miniature crabs.

D. **Management**

1. **For pubic infestation,** treatment with gamma benzene hexachloride (lindane [Kwell]), a solution of pyrethrins with piperonyl butoxide (RID), or a 1% permethrin creme rinse (Nix) is equally effective.

    a. **Lindane** is available by prescription only, is absorbed through the skin, and can cause CNS toxicity (although this has been described only when it was used improperly or taken orally). It should **not be used in pregnant or lactating women or on children** younger than 2 years. The lotion is applied to the affected area, left on for 12 hours, and repeated in 1 week. The shampoo is massaged into the pubic hair and worked into a lather, left on for 4 minutes, and washed off. It is usually not necessary to repeat the application. Nits remaining after either treatment can be removed with forceps or a fine-toothed comb.

    b. **The pyrethrin solution** is available without prescription and is poorly absorbed through intact skin, so it is apparently free of toxicity. Two ounces are massaged into dry pubic hair, left on for 10 minutes, and washed off. One treatment is all that is necessary, and remaining nits can be removed in the manner described previously. **This is the treatment of choice in pregnancy** and lactation.

    c. **1% permethrin creme rinse** is available by prescription only. It should be applied to pubic hair and washed off after 10 minutes. This treatment should be repeated in 10 days, and remaining nits can be removed as discussed previously.

2. **For infestation of the eyelashes,** apply petrolatum bid for 8 days and remove the nits by hand.

3. Even though **fomite transmission** rarely (if ever) occurs, patients should be advised to **wash and dry sheets, bedding, and clothing** in the hot cycle. Sprays are available for use on inanimate objects, but are unnecessary and potentially dangerous and their use should be discouraged.

4. **All sexual contacts** should be treated simultaneously, and the patient should be examined for the presence of other STDs, including hepatitis B and HIV, **since one third to one half of all patients have another STD.**

5. Follow-up after 1 week if symptoms persist. Nonresponders should be retreated with an alternative regimen.

IX. **Scabies infestation** is caused by the mite *Sarcoptes scabiei*. Like the crab louse, its entire life cycle can be completed on humans. The adult female burrows into the skin and remains there for life, approximately 30 days. She rapidly begins laying two to three eggs per day, which become adult mites in 10 days. However, fewer than 10% of the eggs become adults. The average patient with scabies only has 10 to 15 live adult female mites on the body at any time. The mites can survive for only 2 to 3 days at room temperature apart from humans. However, they can survive longer in warm humid areas such as nursing homes than in cool, dry climates.

Several different types of scabies have been described. These include **scabies incognito,** occurring in persons receiving steroids, which alter the clinical presentation; **scabies in the clean,** found in those with good hygiene and in whom physical findings are minimal; and **nodular scabies,** which present as reddish-brown pruritic nodules in the usual scabetic distribution and appear to represent a hypersensitivity reaction; **Norwegian scabies,** which is rare, highly contagious, and usually found in institutions with a propensity for mentally retarded and debilitated persons; and **animal-transmitted scabies,** with dogs as the major source of infection. All of these types are treated the same except the latter. The animal mite cannot complete its life cycle on the human host, so the infestation is self-limited (several weeks), and the animal must be treated to prevent reinfestation.

Transmission is by close personal contact, usually sexual. Scabies are rarely transmitted by fomites or by casual contact. It is more common in men than women.

A. **History.** The **primary symptoms** are **pruritus** and a **rash** that is caused by sensitization to the mite. In primary infestation, it takes 4 to 6 weeks for these to occur, although in reinfestation, symptoms may appear within 24 hours. The pruritus is typically nocturnal. Since the immune system must be intact for a response, patients with a depressed immune system may not itch.

B. **Physical examination.** The rash is usually symmetric and located primarily on the hands (especially finger webs and sides of digits), wrists, elbows, female breasts, waist, penis, and the lower portion of the buttocks. The **pathognomonic lesion** is the burrow, which is a short, wavy, dirty-appearing line. This lesion is seen very infrequently now even though the incidence of scabies is not decreasing. Excoriations of these lesions can lead to secondary infection.

C. **Investigative procedures.** A presumptive diagnosis is made by observing the typical burrows in a symptomatic patient. A definitive diagnosis can be made by demonstrating the mite, the fecal pellets, or the burrow by **special tests.**

   1. A drop of **mineral oil** can be placed on the skin lesions, which are then scraped with a scalpel blade and transferred to a slide for observation through the microscope.

   2. The lesions can be moistened with alcohol, then scraped and transferred to a microscopic slide. Adding 20% potassium hydroxide to the slide and heating gently aids in clearing epidermal debris.

   3. In the **tetracycline test,** a liquid tetracycline solution is applied to areas where burrows are usually found. After drying, the area is cleaned vigorously with isopropyl alcohol and then observed with a Wood's lamp. Burrows that have retained the tetracycline appear as yellow-green lines.

   4. The **ink test,** similar to the tetracycline test, involves rubbing a fountain pen over the suspected area, then cleaning with alcohol, and looking for burrows that the ink has penetrated.

D. **Management**
   1. Several treatments are effective.
      a. **Lindane (1%) lotion** is applied thinly but thoroughly from the neck down and left on for 12 hours. The application is repeated in 1 week **only for those with evidence of treatment failure or reinfestation. Lindane should not be used in pregnancy or lactation or in children younger than 2 years.** Bathing prior to application is not recommended since it can potentiate absorption of the drug. The usual amount needed for adults is 30 mL.
      b. **Permethrin,** 5% cream (Elimite), is an excellent scabicide and less toxic than lindane. This is used as a single application in the same way as lindane and washed off after 10 hours. **Over-the-counter permethrim** products are lower strength, designed to treat pediculosis, and **are ineffective in the treatment of scabies.**
      c. **Sulfur,** as a 6% solution is applied nightly for 3 nights and washed off 24 hours after each application. Its efficacy and toxicity are not well established, and it is unpleasant to use.

2. Treatment should include brushing the formulation under the ends of the fingernails. In children and elderly patients, the face, head, and especially the postauricular fold should be included in treatment.
3. Bedding and clothing should be decontaminated via washing and hot cycle drying. **Fumigation of living areas is unnecessary.**
4. **All persons in close personal contact** with the patient should also be treated with one of the foregoing regimens.
5. For the pruritus, an oral antihistamine, such as hydroxyzine hydrochloride (Atarax), 25 mg tid; or diphenhydramine (Benadryl), 25 mg qid, as needed can be used simultaneously with the scabicide, or a 1% hydrocortisone cream can be used after treatment.

References

1. Centers for Disease Control. 1998 guidelines for treatment of sexually transmitted diseases. *MMWR* 1998;47(RR-1).
2. Nicholas H. Sexually transmitted diseases. Gonorrhea: symptoms and treatment. *Nurs Times* 1998;94:52.
3. Centers for Disease Control and Prevention. *Chlamydia trachomatis* genital infections—United States, 1995. *JAMA* 1997;277:952.
4. Kuhn GJ, et al. Diagnosis and follow-up of *Chlamydia trachomatis* infections in the ED. *Am J Emerg Med* 1998;16:157.
5. Buckley HB. Syphilis: a review and update of the "new" infection of the '90s. *Nurs Pract* 1992;17:25.
6. Farnes SW, Setness PA. Serologic tests for syphilis. *Postgrad Med J* 1990;87:37.
7. Wasserheit JN. Epidemiological synergy: interrelationships between human immunodeficiency virus infection and other sexually transmitted diseases. *Sex Transm Dis* 1992;19:61.
8. White C, Wardropper AG. Genital herpes simplex infection in women. *Clin Dermatol* 1997;15:81.
9. Kellock DJ, et al. Lymphogranuloma venereum: biopsy, serology, and molecular biology. *Genitourin Med* 1997;73:399.
10. Trees DL, Morse SA. Chancroid and haemophilus ducreyi: an update. *Clin Microbiol Rev* 1995;8:357–375.
11. Ronald AR, Plummer FA. Chancroid and granuloma inguinale. *Clin Lab Med* 1989;9:535.
12. Elgart ML. Pediculosis. *Dermatol Clin* 1990;8:219.
13. Elgart ML. Scabies. *Dermatol Clin* 1990;8:253.

4. HUMAN PAPILLOMAVIRUS

Richard H. Oi

Condylomata acuminata (venereal warts) are among the most common sexually transmitted diseases (STDs) and are caused by the human papillomavirus (HPV). The principal mode of transmission is through skin-to-skin contact, and HPV may enter epidermal or mucosal tissue through inflamed and macerated skin or through microscopic abrasions during sexual intercourse. Sexual transmission is a common route of transmission. Other mechanisms of transmission, although rare, include fomite contact and suspected vertical transmission from infected mother to newborn. Genital or anal warts in children can occur without evidence of sexual contact, but the possibility of abuse must be considered.

A fully functional immune system is necessary to attenuate HPV involvement. There is therefore an increased incidence in patients receiving steroids, in immunosuppressed transplant patients, and in those with HIV disease or malignancy. The relative immunosuppressed state of pregnancy promotes rapid growth of these lesions. Estimates of spread from infected persons to uninfected persons range as high as 70%. The incubation period ranges from 3 weeks to 2 years, with warts appearing on average 2 to 4 months after exposure.

Vaginal and cervical condylomata are not as common as on the vulva. Women with vulvar condyloma often demonstrate associated cervical HPV infection. By using molecular hybridization with labeled HPV DNA, over 70 genotypes of HPV have been identified and approximately 27 are associated with anogenital lesions (2). In the cervix, HPV appears to act preferentially in the tissues of the cervical transformation zone in which active squamous metaplasia is occurring. In one study, 91 % of cervical intraepithelial neoplasia (CIN) lesions contained HPV DNA (4). Low-risk (for malignant transformation) HPV type 6 and 11 are associated with condylomatous lesions or with lesions demonstrating minimal degrees of CIN and very often undergo spontaneous regression. HPV type 16 and 18 however, are considered high-risk HPV types and are more often associated with higher grades of CIN and invasive squamous lesions. These high-risk types demonstrate a greater propensity for malignant progression. Other cofactors, such as smoking, genital herpesvirus, and oral contraceptives may play a role in the development of neoplasia.

After treating visible warts, latent viral infection of adjacent normal tissue contributes to recurrence in 25% to 50% of patients (6). Most recurrences are within 3 months but some occur more than 9 months later.

I. **History.** Those with vulvar lesions often present with the complaint of new growths. Condylomata are often asymptomatic but can be painful, friable, or pruritic. They may be stigmatizing socially and are a reminder of the presence of a STD. Presenting symptoms of vaginal condylomata include **vaginal discharge and pruritus,** probably caused by secondary infection.

II. **Physical examination.** Condylomata acuminata are usually found throughout the external genital region. Their infectious nature is demonstrated by their appearance in opposing positions on both sides of the perineum. Diagnosis is usually made by clinical examination of characteristic discrete papillomatous lesions that may coalesce into a plaque-like appearance. Lesions are often multifocal and it is important to examine the entire lower genital tract prior to treatment. Evaluation for intraanal warts by anoscopy is indicated for men and women with recurrent perineal warts and/or a history of receptive anal intercourse.

III. **Investigative procedures**
   A. Those vulvar lesions that lack the classic appearance of a cauliflower-like growth, fail to respond to therapy, or are recurrent or become ulcerated should be biopsied.

B. Subclinical cervical lesions are usually detected by Papanicolaou (Pap) smears and are evaluated by colposcopy and directed biopsies.

C. Men may be examined with magnification after wrapping the penis with 5% acetic acid (white vinegar) soaked gauze for 5 minutes. However, examination can also be readily accomplished by careful scrutiny with a hand lens. Examination of the mons, scrotum, and perineal and perianal areas should complement the penile examination.

D. Women with vulvar condyloma should be followed with pelvic examinations and Pap smears, anticipating HPV involvement of the cervix.

IV. Management. The primary goal is to eliminate warts that cause physical or psychological symptoms. Treatment may result in wart-free periods but the underlying viral presence may persist. If left untreated, warts may resolve spontaneously, remain unchanged, or increase in size and number. Several methods are available for the treatment and may be either patient-applied or health care provider applied.

A. Vulvar lesions

1. Patient applied

   a. Podofilox solution or gel (0.5%) (Condylox)—an antimitotic agent that causes necrosis of visible wart tissues. It may be used on external warts only and not on mucous membrane lesions.

      (1) The gel is applied directly on wart with fingers or applicator and application to the surrounding normal tissues should be avoided. The gel is allowed to dry before allowing apposing skin surface to contact treated area.

      (2) It is applied twice daily for 3 days, off for 4 days and 7-day cycle is repeated until lesions are no longer present. Treatment should not be extended beyond four cycles.

      (3) Patients should wash hands before and after application and especially avoid introducing the agent into the eye.

   b. Imiquimod cream (5%) (Aldara) is a topically active immune enhancer that stimulates production of interferon-α and other cytokines. It has no direct antiviral activity. *It is not indicated for mucosal warts.*

      (1) It is applied as a thin layer to external genital or perineal wart area and rubbed in until the cream is no longer visible. Occlusive dressings should *not* be used.

      (2) The cream is applied three times a week prior to sleeping hours and left on for 6 to 10 hours after which the area should be cleansed with mild soap and water. The patient should wash hands before and after application.

      (3) Local skin reactions are common. Use should be discontinued until the skin irritation clears, then treatment may be resumed.

      (4) Application is continued until warts are cleared *or* for maximum of 16 weeks.

2. Health care provider applied

   a. Podophyllin in a 25% to 40% solution in alcohol, mineral oil, or benzoin should be applied to the lesions weekly. The average number of treatments to clear the lesions is four applications. Podophyllin should *not* be used on lesions larger than 2 cm and care should be taken to avoid getting it on normal skin. It does not need to be washed off within 6 hours of application unless the patient develops irritation. Podophyllin **should not be used in pregnancy** because fetal death and premature labor have been reported from its use. **Podophyllin should not be used intravaginally or on any mucosal lesions.**

      If the lesions do not show signs of regression after 4 weeks or if they are not gone by 6 weeks, another treatment should be used and/or a biopsy should be considered. When a biopsy is performed, the pathology request should specify that podophyllin was used because histologic changes that can be mistaken for neoplasia can be induced by the agent. It often takes a month after the last treatment for reversal of these changes.

  b. **Bi- or trichloroacetic acid (TCA)** in a 30% to 50% solution may be applied to lesions twice monthly. Compared with podophyllin, it requires fewer treatments, is less painful and less irritating to normal tissue, and can be used to treat a larger volume of lesions. Systemic absorption has not been a problem.

  c. **Fluorouracil** (5-FU) applied topically has been used but does not appear to have advantage over other topical treatments. It is applied daily directly to the lesions until erythematous or vesicular changes occur (usually 7–10 days).

  d. **Cryotherapy** Local freezing of warty lesions can be readily accomplished. An appropriate probe is used and freezing is continued until the entire lesion shows ice formation. It usually does not require anesthesia with focal localized lesions but local infiltration will make the procedure more comfortable.

  e. **Excision or electrodesiccation** after local anesthesia should be reserved for recurrent, very large lesions, or for those that do not respond to cryotherapy. These methods are very effective and leave little scarring because the lesion alone is addressed without subepidermal injury.

  f. **Carbon dioxide laser** treatment is painful, requiring anesthesia, but is effective treatment. There is some concern that laser vaporization may result in HPV particles in the plume generated by the vaporization but there has not been evidence of infectivity in this material.

  g. **Injectable therapy. Interferon,** injected into the lesion twice weekly for 8 weeks, is efficacious in approximately 70% of cases. Side effects such as fever, chills, myalgias, and headache are common (3).

B. Vaginal lesions

  1. **Asymptomatic lesions** can be managed by vaginal cleansing and hygiene, anticipating spontaneous regression. The cervix should be assessed for HPV involvement. The patient may be followed and biopsies taken if the lesions do not resolve.

  2. **Symptomatic lesions**

    a. **TCA,** applied as described, in the absence of a keratinized surface in vaginal mucosa results in effective destruction of the warts (see section IV.A.2.B). *Podophyllin should not be used in the vagina.*

    b. **Cryotherapy** is very effective, though it cannot be used on large warts.

    c. **Carbon dioxide laser** treatments can also be used (see section IV.A.2.f).

C. Cervical lesions

  1. **Cryotherapy** or the carbon dioxide laser can be used to ablate cervical lesions after colposcopically directed biopsy and endocervical curettage confirmation.

  2. **Loop electrosurgical excision** procedure (LEEP). After establishing the diagnosis by directed biopsy, LEEP can be used and has the advantage of removing tissue that can be histologically examined.

D. Lesions during pregnancy

  1. **Bichloracetic acid or TCA** is the treatment of choice for symptomatic minimal vaginal and perineal condylomata acuminata. **Podophyllin is contraindicated in pregnancy.**

  2. **Surgical excision or carbon dioxide laser** may be used during the late second trimester if the lesions become problematic for uncomplicated vaginal delivery.

  3. **Cesarean section.** Although 40% to 60% of children with laryngeal papillomatosis are born of mothers with a history of genital HPV (5), it is

not clear if these are acquired antepartum, intrapartum, or by fomites in the postpartum period. Thus, genital HPV infection, per se, is not an indication for cesarean section.

E. Sexual partners with obvious lesions should be examined and treated.

F. Conditions that are **known to enhance the growth** of condylomata acuminata as well as to interfere with their response to therapy are vaginitis, poor personal hygiene, immunosuppressive drugs, and altered immunologic status (including HIV disease).

G. Patients with condylomata should be examined and tested for the presence of other STDs. Patients with **recalcitrant warts** should be screened for **HIV** and **diabetes.**

H. Patients should be instructed that this is a sexually transmitted infection, that recurrences are common, and that smoking may be a risk factor in neoplastic transformation.

References

1. Arends MJ, Wyllie AH, Bird CC. Papillomaviruses and human cancer. *Hum Pathol* 1990;21:686.
2. Duggan MA. Human papillomaviruses in gynecologic cancer. *Curr Opin Obstet Gynecol* 1996;8:56.
3. Eron LJ. Update: prevention and therapy of genital warts. *Compr Ther* 1988;14:7.
4. Kirby P, Corey L. Genital human papillomavirus infections. *Infect Dis Clin North Am* 1987;1:123.
5. Majmudar B, Hallden C. The relationship between juvenile laryngeal papillomatosis and maternal condylomata acuminata. *J Reprod Med* 1986;31:804.
6. Schiffman MH, et al. Epidemiologic evidence showing that human papillomavirus infection causes most cervical intraepithelial neoplasia. *JNCI* 1993;84:394.
7. Duggan MA, et al. The human papillomavirus status of 114 endocervical adenocarcinoma cases by dotblot hybridization. *Hum Pathol* 1993;24:121.
8. Blackledge D, Russel R. "HPV effect" on female lower genital tract: a community study. *J Reprod Med* 1998;43:929.

5. PELVIC INFLAMMATORY DISEASE

Victor P. Chin

I. **Definition.** Pelvic inflammatory disease (PID) is a general description of inflammation caused by infection in the upper genital tract. Many infectious disease experts support eliminating the term PID in favor of just calling this an upper genital tract infection. Although infection of the fallopian tubes (salpingitis) is the most characteristic and common component of PID, infection of the endometrium (endometritis), ovaries (oophoritis), uterine wall (myometritis), and broad ligament or uterine serosa (parametritis) may also be present. PID is an acute process unless unusual organisms, such as tuberculosis or actinomycetes, are involved.

II. **Etiology.** Ninety-nine percent of cases of acute PID are the result of the ascending migration of organisms from the vagina and cervix. Infection spreads along the mucosal surface of the endometrium to the fallopian tubes. Infection and inflammation may then spread by transtubal extension to the serosal surfaces of the fallopian tubes or through the fimbriated ends of the tubes. Infection of the ovaries, parametrium, and peritoneal cavity (peritonitis, pelvic abscess) may then result. Approximately 10% of these ascending infections are iatrogenic or nonvenereal in origin. **Nonvenereal or iatrogenic PID** occurs as a complication of abortion; dilation and curettage (D & C); endometrial biopsies; and other invasive procedures, such as hysterosalpingogram, sonohysterography, cervical dilation, loop excision procedures and intrauterine device (IUD) insertion. Infectious complications following these procedures are less likely if proper sterile techniques are used. Less than 1% of acute PID is secondary to spread of infection from outside the genital tract. **Secondary PID** is associated with transperitoneal spread of infection from a ruptured appendix or intraabdominal abscess.

III. **Microbiologic features.** Previously, PID was divided into gonococcal versus nongonococcal infection, depending on whether gonococci were isolated from the endocervix. Since about 1970, newer diagnostic techniques have elucidated the polymicrobial nature of PID. Bacteria commonly cultured from tubal fluid of PID patients include *Neisseria gonorrhoeae, Chlamydia trachomatis,* endogenous aerobes and anaerobes, and occasionally genital *Mycoplasma* species.

   A. **N. gonorrhoeae (or gonococcal) infection** is epidemic in many parts of the world. Even though the reported incidence in the United States declined 72% from 1975 to 1997, in 1998 and 1999 the numbers leveled off in women and increased slightly in men. The reported cases in women in 1998 and 1999 were approximately 355,000 or 132/100,000 (36). In addition to pelvic infection, hematogenous spread of the gonococci can result in infection of the heart valves, joints, and perihepatic area.

   1. *N. gonorrhoeae* should be the prime suspect if:
      a. PID occurs within a week of menstruation.
      b. There is no previous history of PID.
      c. The patient's partner has documented gonorrhea.
      d. Endocervical exudate contains intracellular gram-negative diplococci in three or more leukocytes.

   2. Once *N. gonorrhoeae* migrates to the tubes, it causes an intense inflammatory reaction within days.

   3. Swelling of the tubes and tubal obstruction by purulent exudate result in extensive damage.

   B. *Chlamydia trachomatis*

   1. *C. trachomatis* causes a wide clinical spectrum of infection, including trachoma; neonatal pneumonitis; conjunctivitis; and in men, acute epididymitis and nongonococcal urethritis. Since 1980, *C. trachomatis* has

been implicated as the most common primary etiologic agent in PID. In many Western societies, *Chlamydia* **is believed to be the most common cause of acute PID followed by** *N. gonorrhoeae.* Immunologic data implicate chlamydial involvement in up to half of the acute PID patients. Unfortunately, the incidence of chlamydia has been steadily climbing. According to Centers for Disease Control and Prevention (CDC) data, the rate of chlamydia infection in women was approximately 250/100,000 in 1990 and had increased to 400/100,000 in 1999 (36).

   a. If not adequately treated, 20% to 40% of women with chlamydia and 10% to 40% with gonococci will develop PID (31).

   b. Since 70% of patients with chlamydia and 50% of patients with gonococci are asymptomatic, epidemiologists feel that routine screening in the age group most likely to be infected can reduce PID by 60% (36).

   c. The Health Plan Employer Data and Info Set (HEDIS) recently implemented routine annual screening of sexually active women between the ages of 15 and 25 as a quality measure in hopes of decreasing PID.

  2. It is speculated that chlamydia ascends from the cervix to cause genital tract damage in much the same way as gonorrhea. However, *C. trachomatis* may remain in the tubes for months following migration. **Chlamydial PID can be an insidious or even a silent illness.** This is particularly disturbing because chlamydial infection often results in more severe inflammatory changes and tubal destruction than other forms of PID. *C. trachomatis* probably destroys the tubal mucosa by an immunopathologic mechanism. Since chlamydial infection tends to be severe and is often associated with abscess formation, **routine screening for chlamydial cervicitis in asymptomatic women is** prudent in women who are at higher risk (i.e., women younger than 25 years old or those with new or multiple sex partners) (2).

C. Anaerobic bacteria. Anaerobic bacteria such as *Bacteroides* species (both *Bacteroides fragilis* and *Bacteroides bivius*), peptostreptococci, and peptococci are almost invariably cultured from pelvic abscesses of patients with acute PID. PID **associated with anaerobic infection is clinically more severe and more resistant to antibiotic therapy.** Anaerobic infection is more likely to occur in women who have had previous episodes of PID. These organisms may be endogenous secondary invaders from the lower genital tract in patients whose tubes have been previously damaged.

D. Aerobic organisms. The most common aerobic organisms cultured from tubal lumina in cases of acute PID are **nonhemolytic streptococci,** *Escherichia coli, Haemophilus influenzae,* **group B streptococci, and coagulase-negative staphylococci** (26).

E. *Mycoplasma hominis* **and T-mycoplasma** *(Ureaplasma urealyticum)* may colonize the lower female genital tract. These organisms have been isolated in 8% and 4%, respectively, of women with PID. There is serologic evidence to suggest a secondary role for *M. hominis* in up to one fourth of all cases of PID. There is no evidence to suggest that *Mycoplasma* alone produces damage to the tubal mucosa.

F. Tuberculous salpingitis. Mycobacterial infection of the fallopian tubes and endometrium is now a rarity in the United States. However, both *Mycobacterium tuberculosis* and *Mycobacterium bovis* remain frequent causes of chronic PID in third-world countries. **There is no strong evidence to support sexual transmission of tuberculous infection.**

  1. *M. tuberculosis* is believed to spread hematogenously from the primary infection in the lung to the pelvis, whereas bovine tuberculosis disseminates to the pelvis by lymphatic or hematogenous spread from the primary infection in the human gastrointestinal tract. Chronic abdominal pain; infertility; abnormal uterine bleeding; and in advanced cases, ascites are the most common presentation of tuberculous salpingitis.

However, some women with culture-proven tuberculous salpingitis are entirely asymptomatic, and up to 50% of women with documented tuberculous salpingitis have a normal pelvic examination.

2. *M. tuberculosis* should be considered as a possible etiologic agent in regions where tuberculosis is prevalent, in an immigrant or visitor, or when a patient fails to respond to conventional antibiotic therapy. If the endometrium is involved (two thirds of cases), appropriate culture and histologic examination of tissue obtained by endometrial biopsy in the late secretory cycle may be diagnostic.

IV. **Incidence.** Accurate estimates are hard to come by since many cases are treated in the office based on clinical findings and not based on laparoscopic procedures. The fact that hospitalizations for PID have decreased over the last two decades has also contributed to less accurate estimates. Nevertheless, in 1998 there were an estimated 238,000 cases treated in emergency departments. Approximately 80,000 cases of PID were hospitalized in 1998 (36). The estimated cost in 1998 of caring for PID and its sequelae was $1.88 billion. The expected lifetime cost per case of PID in 1998 was $1167 (32).

V. **Risk factors**

A. **Age.** The prevalence of acute PID is highest in women younger than 30 years, with one third younger than 20 years and two thirds younger than 25 years. Studies have shown that not only earlier age at first intercourse is a risk factor, but that among adolescents, sex with an older individual is also a risk factor (34,38).

B. **Sexual activity.** Acute PID is extremely rare in women who are not sexually active. However, a small fraction of infections may be endogenous in origin. Multiple sexual partners increase a woman's chance of developing PID three- to fourfold. This is particularly true if exposure to multiple partners occurred within 30 days (34).

C. **Menstruation.** Acute PID is unusual in women who are pregnant, premenarcheal, or postmenopausal. Risk for PID is increased when intercourse occurs during menses (34).

D. **History of PID.** Women who have had one episode of PID are two to three times more likely than other women to have another episode. Recurrence may be partly due to some residual defect in the endometrium's ability to fight infection.

E. **Contraception.** A woman's choice of contraceptive method will markedly influence her subsequent risk **for PID** (19).

1. **Intrauterine devices.** The greatest risk of PID is in the first month after insertion. Beyond the first month, the risk of PID depends on the sexual behavior of the woman and/or her partner. Behavior that increases the risk of STD pathogens will increase the risk of IUD-associated PID. On the other hand, low-risk sexual behavior is associated with an extremely low incidence of PID.

2. **Oral contraceptives.** The relationship between oral contraceptive use and PID is not entirely clear. There are contradictory data in the literature. However, most studies seem to indicate that oral contraceptives exert a protective effect. Whether that protective effect is more against gonorrheal or chlamydial infection is yet to be decided. Furthermore, laparoscopic studies have shown that there is a **decreased inflammatory response in women with PID who are taking oral contraceptives.**

3. **Barrier contraceptives,** such as condoms, diaphragms, and spermicidal jellies and foams, appear to exert significant protective effects against PID. Condoms should be made of a latex material. "Natural" condoms made from sheep intestinal membrane contain small pores that may allow passage of viral particles, including HIV and hepatitis. A recent study among adolescents, however, did not show correlation with PID incidence and condom use (38). Nevertheless, condom use should still be advised as a possible protective device against STDs.

   F. Abortion. The risk of PID following spontaneous abortions is approximately 1%. It is estimated that 0.5% of legal abortions are complicated by acute salpingitis. Postabortion PID usually presents as a febrile illness 5 to 21 days after surgery. Illegal abortion appears to carry a risk of at least 10% for PID.

   G. Recent instrumentation or genital tract invasive procedures. A history of recent (up to 4 weeks prior) instrumentation or genital tract procedures is found in up to 12% of PID cases.

   H. Douching. There are some data to suggest that douching may increase the risk of PID by disturbing the local cervical defenses and increasing bacterial contamination of the endometrium, tubes, and peritoneal cavity (23). However, there are other studies that fail to confirm this association (34).

   I. Other risk factors. Several studies have indicated that the following are also risk factors to consider (34,35,38):

- Involvement with a child protection agency.
- Prior suicide attempts.
- Alcohol before last sex.
- Current or history of chlamydia or gonococcal infection.
- Multiparity.
- Less than 12 years of education.
- Illegal drug use.

VI. Diagnosis. Acute PID can be difficult to diagnose. Studies reveal that the clinical diagnoses of PID are confirmed during laparoscopy in only 30% to 80% of patients. This is true even in women with a previous history of PID (37). Approximately 35% of women in whom acute PID is clinically diagnosed have no evidence of PID on laparoscopy. A recent study showed that the usual clinical and laboratory data used to make the diagnosis of PID have a poor predictive value in distinguishing the severity of the disease (33).

   A. Differential diagnosis

      1. It is essential that every practitioner recognize that the differential diagnosis of PID includes **ectopic pregnancy. An immediate pregnancy test should be obtained in every case of suspected acute PID.**

      2. Other diseases commonly misdiagnosed as PID include **appendicitis, mesenteric adenitis, pelvic endometriosis,** or **conditions resulting from previous acute PID** (chronic salpingitis and adhesions).

      3. **The CDC guidelines** for diagnosis are listed in Table 5.1. These guidelines were designed to include women with mild PID, while excluding those with diseases commonly confused with PID. It is hoped that use of more specific **diagnostic criteria** will **result** in **earlier** and **more accurate diagnosis and treatment.**

   B. History

      1. The symptoms of acute PID most often begin **during or immediately after menstruation,** regardless of microbiologic etiology.

      2. The **presenting complaint of constant and dull lower abdominal pain** and tenderness is found in 90% of PID patients. The pain is usually of less than 7 days duration and is exacerbated by movement or sexual intercourse.

      3. **Increased vaginal discharge** is noted in 55% of patients.

      4. **Fever or chills** are noted in 40% of patients. However, chlamydial PID patients are more often afebrile.

      5. **Nausea, vomiting, and anorexia** associated with marked pelvic peritonitis occur in only 25% of cases.

      6. **Fitz-Hugh-Curtis (FHC) syndrome** occurs in 5% to 10% of cases of PID. It is associated with symptoms of pleuritic **right upper quadrant abdominal pain** referred to the corresponding shoulder or **perihepatitis with mild liver function test abnormalities.**

Table 5.1. Criteria for the diagnosis of acute salpingitis

MINIMUM CRITERIA

Empiric treatment for pelvic inflammatory disease (PID) should be instituted on
the basis of the presence of **all of the following and** in the **absence of an
established cause other than PID:**
- Lower abdominal tenderness
- Adnexal tenderness
- Cervical motion tenderness

ADDITIONAL CRITERIA

These additional criteria may be used to increase the specificity of the diagnosis:
- Oral temperature >38.3°C (>101°F)
- Abnormal cervical or vaginal discharge
- Elevated sedimentation rate
- Elevated C-reactive protein
- Laboratory documentation of cervical infection with gonorrhea or chlamydia

DEFINITIVE CRITERIA

- Histopathologic evidence of endometritis on endometrial biopsy
- Transvaginal sonography or other imaging techniques showing thickened fluid-
  filled tubes with or without free pelvic fluid or tuboovarian complex
- Laparoscopic abnormalities consistent with PID

From: Centers for Disease Control and Prevention: 1998 sexually transmitted diseases treatment
guidelines. *MMWR* 1998;47(RR-1), with permission.

        a. FHC syndrome is secondary to either gonococcal or chlamydial in-
        fection spreading from the fallopian tubes along the paracolic gut-
        ters to the upper abdomen.

        b. A prompt response to antibiotics and the recognition of concurrent
        PID help distinguish FHC syndrome from cholecystitis.

C. Physical examination

    1. **Lower abdominal and pelvic tenderness** remains the most consis-
    tent finding in PID. Cervical motion tenderness is a very frequent find-
    ing but is not specific for PID.

    2. **Swelling of the adnexa or a true adnexal mass** is noted in 10% of
    PID patients.

    3. **Rebound lower abdominal tenderness** suggesting pelvic peritoni-
    tis occurs in only 25% of PID patients.

    4. **Perihepatitis or FHC syndrome,** characterized by upper quadrant
    abdominal tenderness, is found in 5% to 10% of all gonococcally medi-
    ated PID, but may be even more common with chlamydial PID.

D. Investigative procedures

    1. Cultures

        a. **Cervical, urethral, and rectal specimens** should be obtained as
        indicated by history and physical examination

        b. Anaerobic cultures are not helpful in determining PID etiology since
        many anaerobes are normal cervical flora.

        c. Rapid enzyme tests are available for office use for the diagnosis of
        chlamydial and gonococcal infections.

    2. **A Gram stain** of the endocervical secretions for inflammatory cells can
    be helpful.

        a. The presence of gram-negative intracellular diplococci implicate
        N. gonorrhoeae as the causative agent.

        b. Although finding evidence of gonococcal or chlamydial infection on
        a Gram stain is helpful, it is not a prerequisite for diagnosis. The

complete absence of white blood cells in a vaginal Gram-stained preparation, however, is rare in a patient with acute PID.

3. **Giemsa-stained or iodine-stained cervical smears** may be used to identify the intracytoplasmic inclusions of chlamydiae.

4. **Pregnancy testing. Radioreceptor assays** for human chorionic gonadotrophin (hCG) and **radioimmunoassay** (RIA) for the beta subunit of hCG are invaluable in the diagnostic evaluation of women presenting with acute pelvic pain. Approximately 4% of those admitted to the hospital with a diagnosis of acute PID have an ectopic pregnancy. **All women with suspected PID should have an immediate urine or serum pregnancy test to exclude ectopic pregnancy.**

5. **A white blood cell count and erythrocyte sedimentation rate** are neither sensitive nor specific for diagnosis of PID.
   a. Fewer than 50% of women with documented acute PID have an elevated white blood cell count, although this is included as a subcriterion for diagnosis.
   b. A normal erythrocyte sedimentation rate (<15 mm/hr) was found in 24% of women with laparoscopically proven PID.

6. **Ultrasound evaluation** is of limited value in diagnosing acute PID. However, it is 95% accurate for detecting pelvic abscesses and can help monitor response to medical therapy.

7. **Laparoscopy or laparotomy** provides immediate and accurate diagnosis. Laparoscopy offers the chance to inspect the tubes directly, to assess the severity of the inflammatory reaction, and to obtain biopsy and culture specimens. Laparoscopy is usually indicated for a patient being appropriately treated for acute PID who fails to respond to medical therapy or when the diagnosis is too uncertain to begin empiric antibiotic therapy.

8. **Culdocentesis** is occasionally helpful in the evaluation of acute pelvic pain. Culdocentesis is a safe and quick technique, but should not be performed if there is a mass in the cul-de-sac or if the uterus is markedly retroflexed.
   a. Peritoneal fluid that contains more than 30,000 white blood cells per milliliter supports the diagnosis of acute PID.
   b. The aspiration of nonclotting bloody fluid strongly suggests ectopic pregnancy.
   c. When clear serous fluid is found on culdocentesis, a diagnosis of ruptured ovarian cyst should be considered.
   d. All fluids obtained at culdocentesis should be cultured.

VII. Management. The goals of antibiotic therapy in PID are to maintain tubal patency and to relieve discomfort. In general, patients with acute PID can be treated as outpatients, with reexamination within 48 to 72 hours.

A. **Outpatient management**
   1. **Antibiotic therapy** is the cornerstone of therapy for acute PID. After appropriate cultures have been obtained, antibiotic therapy should be initiated **against the broadest range of known pathogens.** The CDC has recently published a set of combination regimens with broad activity against major PID pathogens for both ambulatory and inpatient treatment (6).
      a. **Ofloxacin, 400** mg PO bid for 14 days, **PLUS metronidazole,** 500 mg PO bid, for 14 days.
         OR
      b. **Ceftriaxone,** 250 mg IM once **PLUS doxycycline,** 100 mg PO bid for 14 days.
         OR
      c. **Cefoxitin,** 2 g IM, plus **probenecid,** 1 g PO concurrently; **PLUS doxycycline,** 100 mg PO bid for 14 days.
         OR

   d. 3rd generation cephalosporin (e.g., ceftizoxime or cefotaxime) **PLUS doxycycline,** 100 mg PO bid for 14 days.
2. **Supportive measures**
   a. **Bedrest, sexual abstinence** (until the results of pelvic examination become normal), **hydration,** and **analgesics** should be encouraged.
   b. **An IUD should be removed after antibiotic therapy has been initiated.** Contraceptive counseling should be offered at the time of IUD removal.
3. **Follow-up**
   a. **Outpatients** should be **reexamined in 48 to 72 hours after initiation of antibiotic therapy.** Those not responding favorably should be hospitalized for intravenous antibiotic therapy.
   b. **Repeat cultures** may be obtained **2 weeks after therapy is** completed to document clinical cure. If more sensitive tests are used such as polymerase chain reaction or ligase chain reaction, rescreening should wait for 1 month.
   c. Sexual partners of patients with PID with contact within the past 60 days should be examined for sexually transmitted diseases, cultured, and appropriately treated.
   d. Tests for syphilis (rapid plasma reagin [RPR]), HIV, and hepatitis B (HBsAg) should be obtained.
B. **Inpatient management**
   1. **Hospitalization** should strongly be considered with any of the following:
      a. The diagnosis is uncertain, such as when appendicitis or ectopic pregnancy cannot be excluded.
      b. A pelvic abscess is suspected.
      c. The patient is an adolescent or is believed to be unreliable.
      d. The patient is pregnant.
      e. An IUD is in place.
      f. The patient is unable to keep down oral medication secondary to nausea and vomiting.
      g. There is generalized peritonitis or severe illness.
      h. Outpatient therapy fails.
      i. Clinical reevaluation in 48 to 72 hours cannot be arranged.
      j. Patient is immunodeficient (i.e., has HIV with low CD4 counts, is taking immunosuppressive drugs, or has another disease).
   2. **Surgical intervention** is indicated if the tenderness and size of an adnexal mass do not abate, despite adequate antibiotic therapy. Operations are much less frequent in cases of acute PID than they were in the past. Persistent pelvic abscess, ruptured tuboovarian abscess, or cases of life-threatening infection require surgical consultation.
   3. **Antibiotic therapy.** The CDC guidelines for recommended treatment are:
      a. **Regimen A**
         (1) **Cefoxitin,** 2 g IV q6h, **plus doxycycline,** 100 mg IV or PO q12h.
            OR
         (2) **Cefotetan,** 2 g IV q12h, **plus doxycycline,** 100 mg IV or PO q12h.
         (3) This should continue until the patient has improved for 48 hours. The patient should continue with the doxycycline for a total of 14 days.
      b. **Regimen B**
         (1) **Clindamycin,** 900 mg IV q8h, **plus gentamicin** loading dose IV or IM (2 mg/kg of body weight), followed by a maintenance dose (1.5 mg/kg) q8h. A single daily dose may be substituted. This regimen should be continued until the patient has improved for at least 48 hours, after which time she should

continue to receive either doxycycline 100 mg bid or clindamycin 450 mg qid to complete a total of 14 days of treatment.
When an abscess is present, it may be better to use clindamycin instead of doxycycline.

  c. **Alternative parenteral regimens**
    (1) **Ofloxacin** 400 mg IV q12h **plus metronidazole** 500 mg IV
        q8h.
        OR
    (2) **Ampicillin/sulbactam** 3gm IV q6h **plus doxycycline** 100mg
        q12h.
        OR
    (3) **Ciprofloxacin** 200 mg IV q12h **plus doxycycline** 100 mg
        q12h **plus metronidazole** 500 mg IV q8h.

VIII. Sequelae
  A. Chronic pelvic pain is defined as pelvic pain lasting longer than 6 months
    that causes the patient to seek medical advice. Approximately 20% of all
    post-PID patients develop this problem. Chronic pelvic pain is often associ-
    ated with infertility as well as deep dyspareunia. This may be secondary to
    hydrosalpinx or a collection of sterile fluid in the fallopian tube following
    treatment of pyosalpinx or paraovarian adhesions (see Chapter 15).
  B. Ectopic pregnancy. The number of ectopic pregnancies in this country has
    doubled in the past decade. This increase parallels the increased incidence
    of acute PID. Fifty percent of patients with ectopic pregnancy have evidence
    of previous tubal infection. It has been estimated that a single episode of
    PID increases a woman's chance of ectopic pregnancy sixfold.
  C. Infertility as a result of PID affects more than 60,000 women annually in
    the United States. Infertility caused by tubal closure increases in frequency
    with the severity and number of pelvic infections. Following one episode of
    PID, the risk of infertility is 13%, and after two episodes the incidence rises
    to 35%.
  D. Tuboovarian abscess. Intraabdominal rupture of a tuboovarian abscess
    is one of the most serious complications of pelvic infection. Attempts to man-
    age patients medically with a ruptured tuboovarian abscess have been as-
    sociated with a mortality of 5% to 10%. **Total abdominal hysterectomy
    and bilateral salpingo-oophorectomy are the treatments of choice**
    and are reported to result in a sevenfold decrease in deaths.

References
1. Alary M, et al. Strategy for screening pregnant women for chlamydial infection in
   a low-prevalence area. *Obstet Gynecol* 1993;82:399.
2. Becker T, et al. Sexually transmitted diseases and other risk factors for cervical
   dysplasia among Southwestern Hispanic and non-Hispanic white women. *JAMA*
   1994;271:1181.
3. Burkman RT Jr. Preventing unintended pregnancy: the role of hormonal contraceptives: noncontraceptive effects of hormonal contraceptives: bone mass, sexually transmitted disease and pelvic inflammatory disease, cardiovascular disease,
   menstrual function, and future fertility. *Am J Obstet Gynecol* 1994;170[Suppl]
   1569–1575.
4. Carson SA, Buster JE. Current concepts: ectopic pregnancy. *N Engl J Med* 1993;
   329:1174.
5. Cates W Jr, Joesoef MR, Goldman MB. Atypical pelvic inflammatory disease: can
   we identify clinical predictors? *Am J Obstet Gynecol* 1993;169:341.
6. Centers for Disease Control and Prevention. 1998 sexually transmitted diseases
   treatment guidelines. *MMWR* 1998;47(RR-1).
7. Centers for Disease Control and Prevention. Leads from the *Morbidity and
   Mortality Weekly Report,* Atlanta: 1993 revised classification system for HIV infection and expanded surveillance case definition for AIDS among adolescents and
   adults. *JAMA* 1993;269:729.

8. Centers for Disease Control and Prevention. Leads from the *Morbidity and Mortality Weekly Report,* Atlanta: evaluation of surveillance for *Chlamydia trachomatis* infections in the United States, 1987 to 1991. *JAMA* 1993;270:1676.
9. Centers for Disease Control and Prevention. Leads from the *Morbidity and Mortality Weekly Report,* Atlanta: update: barrier protection against HIV infection and other sexually transmitted diseases. *JAMA* 1993;270:933.
10. Herbst AL, et al. *Comprehensive gynecology.* St. Louis: Mosby, 1992.
11. Hill GB. Bacterial vaginosis: the microbiology of bacterial vaginosis. *Am J Obstet Gynecol* 1993;169[Suppl]:450.
12. Hill GB. *Eubacterium nodatum* mimics actinomyces in intrauterine device-associated infections and other settings within the female genital tract. *Obstet Gynecol* 1992;79:534.
13. Hillis SD, et al. Delayed care of pelvic inflammatory disease as a risk factor for impaired fertility. *Am J Obstet Gynecol* 1993;168:1503.
14. Howard FM. The role of laparoscopy in chronic pelvic pain: promise and pitfalls. *Obstet Gynecol Surv* 1993;48:357.
15. Jewett JF, Hecht FM. Preventive health care for adults with HIV infection. *JAMA* 1993;269:1144.
16. Lindsay MK, et al. Human immunodeficiency virus infection among patients in a gynecology emergency department. *Obstet Gynecol* 1993;81:1012.
17. Livengood CH III, Hill GB, Addison WA. Pelvic inflammatory disease: findings during inpatient treatment of clinically severe, laparoscopy-documented disease. *Am J Obstet Gynecol* 1992;166:519.
18. McCormack WM. Current concepts: pelvic inflammatory disease. *N Engl J Med* 1994;330:115.
19. McGregor JA, Hammill HA. Contraceptive choices for women with medical problems: contraception and sexually transmitted diseases: interactions and opportunities. *Am J Obstet Gynecol* 1993;168[Suppl]:2033.
20. Pearlman MD, McNeeley SG. A review of the microbiology, immunology, and clinical implications of *Chlamydia trachomatis* infections. *Obstet Gynecol Surv* 1992; 47:448.
21. Rosenberg MJ, et al. Barrier contraceptives and sexually transmitted diseases in women: a comparison of female-dependent methods and condoms. *Am J Public Health* 1992;82:669, 674.
22. Safrin S, Schachter J, Dahrouge D, et al. Long-term sequelae of acute pelvic inflammatory disease: a retrospective cohort study. *Am J Obstet Gynecol* 1992; 166:1300.
23. Scholes D, et al. Vaginal douching as a risk factor for acute pelvic inflammatory disease. *Obstet Gynecol* 1993;81:601.
24. Silverman NS, et al. A randomized, prospective trial comparing amoxicillin and erythromycin for the treatment of *Chlamydia trachomatis* in pregnancy. *Am J Obstet Gynecol* 1994;170:829.
25. Soper DE, Brockwell NJ, Dalton HP. Microbial etiology of urban emergency department acute salpingitis: treatment with ofloxacin. *Am J Obstet Gynecol* 1992;167:653.
26. Soper DE, Brockwell NJ, Dalton HP, et al. Observations concerning the microbial etiology of acute salpingitis. *Am J Obstet Gynecol* 1994;170:1008.
27. Steege JF, Stout AL, Somkuti SG. Chronic pelvic pain in women: toward an integrative model. *Obstet Gynecol Surv* 1993;48:95.
28. Sweet RL. Bacterial vaginosis: new approaches for the treatment of bacterial vaginosis. *Am J Obstet Gynecol* 1993;169[Suppl]:479.
29. Washington AE, Katz P. Cost of and payment source for pelvic inflammatory disease. *JAMA* 1991;266:2565.
30. Zenilman JM, et al. Effect of HIV post-test counseling on STD incidence. *JAMA* 1992;267:843.
31. Platt R, Rice PA, McCormack WM. Risk of acquiring GC and prevalence of abnormal adnexal findings among women exposed to GC. *JAMA* 1983;250:3205.
32. Rein DB, Kessler WI, Irwin KL, et al. Direct medical cost of pelvic inflammatory disease and its sequelae: decreasing, but still substantial. *Obstet Gynecol* 2000; 95:397.

33. Eschenbach DA, Wolner-Hanssen P, Hawes SE, et al. Acute pelvic inflammatory disease: associations of clinical and laboratory findings with laparoscopic findings. *Obstet Gynecol* 1997;89:184.
34. Jossens MO, Eskenazi B, Schacter J, et al. Risk factors for PID: a case control study. *Sex Transm Dis* 1996;23:239.
35. Aral SO, Wasserheit JN. Social and behavioral considerations of pelvic inflammatory disease. *Sex Transm Dis* 1998;25:378.
36. Department of Health Services Center for Disease Control and Prevention. Division of STD Prevention 2000. *Sexually transmitted disease surveillance 1999.* www.cdc.gov.
37. Cibula D, Kuzel D, Fucikova Z. Acute exacerbation of recurrent pelvic inflammatory disease: laparoscopic findings in 141 women with a clinical diagnosis. *J Reprod Med* 2000;46:49.
38. Suss AL, Homel P, et al. Risk factors for pelvic inflammatory disease in inner-city adolescents. *Sex Transm Dis* 2000;27(5):289.

6. HIV INFECTION AND AIDS

Mary K. Miller

We are now beginning the third decade of the **AIDS epidemic** in this country since the first report on the United States epidemic occurred June 5, 1981. In spite of all the wonderful advances in therapy, patients continue to die every day. The only hope of stopping this epidemic is **prevention** and the only means of slowing the death rate is through **early detection and intervention.**

Women account for 32% of the HIV cases reported through June 2000; black men and women and Hispanic women represent 77% of cases. AIDS is the third leading cause of death in black women aged 25 to 44. **Persons aged 13 to 24 years account for 15% of reported HIV cases, and young women account for 49% of cases** in this age group. Among newborns there has been a **steep decline in perinatally acquired AIDS** from a peak of over 200 cases per year in the early 1990s, to approximately 50 cases per year by the end of 1998. The **worldwide numbers show that approximately 16.4 million women and 1.4 million children (<15 years of age) are living with HIV or AIDS and over 9 million women and 4.3 million children have died** since the beginning of the epidemic. A chilling reminder about the seriousness of this disease comes from the UNAIDS December 2000 update.

The human immunodeficiency virus (HIV) which causes AIDS has brought about a global epidemic far more extensive than what was predicted even a decade ago. UNAIDS and WHO now estimate that the number of people living with HIV or AIDS at the end of the year 2000 stands at 36.1 million. This is more than 50% higher than what WHO's Global Programme on AIDS projected in 1991 on the basis of data then available.

I. **Pathogenesis. HIV** was **first isolated in 1983.** It belongs to the lentivirus subgroup of retroviruses. Retroviruses are unique in that they code for the enzyme reverse transcriptase, which allows viral RNA to be transcribed into a DNA copy, which, in turn, is incorporated into the host's cellular genomic machinery. From there, HIV takes over the machinery and efficiently produces copies of itself. This viral replication is met with the new production of host $CD4^+$ T-lymphocytes to fight the HIV infection. HIV and host $CD4^+$ cells may reach an unofficial equilibrium. However this balance is fragile and can be broken leading to **increased viral loads and falling $CD4^+$** counts in the human host.

II. **Modes of transmission. HIV is transmitted from person to person by exchange of blood or other bodily fluids (semen, vaginal fluids, and breast milk)** during sexual contact, injectable drug use with shared needles, or through transfusions of blood or blood clotting factors. In addition, health care workers may be exposed to HIV via contact with cerebrospinal fluid (CNS), synovial fluid, or amniotic fluid. Most women are exposed to HIV through heterosexual contact. The second most common mode of transmission is injectable drug use.

III. **Natural history of HIV infection**

   A. **Primary infection.** Between 40% and 90% of individuals who become infected with HIV develop a mononucleosis-like illness from 3 days to 3 months after infection, which generally lasts less than 14 days. Fever, sweats, myalgias, malaise, headache, sore throat, lymphadenopathy, fatigue, and a maculopapular rash are prominent symptoms. The signs and symptoms of primary HIV infection generally occur 2 to 4 weeks after exposure to the virus.

This is a revision of the third edition chapter by Ruth M. Lawrence.

B. Chronic asymptomatic phase. The primary HIV infection is followed by a seemingly quiescent clinical phase (median time of 10 years), whereby signs and symptoms of overt illness are missing. This is the period in which HIV and host CD4+ cells reach an unofficial equilibrium. However, the virus remains busy. Eventually, HIV takes over the immune system as evidenced by increasing viral loads and falling CD4+ counts.

C. Overt AIDS. Overt AIDS is the final stage of HIV infection. It is diagnosed when an infected person develops a serious opportunistic infection or malignancy or when the number of CD4+ lymphocytes falls to 200/μL or fewer. If the patient does not obtain antiretroviral therapy, death will usually occur within 2 to 3 years. The Centers for Disease Control (CDC) case definition for AIDS-indicator conditions includes a positive HIV test with any of the following:

1. Candidiasis of bronchi, trachea, or lungs.
2. Candidiasis, esophageal.
3. Cervical cancer, invasive.*
4. Coccidioidomycosis, disseminated or extrapulmonary.
5. Cryptococcus, extrapulmonary.
6. Cryptosporidiosis, chronic intestinal (>1-month duration).
7. Cytomegalovirus (CMV) disease, other than liver, spleen, or lymph nodes.
8. CMV retinitis.
9. Encephalopathy, HIV-related.
10. Herpes simplex; chronic ulcer(s) (>1-month duration); bronchitis, pneumonitis, or esophagitis.
11. Histoplasmosis, disseminated or extrapulmonary.
12. Isosporiasis, chronic intestinal (>1 month).
13. Kaposi's sarcoma.
14. Lymphoma, Burkitt's immunoblastic, or primary of brain.
15. *Mycobacterium avium-intracellulare* complex or *Mycobacterium kansasii,* disseminated or extrapulmonary.
16. *Mycobacterium tuberculosis,* any site (pulmonary* or extrapulmonary).
17. *Mycobacterium,* other species, disseminated or extrapulmonary.
18. *Pneumocystis carinii* pneumonia.
19. Pneumonia, recurrent.*
20. Progressive multifocal leukoencephalopathy.
21. *Salmonella* septicemia, recurrent.
22. Toxoplasmosis of the brain.
23. Wasting syndrome caused by HIV.
    *Added in the 1993 expansion of the AIDS surveillance case definition.

IV. Screening. Who's at risk? Unfortunately, **everyone** who has **unprotected sex** with an **infected partner** or contact with someone else's **infected blood** is at risk for HIV. **HIV-infected mothers** can pass the virus to their fetuses during pregnancy, delivery, or through breast-feeding. The difficulty for providers is knowing who is infected since looking for physical clues is rarely helpful. **Serologic testing must be performed.** A provider's threshold for offering HIV tests should be extremely low. HIV testing should be offered to all women who:
- Present for STD checks or for any pregnancy-related issues.
- Request an HIV test.
- Have drug abuse histories (especially needle sharing).

Providers involved in gynecologic and/or obstetrical care for women should aggressively (but politely) offer HIV testing to their patients.

V. Diagnosis of HIV infection

A. History. The history can provide valuable information about the likelihood of HIV infection.

1. The **sexual history** should include information about partners who are:
   - Drug users.
   - Bisexual.

- Hemophiliac.
- Experienced as a prostitute.
  Inquiries must also be made regarding sexual practices such as anal intercourse and previous treatment for STDs.
2. Inquiry about receipt of **blood or blood products** and **injectable drug abuse** with needle sharing should be made.
3. Specific symptoms to be included in the review of systems include:
   - Presence of **weight loss** not explained by diet.
   - **Fevers.**
   - **Night sweats.**
   - **Lymphadenopathy.**
   - **Rash.**
   - **Oral lesions.**
   - **Cough and dyspnea.**
   - **Myalgias and arthralgias.**
   - **Personality changes.**
   - **Depression.**
   - **Cognitive difficulties.**
   - **Paresthesias or weakness.**
   - **Changes in visual acuity.**
B. **Physical examination**
   1. The **general physical examination** should include special attention to the ocular fundi for evidence of CMV retinitis (consider an ophthalmology consult), oral mucosa (white patches of oral candidiasis or hairy leukoplakia), lymph nodes, lungs, skin (severe seborrhea, lesions of Kaposi's sarcoma, lesions of secondary syphilis), and neurologic system (dementia, neuropathy, signs of meningoencephalitis or mass lesions).
   2. The **screening pelvic examination and Papanicolaou (Pap) test** should include a search for signs of STDs including syphilis, gonorrhea, chlamydial infection, chancroid, herpes simplex virus, and human papillomavirus (HPV) infection as well as evaluation for cervical and lower genital tract neoplastic changes.
C. **Laboratory diagnosis of HIV infection**
   1. **When to test for HIV?** When patients request an HIV test, even if they do not relate it to a specific exposure, order it as a baseline. Most people develop detectable antibodies within 3 months after infection (average 25 days) but this process **can** take up to 6 months. Therefore, the CDC currently recommends testing 3 months after the last possible exposure (unprotected vaginal, anal, or oral sex or sharing needles). If a patient is exposed to a known HIV-infected partner or there is provider and/or patient concern, a second repeat test may be considered at or after 6 months from the exposure. In between HIV tests, it is important to encourage patients to use safer sex practices.
   2. The enzyme-linked immunosorbent assay (ELISA) **test** detects **antibodies** to HIV in the serum or plasma. If the ELISA test is reactive, it is repeated on the same blood sample. If the sample itself is repeatedly reactive, the results generally undergo the more expensive **Western blot test for confirmation**.
   3. The Western blot test is more specific and can differentiate between HIV antibodies and other antibodies that may react to the ELISA test.
   4. There are other Food and Drug Administration (FDA) approved HIV test technologies in the U.S. using urine and oral fluids (less invasive), however the "gold standard" continues to be the traditional ELISA method described previously.
   5. HIV viral loads or culture and p-24 antigen assays are available, but they are usually not intended for routine screening in clinic settings.
   6. Undergoing testing for HIV infection is a highly charged matter for many patients. Counseling regarding the testing procedures, the meaning of both positive and negative results, education on prevention of

infection in the future, the need to notify sexual partners, and planning for follow-up appointments should be included at the time of testing.

VI. Course and treatment of the HIV-infected woman

   A. Once the diagnosis of HIV infection is established, the **goals of care** include maintenance of general health as long as possible; treatment with antiviral agents active against HIV; anticipation, prevention, and treatment of secondary opportunistic infections; and prevention of further spread of infection to sexual partners and offspring.

   B. **In general, the course of HIV infection in women is the same as in men when controlled for access to health care.** However, recent studies are showing that **women have lower plasma viral loads** (30%–50% less) when compared with men with similar CD4 counts. Possible explanations for this difference may be due to the effects of estrogen or progesterone, however the exact mechanisms are unknown. The clinical implications are also unknown.

   C. Some common early manifestations of HIV infection in women include **severe viral** and **fungal infections** of the **genitalia** with organisms such as **herpes simplex, human papillomavirus (HPV),** and *Candida albicans.* These infections are often more refractory to treatment than in uninfected women and may be recurrent. Also, **pelvic inflammatory disease** (PID) tends to be **more severe** in HIV-infected women.

   D. **Wasting** caused by **HIV** has been reported to be **more common in women** than in men. **Kaposi's sarcoma** is unusual in women but can occur and can be **more aggressive** than in men.

   E. A major problem for women with HIV infection is the increased risk of **lower genital tract neoplasia.** Although HIV infection is clearly associated with the risk of malignancy, it is unclear if HIV itself plays an independent role. However, as immunodeficiency worsens, higher grades of squamous intraepithelial neoplastic changes in the cervix, vagina, and vulva are seen. **Pap smears should be obtained every 6 months.** However, the Pap smear is only a screening tool, hence **liberal use of cervical colposcopy with biopsy is suggested** (see section VII.E.).

   F. Whenever possible, a provider with expertise in HIV should supervise all treatment decisions. Treatment should be offered to
   - All patients with the acute HIV syndrome.
   - Those within 6 months of HIV seroconversion.
   - All patients with symptomatic HIV infection.

   Recommendations on starting antiretroviral therapy in asymptomatic patients are dependent on immunologic and virologic factors.

   1. Generally, treatment should be offered to patients with fewer than 500 CD4$^+$ T cells/mm^3 or plasma HIV RNA levels greater than 10,000 copies/mL (bDNA assay) or 20,000 copies/mL (RT-PCR assay).

   2. Specific information and updates regarding antiretroviral use can be found in the *Guidelines for the Use of Antiretroviral Agents in HIV-infected Adults and Adolescents* a living document available on the HIV/AIDS Treatment Information Service Web site (http://www.hivatis.org).

   G. **Prophylaxis against** *P. carinii* **pneumonia** is given when CD4$^+$ counts fall below 200/μL or if the patient gives a history of oropharyngeal candidiasis.

   1. **Trimethoprim-sulfamethoxazole,** one double-strength tablet by mouth daily or three times per week, is used as first-line prophylaxis. Unfortunately, allergic reactions to the sulfa component are common in HIV-infected patients and the drug may not be tolerated.

   2. Chemoprophylaxis for *P. carinii* pneumonia should be administered to pregnant women. Because of theoretical concerns regarding possible teratogenicity associated with drug exposures during the first trimester, providers may choose to withhold prophylaxis during this time. In such cases, aerosolized pentamidine may be considered because of its lack of systemic absorption.

3. Generally, alternative prophylactic agents include **pentamidine ise-thionate,** 300 mg given by inhalation once monthly and **dapsone,** 50 to 100 mg/day PO if the patient is allergic to sulfa.

H. **Treatment of opportunistic infections** may be relatively simple (as in using antifungal troches for oral candidiasis) or complicated (multiple drug regimens for *M. avium-intracellulare* or *M. tuberculosis* infections). Referral to an infectious disease specialist for the diagnosis and treatment of opportunistic infections and decisions regarding discontinuation of prophylaxis against specific opportunistic infections when the CD4+ count increases is mandatory. Additional information on opportunistic infections can be found on the HIV/AIDS Treatment Information Service Web site (http://www.hivatis.org).

VII. **How do women differ?**

A. **Sexual transmission.** Most women with AIDS are infected through heterosexual exposure, followed by injection drug use. **Receptive vaginal and rectal intercourse** present the greatest risk for infection **(0.1%–0.2% and 0.1%–3% respectively, per episode of intercourse).** Infectious HIV may be found in the semen and cervicovaginal secretions of infected individuals. HIV transmission from male to female is more efficient than female to male secondary to the high concentration of HIV in seminal fluid. The **factors that increase the likelihood of heterosexual transmission** include **lack of condom use, multiple sexual partners, presence of advanced HIV disease in a partner, anal intercourse,** and the presence of **genital ulcers** or **inflammation** (including nonulcerative diseases such as gonococcal or chlamydial cervicitis, bacterial vaginosis (BV), and trichomonal vaginitis).

B. **Gynecologic concerns.** The most common gynecologic infections in HIV-infected women are candidiasis, BV, and trichomoniasis. BV, trichomoniasis, and ulcerative lesions are treated in the same manner as in women who are not infected with HIV (i.e., metronidazole, acyclovir, etc.). Nonulcerative and ulcerative STDs are associated with an increased likelihood of HIV transmission.

1. **Vulvovaginal candidiasis** (VVC) is caused by *C. albicans* and on occasion other less common atypical yeasts. VVC can be clinically suspected when the patient presents with symptoms of erythema, pruritus, and a white discharge in the vulvovaginal area. The diagnosis is usually made by wet preparation demonstrating pseudohyphae or by positive culture. Treatment with **intravaginal azoles** is more effective than with nystatin products. Oral fluconazole (150 mg) can be taken as a single dose.

   Chronic recurrent vaginal candidiasis is frequent in HIV-infected women. The severity of the infection is usually related to the degree of immunosuppression. Symptomatic infection can be treated initially with intravaginal and topical antifungals. If this fails, oral fluconazole 100 mg qd for 14 days can be tried. For frequent relapses, fluconazole 150 mg PO once weekly may suppress recurrences.

2. HIV infection is associated with severe **PID.** Fever, palpable pelvic mass, cervical friability and cervical motion tenderness are common symptoms found in PID. HIV-infected women are more likely to be hospitalized and require surgical intervention, but the overall response to standard antibiotic treatment 48 to 72 hours after diagnosis is similar to women without HIV (see Chapters 3 and 5).

C. **Menstrual irregularities.** Not much is known about HIV and the menstrual cycle. Hormonal fluctuations (estradiol and progesterone) in HIV-infected women with "normal menstrual cycles" are similar to HIV-negative women. It appears however, that HIV-infected women who are healthy with high CD4+ counts, low viral loads, no wasting, and no drug abuse history are less likely to have menstrual irregularities. Women with less than 200 CD4+ cells are more likely to have longer cycles >40 days and those with a viral load >150,000 show the most variability in cycle length (i.e., shorter and longer cycles).

HIV-infected women with menstrual irregularities such as amenorrhea, dysmenorrhea, dysfunctional uterine bleeding, menorrhagia, perimenopausal or menopausal symptoms, etc. should be evaluated by a **gynecologist.** These conditions are treated in the same manner as HIV-negative women, however close attention must be paid to CD4+ counts, viral loads, highly active antiretroviral therapy (HAART) regimens and drug interactions with hormonal agents in HIV-infected patients.

D. **Contraception issues.** There are several **contraceptive choices** for HIV-infected women: male or female condoms preferably with spermicide, diaphragm with spermicide, medroxyprogesterone acetate (Depo-Provera) injection (every 3 months), levonorgestrel implant (Norplant) (every 5 years), oral contraceptives, sterilization, and abstinence. Intrauterine devices are not recommended due to the risk of PID. No matter what contraceptive choice patients make, it is important to always ask about and to encourage safer sex practices.

Certain **antiretrovirals can affect the metabolism of oral contraceptives** (OC) (especially estrogen). Nevirapine, nelfinavir, and ritonavir significantly decrease serum estrogen levels, resulting in a decreased contraceptive effect. An increase in the OC estrogen-component may be necessary and/or use of an additional barrier method. Indinavir and efavirenz can increase OC serum estrogen levels. In addition, hormone replacement therapy for perimenopausal or menopausal HIV-infected women may need adjustments depending on the antiretroviral regimen.

E. **Lower genital tract neoplasia.** HIV-infected women have an **increased frequency of HPV-related lower genital tract dysplasias that are more difficult to treat.** HPV can infect the vulva, vagina, cervix, and perianal regions.

Approximately 20% to 50% of HIV-infected women have cervical intraepithelial neoplasia (CIN). Women with HIV and CIN can have higher-grade lesions; more extensive cervical and endocervical involvement; and multisite vulvar, vaginal, and perianal HPV lesions. An association between advanced cervical neoplasia, declining CD4+ counts, and advanced HIV disease is common. Invasive cervical cancer is considered an AIDS-indicator condition.

The American College of Obstetrics and Gynecology (ACOG) recommends a **Pap smear for HIV-infected women to be performed every 6 months.** Pap smears, if done correctly and expertly read, are still sufficiently sensitive and specific to detect cervical dysplasia in HIV-infected women. The newer "Thin Prep" tests and computer-assisted Pap interpretation products and HPV DNA tests are gaining acceptance, but currently are not routinely used in HIV care. Abnormal results should be referred to a gynecologist, preferably with HIV-experience, for further evaluation. Colposcopy and biopsy may be indicated to evaluate abnormalities. Treatment options for CIN (depending on severity) may include: close observation (i.e., satellite lesions), cryotherapy, LEEP, cold-knife cone, and laser vaporization. Patients with CIS, cervical, vulvar, vaginal, or perianal cancers should be referred immediately to a gynecologic oncologist for further evaluation and treatment.

External genital warts can be treated topically using patient-applied therapies (i.e., podofilox and imiquimod) or provider-administered therapies (i.e., cryotherapy, podophyllin resin, trichloroacetic acid [TCA], bichloracetic acid [BCA], interferon, and excision). Close attention and follow-up is indicated to monitor for severe inflammation, infection, and ulceration. The safety of podophyllin in pregnancy has not been established.

Patients with extensive vaginal warts should be referred to a gynecologist for treatment. 5-fluorouracil (5-FU) can be used for vaginal condyloma and more recently, after "standard surgery for high-grade (cervical) lesions" to reduce the recurrence of CIN in HIV-infected women. A gynecologic consult should be obtained before starting any intravaginal 5-FU therapy.

F. **Lipodystrophy issues.** Lipodystrophy, an abnormal distribution of fat, can occur in both HIV-infected men and women, but there do appear to be gender differences. Women develop fat accumulation in the breasts and abdominal areas as opposed to the neck. Lipid metabolism abnormalities in general are reported less frequently. The exact pathogenesis of lipodystrophy is unclear. Protease inhibitors were originally suspect, however other antiretroviral agents, length of therapy, and HIV disease progression do play a role. A current hypothesis implicates mitochondrial toxicity and lactic acidosis, but this has not been proven as yet. Many women are devastated by the change in body image in severe cases. Treatment of lipodystrophy in women is evolving. Some HIV experts may change antiretroviral therapy, consider recombinant human growth hormone, encourage exercise, and treat lipid abnormalities with statin and fibrate agents. Metformin may improve visceral adipose tissue distribution, insulin resistance, and elevated triglycerides.

G. **Pregnancy and perinatal concerns.** Women of **childbearing age** should be counseled about the risks of transmitting HIV to their infants, advised to avoid pregnancy, and encouraged to use contraception and safer sex practices. Pregnancy termination services should be available to those patients who desire an abortion, if an unintended pregnancy occurs. That said, **pregnancy does not seem to have an adverse effect on the course of HIV infection.** However vertical transmission issues are critical.

In February 1994, the results of the **Pediatric AIDS Clinical Trials Group (PACTG) Protocol 076** showed that **zidovudine (ZDV, also known as AZT) chemoprophylaxis reduced perinatal HIV transmission by nearly 70%.** The placebo group in this study had a perinatal HIV transmission rate of nearly 23%, compared with **7.6% for the ZDV-treated group.** Since 1994, studies have established that the magnitude and rapidity of viral turnover during all stages of HIV infection is much greater than previously recognized. It is estimated that plasma virions have a mean half-life of only 6 hours. Therefore, current treatments now focus on early aggressive combination therapy to suppress viral replication, preserve immune function, and reduce resistance. ZDV chemoprophylaxis alone has done much to reduce the risk of perinatal transmission, however antiretroviral monotherapy is now considered suboptimal treatment. **The current standard of care for antiretroviral chemoprophylaxis requires combination therapy.** Some women may choose to reduce fetal exposure to multiple antiretroviral medications and just go for the three-part ZDV chemoprophylaxis. If they chose ZDV chemoprophylaxis and additional antiretroviral drugs (combination therapy), then ZDV should be included in the regimen (if possible), since ZDV in pregnancy has been more widely studied. Women in the first trimester of pregnancy, may consider postponing therapy until after 10 to 12 weeks gestation.

1. **Combination antiretroviral therapy,** usually consists of two nucleoside analog reverse transcriptase inhibitors and a protease inhibitor. Information about the safety of drugs in pregnancy is derived from animal toxicity studies, anecdotal experience, clinical trials, and registry data. Even so, only minimal data are available regarding the safety and pharmacokinetics of antiretrovirals other than ZDV during pregnancy. Providers who are treating HIV-infected pregnant women and their newborns are encouraged to report cases of prenatal exposure to antiretroviral drugs to the **Antiretroviral Pregnancy Registry,** 1410 Commonwealth Drive, Wilmington, NC 28403, telephone 1-800-258-4263, Fax 1-800-800-1052.

2. The **mechanism of action for ZDV in the PACTG 076 study is not completely understood.** The effect of ZDV on maternal HIV-1 RNA does not fully explain the observed efficacy of ZDV in reducing transmission. Perhaps fetal pre-exposure prophylaxis plays a big role in protection, and if so, transplacental passage of antiretroviral drugs would be a critical factor for prevention of HIV transmission. Luckily, it appears that ZDV is metabolized into the active triphosphate form within the placenta, thus providing additional protection to the fetus. As for

the other antiretrovirals administered during pregnancy, combination therapy may have considerable benefit to the mother, but unknown benefits to the fetus. Many researchers believe that potent combination antiretroviral regimens may provide enhanced protection against perinatal transmission, however this benefit is not yet proven.

3. According to latest *Public Health Service Task Force Recommendations for Use of Antiretroviral Drugs in Pregnant HIV-1-Infected Women for Maternal Health and Interventions to Reduce Perinatal HIV-1 Transmission in the United States* (November 2000).

   "Decisions regarding the use and choice of an antiretroviral regimen should be individualized based on discussion with the woman about a) her risk for disease progression and the risks and benefits of delaying initiation of therapy; b) potential drug toxicities and interactions with other drugs; c) the need for adherence to prescribed drug schedule; and d) pre-clinical, animal, and clinical data relevant to use of the currently available antiretrovirals during pregnancy" (14).

4. In summary, monotherapy is generally, not used except when the patient refuses combination therapy. Minimally, all HIV-infected pregnant women should receive the three-part ZDV chemoprophylaxis (Table 6.1). Better yet, pregnant patients should be on combination therapy that includes ZDV (if possible), even though the benefit of combination therapy is not yet proven. Current **recommendations for antiretroviral use and mode of delivery for HIV-infected pregnant women** are provided in Tables 6.2 and 6.3.

5. It is important to provide the best obstetric, gynecologic and HIV care possible to women infected with the AIDS virus. By teaming up with HIV specialists, patients will receive up-to-date therapies and treatments, have access to large-scale studies, and receive adequate case management and psychosocial support.

VIII. **Prevention of HIV infection**
   A. **Education** about modes of transmission, types of preventive measures, and importance of early diagnosis and treatment remains the cornerstone of any program of prevention. Testing and counseling should be offered to women attending clinics for STDs and to other women identified as high risk.
   B. The importance of **safer sexual practices** should be emphasized. Women need to know the sexual and drug-using histories of their partners and avoid

(*text continues on page 63*)

Table 6.1. PACTG 076 zidovudine (ZDV) protocol

Time of ZDV administration	Regimen
Antepartum Begin at week 14–34, continue throughout pregnancy	ZDV 200 mg PO tid or 300 mg bid (previously 100 mg PO 5 times a day)
Intrapartum	During labor, provide an initial 1-hour IV infusion of ZDV 2mg/kg followed by continuous IV infusion of ZDV 1mg/kg till delivery
Postpartum Newborn administration should begin within 8–12 hours of delivery and be continued for 6 weeks. (IV dosage can be used for NPO infants)	ZDV syrup 2mg/kg PO q6h **or** ZDV 1.5mg/kg IV q6h

Table 6.2. Recommendations for antiretroviral use in pregnant women

Clinical scenario	Recommendations
HIV-infected pregnant woman with **no previous** history of **antiretroviral therapy**	• Choice of therapy is based on immunologic and virologic parameters and is similar to non-pregnant individuals • AZT per PACTG 076 protocol should be strongly recommended • Combination therapy should be provided after counseling about the potential risks and benefits • Women in their first trimester of pregnancy may consider delaying initiation of therapy until after 10–12 weeks gestation
HIV-infected pregnant woman **receiving antiretroviral** therapy during the **current pregnancy**	• Continue therapy after counseling about the risks and benefits of treatment if pregnancy is identified after first trimester • If pregnancy is identified during first trimester, the mother should be counseled regarding the benefits and potential risks of ARV administration during this period, and continuation of therapy should be considered. If the decision is to discontinue therapy then all drugs should be stopped and restarted simultaneously after the first trimester • If the current regimen does not contain ZDV, the addition of ZDV or substitution for another nucleoside analogue ARV is recommended after 14 weeks gestation. ZDV administration is recommended during the intrapartum period and for the newborn, regardless of the antipartum ARV regimen

HIV-infected woman in **labor** with **no prior therapy**	• There are several effective regimens available:
	  1. Single dose nevirapine at the onset of labor followed by a single dose of nevirapine for the newborn at age 48 hours
	  2. Oral ZDV and 3TC during labor, followed by one week of oral ZDV/3TC for the newborn
	  3. Intrapartum intravenous ZDV followed by 6 weeks of ZDV for the newborn
	  4. 2-dose nevirapine regimen combined with intrapartum intravenous ZDV and 6 week ZDV for the newborn
	  5. Assess mother's HIV antiretroviral needs postpartum

Infant born to mother who has not received antiretroviral therapy during pregnancy or intrapartum	• The 6-week neonatal ZDV chemoprophylactic regimen should be discussed with the mother and offered for the newborn • ZDV should be initiated as soon as possible after delivery—preferably within 12–24 hours of birth • Some clinicians may choose to use ZDV in combination with other ARV drugs, particularly if the mother is known or suspected to have ZDV-resistant virus. However, the efficacy of this approach for prevention of transmission is unknown, and appropriate dosing regimens for neonates are incompletely defined • Assess mother's HIV antiretroviral needs postpartum

Table 6.3. Mode of delivery recommendations for HIV-infected pregnant women

Clinical scenario	Recommendations
HIV-infected woman **presenting after 36 weeks not receiving ARVs** and with **HIV RNA levels and lymphocyte subsets pending but not available before delivery**	• Choice of therapy is based on immunologic and virologic parameters and is similar to non-pregnant individuals • ZDV per 076 protocol should be started • Combination therapy should be provided after counseling about the potential risks and benefits • Counsel that scheduled cesarean section is likely to reduce the risk of transmission to her infant • Counsel that there are increased risks of postop infection, anesthesia risks, and other surgical risks with cesarean section • If cesarean section is chosen: schedule at 38 weeks based on best clinical information; ZDV infusion 3 hours prior to surgery **with** infant receiving 6 weeks of ZDV therapy after birth • Options for continuing or initiating combination therapy after delivery should be discussed with patient as soon as viral load and lymphocyte subset results are available
HIV-infected woman with **late prenatal care (early 3rd trimester) on HAART with initial virologic response but with viral load still substantially over 1,000 copies/mL at 36 weeks gestation**	• Continue HAART • Counsel that although she is responding to ARVs, it is unlikely that her HIV RNA level will fall below 1,000 copies/mL before delivery • Counsel that cesarian section may provide additional benefit in preventing intrapartum transmission of HIV • Cesarian section timing, risks, 076 ZDV protocol, postpartum therapy, etc. are the same as above • HAART should be continued on schedule as much as possible before and after surgery
HIV-infected woman **on HAART with an undetectable HIV RNA level at 36 weeks gestation**	• Counsel risk of perinatal transmission with a persistently undetectable HIV RNA level is low, probably 2% or less, even with vaginal delivery • No information is available to evaluate whether performing a scheduled cesarean section will further lower risk
HIV-infected woman **scheduled for cesarean section presenting in early labor or shortly after rupture of membranes**	• ZDV should be started immediately • If labor is rapidly progressing, allow vaginal delivery • If cervical dilatation is minimal and a long labor is anticipated: consider ZDV intravenous loading dose **and** proceeding to cesarean section **OR** consider piton augmentation • No scalp electrodes or other invasive monitoring if possible • Treat infant with 6 weeks of ZDV

partners whose behavior has placed them at high risk of acquiring infection. Use of **latex condoms with nonoxynol-9 spermicide, water-based lubricants** rather than petroleum-based products and **contraceptive sponges impregnated with nonoxynol-9** adds a measure of safety **but** is by no means infallible.

C. The **hazards of injectable drug use** must be explained. Women who are using injectable drugs should be offered treatment. Failing abstinence, use of solutions of household bleach to clean drug paraphernalia or clean-needle exchange programs can help reduce transmission of the virus.

D. Several different approaches to **vaccine development** are under way, but a vaccine for HIV is years away. Until that time, safer sexual practices, mutually monogamous relationships, and avoidance of injectable drug use are essential.

References

1. Anastros K, Gange SJ, Lau B, et al. *The women's interagency HIV study (WIHS) and the multicenter AIDS cohort study (MACS). Gender specific differences in quantitative HIV-RNA levels.* Paper presented at the 6th Conference on Retroviruses and Opportunistic Infections, Chicago, 1999.

2. Blair J, Hanson D, Jones J. *Do gender differences in viral load predict differences in HIV disease progression?* Program and abstracts of the 7th Conference on Retroviruses and Opportunistic Infections, Jan. 30–Feb. 2, 2000, San Francisco. Abstract 195.

3. Centers for Disease Control and Prevention. *Revised guidelines for HIV counseling, testing, and Referral (DRAFT),* Oct. 17, 2000:1–93.

4. Centers for Disease Control and Prevention. *HIV/AIDS surveillance report,* 2000; 12(No. 1):1–43.

5. Centers for Disease Control and Prevention. *HIV/AIDS surveillance report,* 1999; 11(No. 2):1–44.

6. Centers for Disease Control and Prevention. 1999 USPHS/IDSA guidelines for the prevention of opportunistic infections in persons infected with human immunodeficiency virus: U.S. Public Health Service (USPHS) and Infectious Diseases Society of America (IDSA). *MMWR* 1999;48(No. RR-10):1–66.

7. Centers for Disease Control and Prevention. 1993 revised classification system for HIV infection and expanded surveillance case definition for AIDS among adolescents and adults. *MMWR* 1992;41(No. RR-17).

8. Centers for Disease Control and Prevention. *Pneumocystis* pneumonia—Los Angeles. *MMWR* 1981;30:250–252.

9. Farzadegan H, Hoover D, Astemborski J, et al. Sex differences in HIV-1 viral load and progression to AIDS: infectious HIV burden among injecting drug users. *Lancet* 1998;353:589–590.

10. Junghans C, Ledergerber B, Chan P, et al. Sex differences in HIV-1 viral load and progression to AIDS. *Lancet* 1999;353:589.

11. Maiman M, Watts DH, Andersen J, et al. Vaginal 5-fluorouracil for high-grade cervical dysplasia in human immunodeficiency virus infection: a randomized trial. *Obstet Gynecol* 1999;94:954–961.

12. Moroni M. Sex differences in HIV-1 viral load and progression to AIDS. *Lancet* 1999;353:589.

13. Panel on Clinical Practices for Treatment of HIV Infection. *Guidelines for the use of antiretroviral agents in HIV-infected adults and adolescents.* Online: http://www.hivatis.org/. January 28, 1999.

14. Perinatal HIV Guidelines Working Group. *Public Health Service Task Force recommendations for use of antiretroviral drugs in pregnant HIV-1-infected women for maternal health and interventions to reduce perinatal HIV-1 transmission in the United States.* Online: http://www.hivatis.org/. November 3, 2000.

15. UNAIDS/WHO. *AIDS epidemic update,* December, 2000:1–24.

7. URINARY TRACT INFECTIONS

Raymond Frink

At least 10% to 20% of women in the general population will develop one or more cases of urinary tract infection (**UTI**) during their lifetime. UTI is the **most common bacterial infection affecting women throughout their life span,** generating approximately 6 million office visits per year. UTIs in women from menarche through their menopausal years are discussed. This chapter provides a practical approach to UTIs and a starting point for further knowledge.

I. **Clinical aspects of UTI.** The clinical spectrum of UTI includes three categories with some overlap.
   A. **Asymptomatic bacteriuria,** in which patients have **no symptoms.**
   B. **Lower tract infection,** which is characterized by various combinations of **dysuria, frequency, nocturia, urgency, suprapubic discomfort and tenderness,** and sometimes **hematuria.** This clinical syndrome can be caused by the following:
      1. **Bacterial infection of the bladder** (traditionally classified as $\geq 10^5$ bacteria per milliliter of urine) with or without silent renal involvement. This can occur as an isolated infection, an unresolved infection indicating that the initial therapy was **not** adequate, **or** a recurrent UTI resulting either from reinfection or bacterial persistence.
      2. Patients whose symptoms are **indistinguishable from cystitis in** women, but not meeting traditional bacteriuria levels, can be defined in **three subgroups:**
         a. **Those with bladder bacteriuria with less than 10^5 bacteria/ mL** (usually accompanied by pyuria of >10 white blood cells [WBCs]/ mL of voided unspun urine). In most populations, this group constitutes the **majority of women with urethritis.** It is **difficult** to **differentiate** between **urethritis** and **cystitis in women,** but **inflammation isolated only** to the **urethra** is **rare.**

            The **traditional criteria** for a **positive urine culture** of colony counts of 10^5mL **has two important limitations.** Women with **symptomatic UTI** can be **cultured with colony counts of 10^2 to 10^4 colony forming units** (cfu)/mL **20% to 40 % of the time. Thus greater than 10^2 cfu/mL** of a **known pathogen in a dysuric patient** should alert the examiner to **significant bacteriuria requiring treatment.** Secondly, women who are susceptible to infection often carry large numbers of pathogenic bacteria on the perineum. This may contaminate an otherwise sterile urine sample.
         b. **Those with pyuria** (as described in a.) **and no bacteriuria.** This is associated with a high rate of sexually transmitted disease (STD) in young women and should prompt an investigation for *Chlamydia trachomatis, Neisseria gonorrhoeae,* or herpes simplex infection.
         c. **Those with no bacteriuria or pyuria, who usually have no identifiable cause of symptoms.** Hypoestrogenic urethra, detrusor instability, and urethral dysfunction should be ruled out.

            Urethral syndrome is a term often applied to symptoms of frequency, urgency, dysuria, suprapubic discomfort, and voiding difficulties in the absence of any infectious process or interstitial cystitis and should not be applied to I.B.2.a.or b. In the absence of these two processes, dysfunctional voiding or an emotional basis for symptoms should be considered. Urodynamic testing may be useful in these cases.

C. **Acute pyelonephritis, with costovertebral angle** (CVA) **pain and tenderness, fever, rigors,** and sometimes **accompanying symptoms and signs of cystitis.**

II. **Asymptomatic bacteriuria** must be **treated only if it has been shown to predict occurrence of symptomatic UTI and treatment has been shown to be effective in preventing morbidity.** In general, this statement **implies that asymptomatic bacteriuria in adult women requires treatment only during pregnancy,** for which numerous studies have shown a significant reduction in risk of pyelonephritis and low birth weight infants. Although certain large-scale epidemiologic studies have associated asymptomatic bacteriuria with an increased overall mortality in adult women and in the geriatric population, a causal link has not been established. The significance of asymptomatic bacteriuria in older adults is unclear. It appears to be a marker for poor health rather than a causal factor for increased mortality.

III. **History and physical examination.** Clinical diagnosis is fraught with problems in the categorization of UTI. The reasons include the facts that **history and physical examination do not reliably discriminate between patients** with urethritis and other forms of UTI (i.e., cystitis) and that it is **not possible to differentiate between upper tract and lower tract infection** on clinical grounds alone. Furthermore, up to 50% of all patients with bacteriuria have been shown **by localization techniques to have silent renal infection.**

A. **History.** The characteristic history for a **lower tract infection** might include the **sudden onset of dysuria, frequency, urgency, suprapubic discomfort, and sometimes hematuria** in a previously healthy woman. Microscopic hematuria is found in 40% to 60% of cases of cystitis and is uncommon in other conditions causing similar symptoms.

1. **Acute pyelonephritis** may include any of the previously mentioned symptoms in addition to a **history of CVA pain, fever, nausea, vomiting, and rigors.**
2. In women **presenting with dysuria,** a diagnosis of **vaginitis is at least as likely** as a diagnosis of UTI.
3. If the **dysuria is internal** and there is **no vaginal irritation or discharge,** there is a lower probability of vaginitis and a **higher probability of UTI.**
4. If there is **external dysuria and vaginal discharge or irritation,** the **probability of vaginitis is higher** than that of UTI.
5. These distinctions have been **useful** in the hands of some practitioners but are certainly **not foolproof.**

B. **Physical examination**
1. In women with **lower tract infection, suprapubic tenderness** may be the only physical finding.
2. **With acute pyelonephritis, temperature elevation and CVA tenderness** are often found. In addition, the patient may appear **pale, ill, and in great pain.**

IV. **Investigative procedures.** Initial laboratory evaluation in all women with suspected UTI should include at least **microscopic examination of unspun urine and quantitative culture of freshly voided urine** obtained as a clean-catch, midstream sample.

A. **Dipstick.** No **chemical abnormality** is consistently found on dipstick analysis of urine of women with UTI. The finding of **bacteriuria (nitrates) or pyuria (leukocyte esterase)** is clinically useful, but less accurate than microscopic examination of the urine. **Occult blood** and proteinuria are also **commonly found.**

B. **Microscopic studies.** Elements consistent with UTI include **leukocytes, erythrocytes,** and **bacteria** in unspun urine.
1. The **absence of any or all of these elements does not rule out UTI.**
2. **Leukocyte casts,** if present, **confirm** the presence of **renal infection.**
3. In uncomplicated UTIs, **aerobic gram-negative coliforms are the most common etiologic agent,** with *Escherichia coli* being responsible

for 80% to 85% and *Staphylococcus saprophyticus* responsible for 5% to 15% of uncomplicated UTIs in young women.

4. Microscopic examination of urine may be facilitated by **Gram staining of specimens.** Clinicians may find this a useful adjunct procedure in the diagnosis of UTI.

C. **Urine culture.** In interpreting results of urine culture, it should be noted that the definition of **significant bacteriuria** has recently undergone radical change. The traditional criterion of greater than 10^5 bacteria/mL only identifies half of symptomatic women with proven coliform infection of the bladder. Among symptomatic women, the **criterion of greater than 10^2 coliforms/mL of clean voided urine has a high sensitivity** (0.95), **specificity** (0.85), and **predictive value** (0.88), and is **preferable to previous criteria.** In addition, many symptomatic women with mixed culture results in which one of the isolates is a coliform have a true bacterial infection of the bladder. **With mixed or lower-level (<10^5/ml) culture results, the likelihood of true infection is increased when pyuria is present.**

V. **Drug therapy.** A wide variety of antibiotic regimens will cure the great majority of acute, uncomplicated UTIs. In fact, the high concentration of many antibiotics in the urine results in eradication of many organisms with *in vitro* drug resistance. In evaluating antibiotic treatment of UTI, it must be remembered that studies using placebo treatment have shown that **most nonpregnant women with acutely symptomatic UTI eventually have sterile urine without antibiotic therapy.**

A. **Urethritis and cystitis**

1. When coliforms are the offending organism, most women with urethritis or uncomplicated acute cystitis can be managed with either **single-dose** or **short-course therapy.** Trimethoprim-sulfamethoxazole (two double-strength tablets), 2 g oral sulfisoxazole, or kanamycin 500 mg intramuscularly are the medications of choice for **single-dose therapy.** The **use of single-dose therapy is controversial.** Short-course therapy has been effective for some patients. For a 3-day course of treatment, cephalexin 250 mg or 500mg qid, or trimethoprim-sulfamethoxazole double-strength bid is used.

2. **Patients not suitable for single-dose or short-course therapy include:**
   a. Teenagers.
   b. Diabetics.
   c. Immunosuppressed patients.
   d. Patients older than 55 years.
   e. Women with frequent or recurrent UTIs despite antibiotic therapy.
   f. Patients who are febrile with or without flank pain (upper tract infection).
   g. Those with symptoms for more than 7 days.
   h. Those with history of pyelonephritis.
   i. Patients with symptoms of vaginal discharge or STD.
   j. Patients with coliform infection not eradicated by single-dose therapy.
      If contraindications for single-dose or short-course therapy exist or if a coliform infection is not eradicated by single-dose or short course therapy, a 7- to 14-day course of antibiotic therapy is indicated.

3. Urethritis caused by *Chlamydia* or *N. gonorrhoeae* should be treated according to Centers for Disease Control and Prevention (CDC) guidelines for STD treatment (see Chapter 3). Sexual partners should be treated.

4. **Symptomatic women without pyuria** should receive therapy appropriate to the underlying condition.

B. **Extended regimens**

1. **Abbreviated regimens are not recommended** for women with **any** of the aforementioned **contraindications** (see section V.A.2.) or for **clinically stable patients who have failed therapy,** as evidenced by

persistence of symptoms or positive culture 2 to 3 days after treatment. These patients should **receive a standard regimen for 7 to 14 days.**

2. In an **acutely symptomatic woman,** the standard drug regimen should be started while cultures are pending. If a woman **fails to respond to abbreviated** treatment **or has signs or symptoms of upper tract infection** a 2- to 4-week antibiotic course is indicated.

3. Standard treatment regimens for 7- to 14-days therapy should be **governed by urine culture and sensitivity reports. Empiric therapy,** based on symptoms and urinalysis, include: **nitrofurantoin,** 50 to 100 mg PO qid; **trimethroprim-sulfamethoxazole DS,** one tablet PO bid; **ampicillin,** 250 to 500 mg PO qid; **amoxicillin,** 250 mg PO tid; **cephalexin,** 250 to 500 mg PO qid; **ciprofloxacin,** 250 mg PO bid; and **tetracycline,** 250 to 500 mg PO qid. Ampicillin and amoxicillin are **no longer effective in 30% of all UTIs.** Women with simple acute cystitis who experience resolution of their symptoms do not require post-therapy reassessment.

C. **Pyelonephritis**
1. **Differentiation of upper and lower tract infection can be done quite accurately with bladder washout and ureteral catheterization** but these are expensive and time-consuming techniques. Testing for antibody-coated bacteria has significant false-positive and false-negative result rates.

   a. **The response to single-dose therapy may be the most practical guide to anatomic site of infection.** If bacteriuria is still present 2 to 3 days after single-dose therapy, an upper tract infection or **silent renal involvement** should be assumed and appropriate treatment given. Treatment with 10 to 14 days of a standard antibiotic regimen based on susceptibility testing, is needed. Failure of this regimen is an indication for assessment of **risk factors** for **bacterial persistence or relapse.**

   b. The **failure to seek medical attention within 6 days of the onset of symptoms or findings consistent with upper tract or complicated infection** should alert the clinician to a greater likelihood of upper tract involvement.

2. **Overt pyelonephritis** may require hospitalization for patients who are pregnant; have severe underlying disease; have complications (see section VIII.); are suspected to have poor follow-up or compliance; or have acute disease severe enough to require management of pain, nausea, emesis, or other manifestations of illness.

   a. **Patients hospitalized** for pyelonephritis should have urine and blood cultures done. **Parenteral** antibiotic choice may be empiric with an agent or combination of agents such as **ampicillin, a cephalosporin, or aminoglycoside.** Continued use of aminoglycosides should depend on bacterial susceptibility testing.

   b. Whether patients **require hospitalization or not, a minimum 2-week course of an antibiotic regimen** is indicated for **all** patients with pyelonephritis. Outpatient therapy can be initiated with a **cephalosporin** (cephalexin), 500 mg PO qid; **trimethoprim-sulfamethoxazole DS** bid; or **a quinolone antibiotic** (such as ciprofloxacin), 500 mg PO bid.

   c. Women with community-acquired pyelonephritis who do **not** require hospitalization respond better to trimethoprim-sulfamethoxazole DS than to ampicillin and 2 weeks of therapy has been as effective as 6 weeks of therapy. The **use of amoxicillin** and ampicillin in UTIs **is decreasing,** particularly in single-dose or short-course therapy (see section A.1.) and when silent or overt renal involvement is suspected.

   d. **Follow-up cultures 3 days after starting and 1 week after completion of therapy** are indicated to look for **failure of therapy and early relapse.**

3. **Bacteremia. Blood cultures** should be done on all patients with clinically overt pyelonephritis requiring hospitalization and on selected outpatients since **bacteremia may complicate the course of overt pyelonephritis.** Such episodes are usually not associated with the serious sequelae of gram-negative sepsis (such as septic shock and disseminated intravascular coagulation [DIC]). Persistent bacteremia should lead to intravenous pyelography, renal ultrasound, or both.

D. **UTI recurrence**

1. Recurrence is usually seen within 1 to 2 weeks after completion of treatment and most commonly is a **reinfection** by different bacteria than the initial strain involved. However, ascending infection from the vaginal introital area is still the most common source of the offending bacteria.

2. Less commonly, **relapse** occurs by reappearance of the original infecting strain. Usually occurring within 2 weeks of completion of therapy, **relapse** can only be differentiated from **bacterial persistence** by documentation of sterile urine after therapy. In either event, efforts should be made to identify correctable abnormalities that are risk factors for recurrence.

   Abnormalities that can contribute to bacterial persistence include stones, ureteral duplication and ectopic ureters, foreign bodies (suture), ureteral diverticulum, infected paraurethral glands, and fistulas. **Failure to respond to treatment** may also be due to patient noncompliance.

3. **Treatment.** A 4- to 6-week course of one of the drug regimens specified in C.1.a. is indicated in patients with **early recurrence** of UTI, **multiple episodes** of UTI that have been difficult to control, **underlying anatomic abnormality, or a history of renal transplantation.** In addition, these patients should be considered candidates for **UTI prophylaxis if they have closely spaced recurrences.** Although many clinicians recommend long initial courses of therapy for diabetics, an initial 7- to 10-day course is justified for acute, uncomplicated infection. Guidelines for selection of women for self-medication have been developed (Fig. 7.1).

E. **Prophylaxis and prevention** is cost-effective and efficacious in these women who have three or more UTIs yearly. Effective regimens include **daily administration** of one-half tablet of trimethoprim-sulfamethoxazole (single-strength); **nitrofurantoin,** 100 mg; or **trimethoprim,** 100 mg. Regimens requiring **thrice weekly or postcoital dosing** of the same antibiotics have also been effective. In all regimens, the **beneficial effect of the antibiotic stops after prophylaxis is withdrawn.** An initial 6-month trial will establish tolerance and effectiveness. Subsequently, treatment is individualized depending on the baseline rate of infection. One reasonable approach is to stop prophylaxis every 6 months to see whether a long-term remission will occur. Periodic prophylaxis for a portion of every year is another reasonable strategy. **Occasional urine cultures during periods of prophylaxis are needed** to be certain of effectiveness.

F. **Symptomatic therapy** may include **antipyretics,** if needed for fever, and **phenazopyridine** (Pyridium), 200 mg PO tid for **no longer** than 2 days, for dysuria.

VI. **General measures: patient education**

A. **Prevention of UTIs may be facilitated by patient education.** Teaching should include issues of perineal hygiene such as wiping front to back, as well as instructions to limit douching and feminine hygiene sprays, avoid deodorized tampons, avoid using petrolatum (Vaseline) as a sexual lubricant, to use cotton panties, and to increase fluid intake.

B. **When being treated for UTI,** women should be advised according to section VI.A. as well as told about the **possibility of yeast vaginitis related to antibiotic therapy.** Daily ingestion of yogurt or cultured milk may help avoid yeast vaginitis. Women should also be instructed to **expect orange discoloration of urine because of phenazopyridine.**

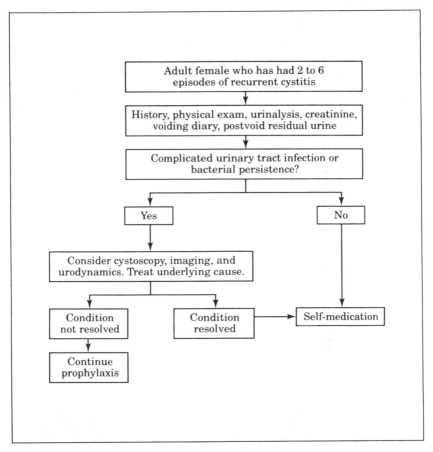

FIG. 7.1. Selecting patients for self-medication. (From Tucker S. Self-medication protocol for UTI patients. *Contemp Obstet Gynecol* 1993;38:75, with permission.)

VII. **Indications for further evaluation.** An **intravenous pyelogram** and perhaps a **voiding cystourethrogram or cystoscopy** appear most useful in adult women with a **history of multiple childhood infections** (if not already evaluated), **possible nephrolithiasis, relapsing infection** (when repeated lack of response of an effective agent can be shown), **diabetes** with relapses, **neurogenic bladder, painless hematuria,** or **pyelonephritis** that does not respond quickly to appropriate therapy.

Recent reports indicate that urologic studies such as **intravenous pyelography, cystoscopy, and cystography** have a **very low yield** and, hence are **not cost-effective for adult women with uncomplicated lower UTIs.**

VIII. Complications
  A. **Catheter-associated UTIs can be minimized by standard guidelines for bladder catheter care.**
    1. If the patient is **asymptomatic,** she should **not be treated until the catheter is removed.**
    2. For women with **chronic indwelling catheters,** treatment should **be reserved for symptomatic UTIs** (e.g., fever, chills, dyspnea,

hypotension) and should include **changing catheters as well as prescribing antibiotics.** Changing long-term indwelling catheters every 8 weeks has been suggested.

3. **All symptomatic patients with indwelling catheters should be treated.**

4. **While urine cultures are pending, choice of antibiotic** should initially be **based on past urine culture and sensitivity reports.**

B. **Population at risk for morbidity.** In general, women at risk for severe morbidity, renal scarring, or both from UTIs include women with the following:

1. **Infection with urea-splitting organisms** (usually *Proteus*), which cause struvite renal stones.

2. **Congenital anomalies** such as duplications of the renal collecting system that become secondarily infected. **Surgery is often required.**

3. **Bacteriuria in the presence of obstruction of the urinary tract** such as that caused by renal stones. This condition requires **emergency drainage of the kidney.**

4. **Analgesic nephropathy** (especially with obstruction from papillary necrosis). **Immediate relief of the obstruction is critical.**

5. **Diabetes** (especially with emphysematous pyelonephritis, a surgical emergency).

6. **Neurogenic bladder.**

7. **Pregnancy, which always requires screening for asymptomatic bacteriuria.**

C. **Perinephric abscess** is often **secondary to coliform-induced UTIs complicated by renal calculi and obstruction.** Onset is insidious, diagnosis is difficult, and the mortality is high.

1. Any patient with pyelonephritis who fails to have a timely response to oral or intravenous antibiotics should have an **ultrasound study of the kidneys. Intravenous pyelogram, gallium scan, or computed tomography** (CT scan) **may be necessary** for diagnosis.

2. **The treatment is surgical.**

IX. **Urinary tract infections in pregnancy.** UTIs occur commonly in pregnant women and are managed **differently** than those in nonpregnant women. **Renal length increases** approximately 1 cm **in pregnancy.** The collecting system undergoes **decreased peristalsis** during pregnancy and **hydroureter** is common in the **third trimester** due both to smooth muscle relaxation and partial obstruction.

A. **Asymptomatic bacteriuria.** All pregnant women should be **screened** for **asymptomatic bacteriuria** since this occurs in **4% to 8% of pregnant** women. This is no different than the nonpregnant patient, however risk of infection and complication is greater.

1. **History.** Patients are asymptomatic.

2. **Physical.** No findings.

3. **Investigative procedures**

a. Urinalysis may be normal.

b. A midstream, clean-catch specimen that is cultured reveals $\geq 10^5$ colonies per milliliter: 80% of infections are caused by *E. coli*; 10% to 15% are caused by *Klebsiella pneumoniae* or *Proteus* species; and 5% or less being caused by group B streptococci, enterococci, or staphylococci.

4. **Management.** Appropriate treatment depends on culture results and any history of allergies.

a. **Nitrofurantoin,** 100 mg PO q12h for 7 days.

b. **Cephalexin** (Keflex), 500 mg PO q6h for 7 days.

c. **Amoxicillin,** 500 mg PO q8h for 7 days (see section V.B.3. for efficacy issues).

d. **Trimethoprim-sulfamethoxazole** and **amoxicillin-clavulanic acid** (Augmentin) should be reserved for refractory infections caused by resistant microorganisms. **Sulfisoxazole** may cause **jaundice** in **preterm** infants.

e. The **quinolones** have **deleterious** effects on **fetal cartilage in animals** and should be **avoided in pregnancy.**

f. **Tetracyclines** are **also** contraindicated in pregnancy secondary to dental staining.

g. A repeat culture should be done after completion of treatment, followed by periodic cultures.

h. **Forty percent will develop pyelonephritis if untreated.**

B. **Acute cystitis.** This disorder occurs in 1% to 3% of pregnant patients.

1. **History.** Patients may have dysuria, urgency, and frequency.

2. **Physical examination.** Normal findings or mild suprapubic tenderness may be noted.

3. **Investigative procedures.** Urinalysis shows a WBC count of **10** WBC per milliliter of voided urine, bacteria, and possibly red blood cells. Culture and sensitivity should be done (see section IX.A.3.b.).

4. **Management.** When empiric therapy must be given (culture pending), amoxicillin should be **avoided** owing to resistance among strains of *E. coli* and *K. pneumoniae.* The risk of recurrent UTI later in pregnancy is 15% to 25% (see section IX.A.4.).

C. **Acute pyelonephritis.** This disorder occurs in 1% to 2% of obstetric patients. **Pregnant women** are particularly **susceptible** due to a **decrease in ureteral peristalsis** and **mechanical obstruction** from the uterus.

1. **History.** The patient may complain of fever, chills, flank pain, urinary frequency, and urgency. She may have had a **prior UTI** or **asymptomatic bacteriuria**.

2. **Physical examination.** The woman may have a fever and flank tenderness. Of the pregnant women with pyelonephritis 70% to 75% have a right-sided infection.

3. **Investigation procedures**

a. **Urinalysis** may reveal WBC casts and bacteria.

b. The **urine culture** is **positive** unless the patient has been taking antibiotics. The most common organisms are **E. coli, K. pneumoniae,** and **Proteus** species.

c. **Blood cultures** are positive in up to **10%** of patients.

4. **Management**

a. Pregnant women with **pyelonephritis** should be **hospitalized.**

b. **Parenteral antibiotics** should be given, such as cefazolin, 1 to 2 g IV q8h and gentamicin, 1.5 mg/kg IV q8h, can be added if the patient appears to be critically ill.

c. **Parenteral antibiotics** should be continued until the patient has been **afebrile** and **asymptomatic** for **24 to 48 hours.** Culture and sensitivity reports should be ready by this time.

d. **On discharge,** the patient should be treated with an appropriate oral antibiotic for another 7 to 10 days.

e. **Monthly urine screens** should be obtained.

f. Some clinicians choose to keep the pregnant patient on prophylactic antibiotics such as nitrofurantoin, 100 mg PO qhs to prevent recurrence.

X. **Urinary tract infection in older women**

A. **Etiology**

1. In older women, the causes of increased susceptibility to **infection are multiple,** including **physiologic changes, acquired abnormalities** of the **urinary tract,** and increased exposure to **environmental risk factors.**

2. If a UTI **relapses or reinfection** occurs, an **evaluation** for urinary tract abnormalities should be performed.

3. **Bacteriuria** is found in **20%** of women **older than** the age of **65 years** however, **only a small number has persistent bacteriuria.**

72 7. Urinary Tract Infections

B. Presentation
1. Symptoms of **lethargy, confusion, anorexia and/or incontinence** commonly occur.
2. A high index of suspicion is warranted, especially when risk factors are present.
3. The absence of pyuria is a good negative predictor for bacteriuria in this population.

C. Management
1. Treatment should follow the guidelines listed previously for uncomplicated cystitis.
2. Older patients, however, are more susceptible to any toxic or adverse effects of antibiotics.

References

1. Boscia JA, Kobasa WD, Knight RA, et al. Epidemiology of bacteriuria in an elderly population. *Am J Med* 1986;80:208.
2. Boscia JA, et al. Asymptomatic bacteriuria in elderly persons: treat or do not treat? *Ann Intern Med* 1987;106:764.
3. Fairley KF, Grounds AD, Carson NE, et al. Site of infection in acute urinary-tract infection in general practice. *Lancet* 1971;2:615.
4. Fowler JE, Pulaski ET. Excretory urography, cystography, and cystoscopy in the evaluation of women with urinary-tract infection. *N Engl J Med* 1981;304:462.
5. Grieco MH. Use of antibiotics in the elderly. *Bull NY Acad Med* 1980;56:197.
6. Hooten TM. Recurrent urinary tract infections in women. *Int J Antimicrob Agents* 2001;17:259–268.
7. Jordan PA, Iravani A, Richard GA, et al. Urinary tract infections cause by *Staphylococcus saprophyticus*. *J Infect Dis* 1980;142:510.
8. Karram MM. Lower urinary tract infection. In: Ostergard DR, ed. *Urogynecology and urodynamics, theory and practice*. Baltimore: Williams & Wilkins, 1991.
9. Kass EH, Platt R. Urinary tract and genital mycoplasmal infection. In: Wald NJ, ed. *Antenatal and neonatal screening*. New York: Oxford University Press, 1984.
10. Komaroff AL. Urinalysis and urine culture in women with dysuria. *Ann Intern Med* 1986;104:212.
11. Kunin C. Duration of treatment of urinary tract infections. *Am J Med* 1981;71:849.
12. MacLean AB. Urinary tract infection in pregnancy. *Int J Antimicrob Agents* 2001;17:273–276.
13. Naber KG. Treatment options for acute uncomplicated cystitis in adults. *J Antimicrob Chemother* 2000;46[Suppl 1]:23–27.
14. Neu HC. Quinolones: a new class of antimicrobial agents with wide potential uses. *Med Clin North Am* 1988;72:623.
15. Patterson TF, Andriole VT. Detection, significance, and therapy of bacteruria in pregnancy: update in the managed health care era. *Infec Dis Clin North Am* 1997;11:593–608.
16. Philbrick JT, Bracikowski JP. Single-dose antibiotic treatment for uncomplicated urinary tract infections: less for less? *Arch Intern Med* 1985;145:1672.
17. Raz R. Postmenopausal women with recurrent UTI. *Int J Antimicrob Agents* 2001;17:269–271.
18. Ronald AR. Optimal duration of treatment of kidney infection. *Ann Intern Med* 1987;106:467.
19. Rubin RH. Infections of the urinary tract. In: Rubenstein E, Federman D, eds. *Scientific American medicine*. New York: Scientific American, 1989: Sec. 7, Chap. 23.
20. Schaeffer AJ. Infections of the urinary tract. In: Walsh PC, Retik AB, Vaughan ED Jr, eds. *Campbell's urology*. Philadelphia: WB Saunders, 1998:548.
21. Stamey T. Urinary tract infections in the female: a perspective. In: Remington J, Swartz M, eds. *Current clinical topics in infectious diseases*. New York: McGraw-Hill, 1981.
22. Stamm WE. Recent developments in the diagnosis and treatment of urinary tract infections. *West J Med* 1982;137:213.

23. Stamm WE, Hooten TM. The management of urinary tract infections in adults. *N Engl J Med* 1993;329:1328–1334.
24. Stamm WE, Raz R. Factors contributing to susceptibility of postmenopausal women to recurrent urinary tract infections. *Clin Infect Dis* 1999;28:723–725.
25. Stamm WE, Wagner KF, Amsel R, et al. Causes of the acute urethral syndrome in women. *N Engl J Med* 1980;303:409.
26. Stamm WE, Counts GW, Wagner KF, et al. Antimicrobial prophylaxis of recurrent urinary tract infection. *Ann Intern Med* 1980;92:770.
27. Stark RP, Maki DG. Bacteriuria in the catheterized patient: what quantitative level of bacteriuria is relevant? *N Engl J Med* 1984;311:560.
28. Tucker SM. Self-medication protocol for UTI patients. *Contemp Obstet Gynecol* 1993;38:75.
29. Waltzer WC. The urinary tract in pregnancy. *J Urol* 1981;125:271.
30. Wigton RS, Hoellerich VL, Ornato JP, et al. Use of clinical findings in the diagnosis of urinary tract infection in women. *Arch Intern Med* 1985;145:2222.

8. URINARY INCONTINENCE

Kenneth Griffis

The proper diagnosis and treatment of urinary incontinence is a very important aspect of women's health care. The National Institutes of Health in 1996 estimated that urinary incontinence may have accounted for as much as $15 billion spent annually in health care delivery, with approximately 13 million women affected by involuntary urine loss.

In **middle-aged to older women,** some studies have reported a **prevalence** as high as 30% to 40%. Despite this high prevalence, some surveys have shown that fewer than half of women with urinary incontinence seek help for their condition. This may be either because of embarrassment or a perception that their symptoms are normal. Experts have suggested that urinary incontinence and related disorders of the pelvic floor may represent one of the largest unaddressed women's health care issues in the United States today.

Incontinence of urine may be defined as **involuntary loss of urine** when urine loss is not only socially or personally unacceptable as perceived by the patient, but also objectively demonstrable to the health care provider. Although stress incontinence is the most common form of involuntary urine loss, it must be emphasized that **no single factor underlies the etiology of all forms of involuntary urine loss.** Appropriate evaluation and diagnosis of the incontinent patient must be completed **before** care can be effected (Fig. 8.1).

    I. **Pathophysiology of urinary incontinence.** In a simplified view, the bladder may be thought of as a balloon-like organ that collects urine passively from the ureters; stores urine; and after a voluntary message is sent, releases the urine at a place and time that is acceptable to the patient. The pressures on and inside the balloon represent expulsive forces, and the squeeze at the level of the balloon neck (the urethra and bladder neck) represents retentive forces (Fig. 8.2).

        A. **The patient is continent** when the **intravesical pressure** (total expulsive force) is **less than** those pressures affecting **maximum urethral pressure** (total retentive force). If **intravesical pressure** (expulsive force) **exceeds urethral pressure** (retentive forces), then urine spills from the bladder.

        B. This overall simple scheme of normal collection, storage, and voiding mechanism requires a complex coordination of neurologic pathways and physiologic and anatomic factors that influence these expulsive and retentive forces (Fig. 8.3). At least four neurologic loops, nerve roots T-10 through S-4, and both parasympathetic and sympathetic pathways are involved with the neurologic aspects of micturition alone. Any part of the function of these systems can malfunction by itself (or in combination with other parts of the system) to lead to incontinence.

        C. The **differential diagnosis** leading to incontinence must take into **account the underlying complexity of micturition.** It is linked to such problems as **pelvic relaxation disorders** (cystocele or prolapse), **detrusor instability,** and **hyperreflexibility** (detrusor dyssynergia, "urethral syndrome"), **systemic disabilities** (diabetes, thyroid disease, systemic lupus erythematosus), **psychofunctional disturbances, infections, anatomic abnormalities** that are either congenital (ectopic ureters, diverticula) or induced (fistulas), **primary neurologic disorders** (multiple sclerosis, cerebral vascular accidents), and **pharmacologic causes of involuntary loss of urine; all of which may coexist,** thereby compounding the diagnosis and treatment (Table 8.1).

    II. There are **several types of incontinence.** The following definitions help to categorize the multiple etiologies for involuntary urine loss.

This chapter is a revision of the third edition chapter by Gregory A. Herrera.

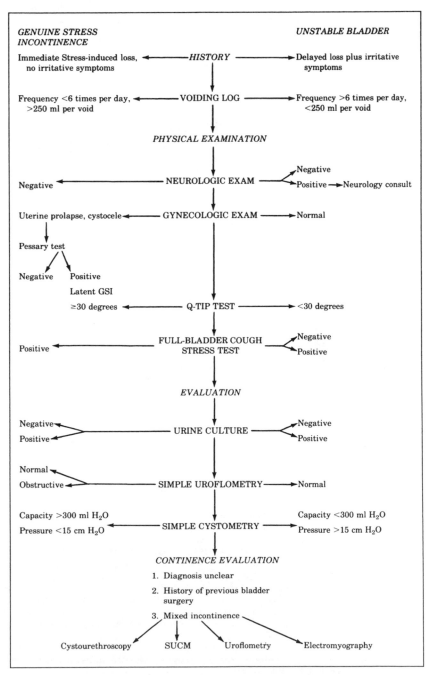

FIG. 8.1. Differential diagnosis of the patient with urinary incontinence. GSI, genuine stress incontinence; SUCM, simultaneous urethrocystometry.

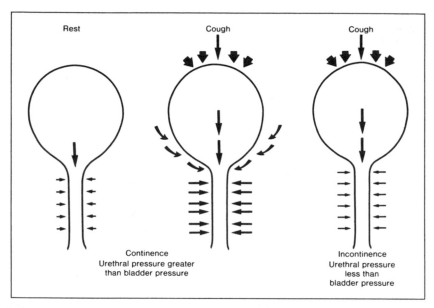

FIG. 8.2. The pressure transmission patterns of the bladder and the urethra. At rest the urethral pressure exceeds the intravesical pressure and no urine leakage occurs. The number and length of the arrows indicate the relative amount of pressure caused by coughing. The normal woman's bladder and urethra both receive the same force with little net difference because of a good pressure transmission capacity ratio. This occurs when the urethra is an intraabdominal organ. When the urethra loses its anatomic supports, it becomes an extraabdominal organ. In this abnormal position it receives less pressure than the bladder. Thus, there is more force applied to the bladder than to the urethra. When this force exceeds urethral resistance, incontinence occurs because of an insufficient pressure transmission capacity ratio. (From Ostergard DR. *Gynecologic urology and urodynamics: theory and practice*. Baltimore: Williams & Wilkins, 1980, with permission.)

> A. **Genuine stress incontinence.** (GSI) is an involuntary **loss of urine in the absence of unstable detrusor contractions.** This is **also called anatomic stress urinary incontinence.** It occurs when the intravesical pressure exceeds the maximum ureteral pressure due to an elevation of intraabdominal pressure. GSI is due to one or more of the following factors:
>   1. **Descent of the urethrovesical junction outside the intraabdominal zone of pressure.**
>   2. **Decrease in urethral pressure.**
>   3. **Short functional length of the urethra.**
> B. **Detrusor instability** includes a diverse group of bladder-filling disorders associated with **urge incontinence,** which is an **involuntary loss of urine** with a strong **desire** to void. Usually, **involuntary bladder contractions** are the **hallmark** of the **diagnosis.**
>   1. **Symptoms** may include **urgency,** increased **frequency, nocturia, loss of urine with coitus,** and **urgency to void with cold weather and/or the sound of running water.**
>   2. **Detrusor instability** is the **most common cause** of urinary incontinence in **older women** and the **second** most common cause of incontinence in women during their **reproductive years.** It occurs in 30% of asymptomatic older women.

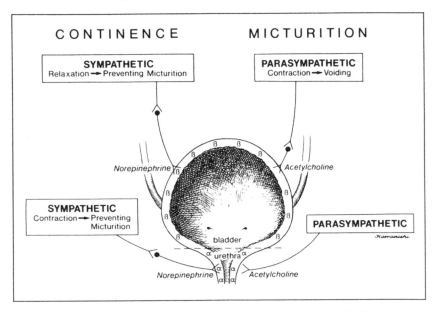

FIG. 8.3. The innervation of the bladder and urethra. Parasympathetic fibers arising in S-2 through S-4 have long preganglionic fibers and pelvic ganglia close to the bladder and urethra. These parasympathetic fibers excrete acetylcholine. Sympathetic fibers that have long postganglionic fibers discharge norepinephrine to beta-adrenergic receptors, primarily in the bladder, and alpha-sympathetic receptors, primarily in the urethra. (From Droegemueller W, et al. *Comprehensive gynecology*. St. Louis: Mosby, 1987, with permission.)

3. **Detrusor instability usually** takes the form of **urge incontinence,** but stress incontinence may also occur. Other symptoms include frequency, nocturia, and urgency. Unfortunately, clinical examination for detection of this bladder abnormality is unrewarding, and the **objective demonstration** of the detrusor contraction can be documented only by **cystometry.**
4. The **etiology** of detrusor instability is **uncertain,** but in the **majority** of cases it is **idiopathic.** It **may be psychosomatic** and, occasionally, there may be an **underlying neurologic abnormality.** *Neurogenic bladder* is a type of bladder instability caused by diseases of the peripheral or central nervous system such as parkinsonism or multiple sclerosis. There is also an increased incidence following incontinence surgery. Local bladder or urethral irritation, foreign bodies, bladder stones, suture material, interstitial cystitis, and infection also can cause detrusor overactivity.
C. **Reflex incontinence** (also known as detrusor hyperrelesia, neurogenic bladder, and motor neuron autonomic bladder) is an **involuntary loss of urine** as a result of abnormal reflex activity at the **spinal cord level.** These patients also have involuntary bladder contractions but without sensations of urgency. Patients with this variant of involuntary urine loss are usually unaware of their incontinence until disturbed by wetness (bedwetting, loss of urine with position changes, and so on).
D. **Overflow incontinence** occurs when the bladder cannot empty normally, becomes overdistended, and the intravesical pressure exceeds the maximum urethral pressure.

Table 8.1. Differential diagnosis of urinary incontinence

GENITOURINARY ETIOLOGY
Filling/storage disorders
    Detrusor hyperreflexia (neurogenic)
    Detrusor instability (idiopathic)
    Genuine stress incontinence
    Mixed types
    Overflow incontinence
Fistula
    Ureteral
    Urethral
    Vesical
Congenital
    Ectopic ureter
    Epispadias

NONGENITOURINARY ETIOLOGY
Cognitive
Environmental
Functional
Metabolic
Mood
Neurologic
Pharmacologic

From Walters MD. Steps in evaluating the incontinent woman. *Contemp. Obstet. Gynecol.* 1992;37:9, with permission.

1. **Symptoms include dribbling of urine, sometimes with constant urine loss.**
2. **Causes include neurologic abnormalities, partial obstruction to the outflow tract (tumors, strictures), and medications.**
   a. Extraurethral or total incontinence occurs with fistulas.
   b. The primary symptom is constant loss of urine.
   c. In industrialized countries, this is usually associated with a history of prior pelvic surgery or irradiation. In developing countries and less so in industrialized countries, fistulas can occur with obstetric trauma.
III. The **history** is paramount and identifies the etiology and subsequent appropriate treatment. To best identify which part of the **voiding mechanism** is defective, the history must include the nature and **character** of the **incontinence, gynecologic data, medical diseases or problems,** and **medications.**
   A. **Involuntary loss of urine history** must include the following:
      1. **Stress incontinence with coughing, sneezing, and/or Valsalva maneuver.**
      2. Symptoms of instability include **dribbling, urgency,** and **increased frequency.**
      3. **Overflow incontinence** includes constant **wetness, incomplete emptying,** and **dribbling.**
      4. **Reflex loss—enuresis.**
      5. **Infection** may result in hematuria and dysuria.
   B. Past surgical history should include any abdominal or pelvic surgery. The potential for trauma or fistulas must be considered.
   C. **Medical, neurologic,** and **endocrine disorders may produce urinary incontinence.** A **history** of the following problems is of particular significance.

       1. **History of infection.**
       2. **Dyssynergic symptoms** and a detailed description of the circumstances under which urine is lost.
       3. Any past **urologic, gynecologic,** or **obstetric** history.
       4. **Neurologic** and **renal** diseases.
       5. **Endocrine** and **metabolic** diseases.
   D. **Pharmacologic history.** There are a number of medications that can cause urinary incontinence. Those that are of particular significance include:
       1. **Psychotropics.**
       2. **Tranquilizers.**
       3. The combination product **hydrocodone and acetaminophen** (Vicodin) and codeine
       4. **Bromocriptine (Parlodel).**
       5. **Antihypertensives.**
IV. The **physical examination** should include a general gynecologic and neurologic examination on every patient with involuntary urine loss. The clinician should not jump to a diagnosis such as cystocele since there **may be multiple causes for any given patient's involuntary urine loss.**
   A. The general **physical** examination should **focus** on signs of **asthma** or **pulmonary disease,** which may aggravate urine loss. The patient's **estrogen state** and **associated signs of atrophy** may contribute to loss of urethral tone.
   B. The **neurologic examination** should include testing for nerve roots **T-10** through **S-4,** and a motor and sensory examination of the lower extremities dependent on these nerve roots is necessary.
       1. **"Anal wink"** reflex, peroneal dermatomes, and flexion-extension tests of the knee, hip, and ankle are easy to do, as well as patellar reflexes and perineal and thigh sensation to pinprick.
       2. **Abnormal neurologic findings require further investigation.**
   C. The **gynecologic examination** should emphasize evaluation for signs of **pelvic relaxation** (cystocele, rectocele, and uterine prolapse), **vaginal infection, urethral diverticula,** and both vulvar and vaginal **atrophy** (hypoestrogenemia). **All** of these have been known to **mimic stress incontinence.**
V. **Investigative procedures** specific to the urogynecologic examination involve tests both simple and very sophisticated. Not all of these tests are a required prelude to treatment, but all of them should at least be considered on a case-by-case basis.
   A. **A urinalysis is always required to rule out obvious infection.**
   B. **Testing** for **diabetes** and **thyroid** disease is appropriate, if indicated by history and/or examination.
   C. **Voiding diary.** One of the first steps in the assessment of the incontinent patient is the voiding dairy. This provides the clinician with a 24-hour history of events and factors that influence or accompany incontinence. The diary should include:
       1. **How many times voided.**
       2. **How many times incontinent.**
       3. **How many episodes of nocturia.**
       4. **How many pads or absorbant underpants used.**
       5. **Whether or not there is presence of urge to urinate with incontinence.**
       6. **Estimated volume of incontinence.**
       7. **Volume voided each time.**
       8. **Intake volume.**
   D. **Stress test.** The patient is asked to **cough with a full bladder** (at least 250–300 mL). This will demonstrate leakage spurts in stress-related incontinence but does not distinguish GSI from other forms of incontinence with stress.
   E. **Cotton swab (Q-Tip)** test is an easy and relatively painless method of determining an abnormal urethrovesical angle and should be included in the initial investigation. Lubricated with an anesthetic (lidocaine jelly), a Q-Tip

is introduced into the urethra to the bladder neck. While in the lithotomy position, patients with significant loss of support to the posterior angle of the urethra and bladder (the bladder neck) should show a deviation greater than 30 degrees from the horizontal axis with straining. These patients may benefit from a bladder neck suspension. "Normal patients" generally show a deviation of less than 30 degrees.

F. **Uroflowmetry** can be accomplished using a stopwatch and a container (a toilet seat "hat") to measure the voiding time for the patient to pass at least 150 to 200 mL of urine. Flow rates should be at least 10 mL/sec, and a residual catheterization should have no more than 50 to 75 mL of urine. Slow flow rates and high residual urine values (>100 mL) are associated with **obstruction** or **neurologic problems** with the bladder.

G. **Cystometry** is a study to demonstrate bladder compliance or pressure-volume relations during the bladder filling. Simple office cystometry uses a two-channel Foley catheter hooked to an IV bottle with saline for infusion and a measuring stick-manometer device to record pressures (Fig. 8.4). Involuntary, uninhibited bladder contractions with filling are consistent with the diagnosis of an unstable bladder or detrusor dyssynergia. A low urethral opening pressure and stable filling rates are more compatible with GSI (Fig. 8.5).

H. **Cystourethroscopy** (with or without multichannel urodynamics) is a urodynamic study that can be performed in the office. It provides visualization of the urethra, the bladder walls (along with the trigone and ureteral orifices), observation and recording of the bladder neck dynamics, and collection of cystometric data.

1. Testing with cystourethroscopy depends on **direct visualization** with **simultaneous pressure recordings** (channels in the bladder, urethra, rectum) while the bladder is filled either with a gas or fluid.

2. The patient is also asked to strain (Valsalva maneuver), cough, and sometimes change position during the examination.

3. **Intrinsic bladder and urethra lesions** (diverticula, trabeculation, fistulas, ectopic ureters, interstitial cystitis, foreign bodies, and tumors) are seen, as well as dynamic disorders related to expulsive and retentive forces demonstrated and recorded by direct visualization (detrusor irritability filling patterns, and/or displacement of bladder neck with straining).

4. Urethral pressure profiles have been considered useful by some clinicians in evaluating the sphincteric integrity of the urethra in relation to bladder and intraabdominal pressure changes.

VI. **Management of urinary incontinence** varies with the cause. It cannot be overemphasized that there may be **multiple causes for urine loss,** and **careful diagnosis is crucial to successful management.** Many, and possibly most, **failures of treatment,** particularly surgical failures, can be **traced to initial misdiagnosis.** Possibly the most commonly used example of such a treatment failure is the repair of a cystocele in a woman with minimal urine loss. A large cystocele can actually afford a patient a degree of protection from incontinence since its bulge may act as a "relief valve" for increased bladder pressures. **Repair of the cystocele alone, without concurrent bladder neck suspension or treatment of other existing conditions, might convert a mostly continent woman into being floridly incontinent,** since other incontinence factors (detrusor dyssynergy, occult bladder neck displacement, chronic cystitis, or others) were not addressed. The medical-legal-ethical implications of this example should be self-evident.

A. **Treat underlying medical conditions first.** Consider the possibility of multiple causes for urine loss, and begin treatments with the simplest, least destructive choices for therapy first, then wait for therapeutic effect. Even patients with mixed disorders improve with various forms of **conservative therapy** in as many as **60% of cases.**

1. Therapy may be tried without first completing urodynamic studies, **if one has made a substantial diagnosis.** This might apply to the el-

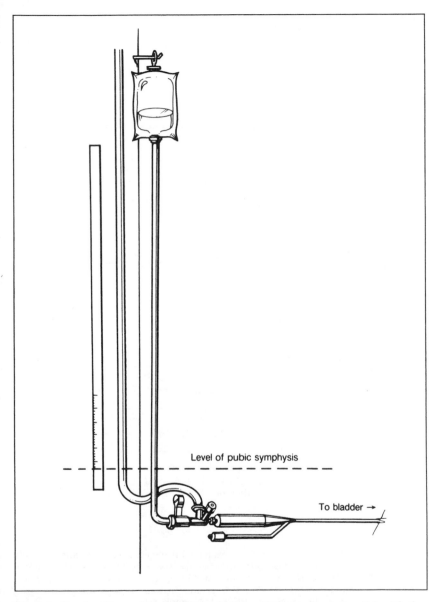

FIG. 8.4. Simple office cystometry using a Foley catheter and a meter stick with the 0 mark positioned at the upper level of the patient's pubic symphysis. Optimally the patient should be in the standing position and fluid infused at a rate of 80 to 100 mL/min. (From American College of Obstetricians and Gynecologists [ACOG]. *Urogynecologic evaluation, endoscopy, and urodynamic testing in the symptomatic female.* ACOG Audiovisual Library. Washington, DC: ACOG, 1990, with permission.)

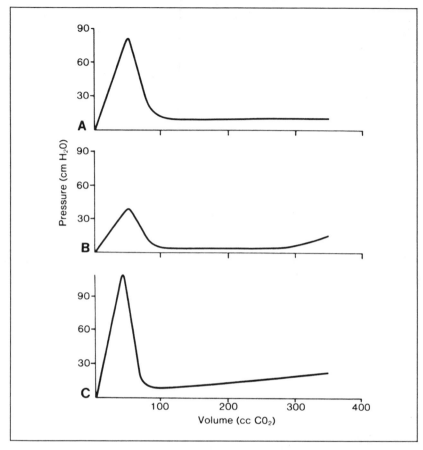

FIG. 8.5. Urethral opening pressures. **(A)** normal, **(B)** genuine stress incontinence, and **(C)** detrusor instability patients. (From Ostergard DR. *Gynecologic urology and urodynamics: theory and practice.* Baltimore: Williams & Wilkins, 1980, with permission.)

derly patient with mostly urge incontinence, who is not a good candidate for surgery or patients with urinary tract infections, and so forth.
2. **Medications** should be **started** in **minimal doses.** This is particularly important when using sedatives, neuroleptics, anticholinergics, cholinergic agonists, and antihypertensives.
B. **GSI can be treated** using **medical** and **nonsurgical therapies** in those patients who are minimally symptomatic. This is an important consideration in women who are poor operative risks or who are still anticipating future childbearing. Surgery still remains the principal treatment for GSI for most patients.
   1. **Pharmacologic agents** for GSI (Table 8.2) may include:
      a. **Estrogen therapy** for the hypoestrogenemia patient with urethral atrophy. Estrogen therapy involves estrogen receptors in the bladder and the urethra and may do more than aid in replenishing epithelial integrity to the urethra. Patients with detrusor instability

Table 8.2. Drugs used in therapy for urinary incontinence

Type	Drug	Usual dose	Mode of action
Anticholinergics	Propantheline (Pro-Banthine)	15–30 mg tid or qid	Competition for cholinergic receptors
	Methantheline (Banthine)	50 mg qd or bid	—
	Oxybutynin chloride (Ditropan)	5–10 mg bid, tid, or qid	Anticholinergic, direct musculotrophic, anesthetic, calcium transport inhibitor
	Tolteridone (Detrol)	1–2 mg qd or bid	—
	Emepronium bromide	200 mg/day	Peripheral and ganglionic anticholinergic
	Terodiline (Bicor)	25 mg bid	Anticholinergic, calcium transport inhibitor
Musculotrophic agents	Dicyclomine hydrochloride (Bentyl)	10 mg qd or tid	Direct musculotrophic and anticholinergic
	Flavoxate hydrochloride (Urispas)	100 mg bid or tid	Direct musculotrophic, minimal anticholinergic
Tricylic antidepressant	Imipramine hydrochloride (Tofranil)	25–50 mg bid or tid	Central antidepressant, central and peripheral adrenergic potentiation, anticholinergic, direct musculotrophic
Calcium antagonists	Nifedipine (Procardia)	10 mg qd or bid	Inhibition of calcium transport
	Flunarizine	20 mg/day	Inhibition of calcium transport
Antiprostaglandins	Indomethacin (Indocin)	50 mg qd or bid	Inhibition of prostaglandin synthesis
	Flurbiprofen	50 mg tid	Inhibition of prostaglandin synthesis
Central nervous system depressants	Diazepam (Valium)	5 mg bid or tid	General sedation, muscular relaxation, partial anticholinergic action
beta-Adrenergic stimulants	Terbutaline (Bricanyl)	2.5–5 mg tid	Beta-adrenergic receptor agonist
Antidiuretic hormone analogs	Desmopressin (DDAVP intranasal spray)	20 mg qhs	Affecting renal water conservation, synthetic analog of 8-arginine vasopressin
alpha-Adrenergic stimulating agents	Phenylpropanolamine (Dexatrim)	75 mg/day	Alpha-adrenergic receptor agonist
Hormones	Conjugated estrogens (Premarin cream)	1 g qhs, taper	Estrogen receptors
alpha-Sympathetic blockers	Phenoxybenzamine (Dibenzylene)	10 mg bid	Relaxes uretheral sphincter
Parasympathetic stimulators	Bethanecol chloride (Urecholine)	10 mg tid	Increases bladder tone

had larger first sensation and maximal bladder capacity after estrogen supplemental therapy. This may represent a beneficial effect of estrogen on the proprioceptive sensory threshold of the lower urinary tract.

    (1) The dose of vaginally applied estrogen cream is 1 g (an applicator full) daily for 1 to 2 weeks, then 1 g twice weekly.

    (2) Significant improvement may take 2 to 4 months.

  b. α-Adrenergic-stimulating agents have increased the tone of the urethral sphincteric factors.

    (1) Pseudoephedrine 120 mg sustained release every 12 hours.

    (2) Phenylpropanolamine has been removed from the market in the United States.

    (3) Imipramine, doses of 10 mg PO bid to tid, can also be used.

  c. Caffeine-containing preparations should be avoided.

2. Kegel exercises (Table 8.3). Like many exercises, the success of Kegels depends on the patient tightening the correct muscles and practice. Kegel exercises can improve urinary control in about 50% of patients.

3. Mechanical devices have been used to aid in pelvic floor support in women with and without involuntary urine loss.

  a. A rubber "donut," fitted rings, and Smith-Hodge pessaries have relieved incontinence and minimized discomfort from cystocele and uterine prolapse. They may enhance continence by compressing the urethra, and perhaps by pressing the bladder neck above the pelvic floor.

  b. Tampons and contraceptive diaphragms may also be useful.

4. Surgery for stress incontinence is primarily intended to **elevate the bladder neck above the pelvic floor.** Exceptions to this concept are those patients with "open drainpipes" of urethras (traumatized, scarred, and usually immobile) for whom urethral sling operations have been devised (compresses the urethra rather than restoring normalized bladder neck dynamics). It is beyond the scope of this discussion to review the techniques and merits of the various types of procedures employed.

  a. The **abdominal retropubic urethropexy** (Burch-type) is currently the most favored, but many surgeons are reporting very good results with needle suspension procedures (modifications of the Pereyra procedure) that can easily be combined with additional vaginal surgery and are approaching outpatient status in management.

  b. The use of **suprapubic catheters** is becoming a standard since they permit early ambulation and early testing of a patient's ability to void postoperatively (without repeated catheterization to check for residual urine values).

  c. Success rates for all types of surgery for properly diagnosed stress incontinence **range from 50% to 70%.**

C. Detrusor instability and reflex incontinence treatments are concentrated on eliminating the source of the involuntary contractions.

Table 8.3. Directions for performing kegel exercises

---

1. To identify the pubococcygeal muscle (PC), try to stop and start the urine flow while voiding. If you can stop and start the stream, you are using the PC muscle.

2. To do the Kegel exercises, tighten the PC muscle and hold it for 3 seconds. Do the exercises in sets of ten, five times daily.

3. Each week increase the number of exercises in a set by five.

4. The exercises should be continued for 3–6 months.

5. In women who cannot identify the right muscle to exercise, a vaginal manometer, known as a **perineometer**, is used, which enables these women to measure the force and efficacy of the perineal muscle contractions.

Pharmacologic treatment, psychotherapy, bladder drills, electrical stimulation, and biofeedback therapy also have been used. **Surgery** for treatment of the unstable bladder is **almost completely contraindicated** but denervation procedures and urinary diversion operations have been described for desperate cases. This is rarely necessary since, for many patients, detrusor instability is a disorder characterized by spontaneous exacerbation and remission.

1. **Pharmacologic treatment** is the most useful therapy for detrusor instability (Table 8.2).

    a. **Anticholinergic drugs** provide the first line of treatment, but produce a cure in only 50% to 60% of patients.

    (1) Oxybutynin chloride (Ditropan), 5 to 10 mg bid, tid, or qid, is the common dosage. It is also available in an extended release formulation for dosing at 5, 10, or 15 mg daily. These drugs bind to acetylcholine receptors on the bladder under parasympathetic stimulation, decreasing tone.

    (2) Tolterodine (Detrol), 1 to 2 mg bid. Some patients may respond to a once daily dose instead of bid. A long acting 4-mg formulation is currently under study for once daily dosing.

    (3) Propantheline (Pro-Banthine) is also used in this way, 15 to 30 mg tid to qid.

       (a) **Anticholinergic drugs** are **contraindicated** in women with glaucoma.

       (b) Minor side effects may include dry mouth, drowsiness, and constipation, which may be minimized by starting with low doses and gradually titrating upward as needed.

    b. Imipramine, a tricyclic antidepressant, is especially effective in those patients with mixed incontinence punctuated by bladder instability. Doses are 10 to 50 mg bid to tid (see section VI.B.1.b).

2. **Psychotherapy** has improved urgency and nocturia. It is not particularly useful for urinary-frequency. As with the other therapies mentioned in the following, patients should be encouraged to **void regularly, avoid caffeine and drinking excess fluids and should be considered for concurrent pharmacologic treatments.** Hypnotherapy can be tried when other therapeutic modalities have failed.

3. **Behavior training,** in the form of bladder drills, biofeedback, and functional electrical stimulation, have a success rate that is dependent on the motivation of the patient and the knowledge and familiarity of the techniques on the part of the health care provider.

    a. **Bladder drills** are based on the assumption that conscious efforts (use of the higher cortical centers) can overcome spinal reflex loops to some degree.

    (1) Patients record the number of episodes of involuntary leaking and nocturia each day to assess the improvement.

    (2) Bladder retraining is not followed at night.

    (3) Follow-up visits are scheduled weekly, and intervals between voidings are increased 30 to 60 minutes accordingly.

    (4) This treatment continues for 4 to 6 weeks.

    b. **Biofeedback** is a way of using these same higher centers through auditory and visual signals to enhance control of micturition.

    c. **Bladder instability** has been treated with electrical stimulation based on the "gate theory" of incoming nerve impulses to diminish bladder contractions and increase bladder volume. Success rates can approach 80%, but only in select patients for whom more pressing anatomic, physiologic, and medical causes have been ruled out.

    d. **Overflow incontinence is best treated by addressing the underlying problem.**

    (1) **Intermittent catheterization** is easily taught to many patients with severe, nonoperative obstructions (often preferred

in patients with drainpipe urethras who have undergone a severe urethral sling procedure as treatment for constant urine drainage).

(2) The **α-sympathetic blocker** (phenoxybenzamine [Dibenzyline], initially 10 mg bid) can relax the urethral sphincter apparatus and sometimes treat obstruction.

(3) **Parasympathetic stimulators** (bethanecol chloride [Urecholine], 10 mg tid) increase bladder tone and can aid in micturition in postoperative patients having difficulty initiating a urine flow.

References

1. Abrams P, Blaivas JG, Stanton SL, et al. The standardisation of terminology of lower urinary tract function. The International Continence Society Committee on Standardisation of Terminology. *Scand J Urol Nephrol* 1988;[Suppl]114:5.
2. Bhatia NN, Bergman A, Karram MM. Effects of estrogen on urethral function in women with urinary incontinence. *Am J Obstet Gynecol* 1989;160:176.
3. Cardozo LD, Stanton SL. Genuine stress incontinence and detrusor instability—a review of 200 patients. *Br J Obstet Gynaecol* 1980;87:18.
4. Herbert DBM, Ostergard DR. Vesical instability: urodynamic parameters by microtip transducer catheters. *Obstet Gynecol* 1982;60:331.
5. Horbach NS. Genuine SUI: best surgical approach. *Contemp Obstet Gynecol* 1992; 37:53.
6. Hurt WG. *Urogynecologic surgery.* New York: Raven, 1992.
7. Klugo RC, Cerny JC. Standard water cystometry and electromyography of the external urethral sphincter. *Clin Obstet Gynecol* 1978;21:669.
8. Morrison JFB. Bladder control: role of higher levels of the central nervous system. In: Torrens M, Morrison JFN, eds. *The physiology of the lower urinary tract.* London: Springer-Verlag, 1987.
9. Ostergard DR. *Gynecologic urology and urodynamics: theory and practice.* Baltimore: Williams & Wilkins, 1980.
10. *Precis V: an update in obstetrics and gynecology.* Washington, DC: American College of Obstetricians and Gynecologists, 1994:234–245.
11. Raz S. *Atlas of transvaginal surgery.* Philadelphia: WB Saunders, 1992.
12. Robertson JR. Evaluation of stress incontinence by endoscopy and carbon dioxide cystometry. *Mediguide Ob/Gyn* 1982;1:1.
13. Rowe JW. The NIH Consensus Development Panel: urinary incontinence in adults. *JAMA* 1989;261:2685.
14. Stanton SL, Tanagho EA. *Surgery of female incontinence.* New York: Springer-Verlag, 1980.
15. Wall LL. The unstable bladder. In: Thompson JD, Rock JA, eds. *Te Linde's operative gynecology updates. Te Linde's operative gynecology,* 7th ed. Philadelphia: Lippincott, 1992:1:10;1–13.
16. Walters MD. Steps in evaluating the incontinent woman. *Contemp Obstet Gynecol* 1992;37:9.
17. Fantl JA, Collins J, et al. *Urinary incontinence in adults: acute and chronic management.* Clinical Practical Guideline, No. 2, 1996 Update. Rockville, MD: U.S. Department of Health and Human Services. Public Health Service, Agency for Health Care Policy and Research. AHCPR Publication No. 96-06-0682, March 1996.

9. BREAST DISEASES

Kara Riley-Paull

I. **Introduction.** Breast cancer is generally the primary concern for a woman presenting to her clinician with a breast sign or symptom. It is important that the provider is sensitive to this concern even if the patient does not volunteer her concern. The physician must be able to recognize and manage benign breast disease and recognize malignant disease for prompt referral. This chapter reviews the breast physiology and breast trauma, infection, and benign and malignant diseases.

According to embryologists, the breast is nothing more than a highly developed sweat gland. However, the breast has developed into a complex organ, subject to a complex series of diseases. The **breast can be involved in any systemic disease,** from chronic eczematoid dermatitis to the vasculitis of the collagen diseases. The focus of this chapter is on **primary disease** of the breast.

Each breast is **composed of six to ten lobes; each lobe is comprised of multiple lobules of breast secretory tissue dispersed in a stroma of fat and loose connective tissue.** Variation in the size of breasts is more the result of variable amounts of fat and stroma than of secretory breast tissue itself. The ducts from the lobules within each lobe coalesce and merge to form one of the six to ten major ducts that course through the breast toward the areola. At the areola, the ducts turn toward the surface at a 90-degree angle to emerge on the nipple as six to ten pinhole openings, each representing the drainage from a single lobe (see section IV.).

The lobes are not equally dispersed around the breast. There are **more lobes in the outer quadrants,** especially in the upper outer quadrant. This is why the breast tissue feels more solid in these areas and why **breast cancer is more common in these areas. Another area of normal thickening is the inframammary ridge from overlap of tissues as a result of upright posture.**

To better understand the diseases of the breast, it is helpful to divide them into groups: those that **affect the breast, irrespective of anatomy** (trauma and infection); those that **affect the major ducts;** and those that **affect the secretory lobules and their adjacent lobular ducts.** Such groupings also separate the diseases into those with common clinical features and set the stage for better differential diagnosis.

II. **Trauma and infection.** Because of its exposed location, the breast is subject to trauma. This usually results in a **mild bruise or soreness,** but occasionally, the trauma is severe enough to **produce a hematoma, rupture cysts, or set the stage for fat necrosis.** Clinically, these present with **sudden onset of pain and tenderness,** with or without erythema. An infection in the breast can cause similar symptoms.

   A. **Hematoma**

      1. **History.** The patient may complain of **trauma,** have a **known bleeding disorder,** or both.

      2. **Physical examination.** There is **localized tenderness** (moderate) and **mild swelling** and there **may be discoloration.**

      3. **Investigative procedures.** In general, **nothing is necessary unless an underlying coagulopathy is suspected.** In this event, the necessary tests are **bleeding time, prothrombin time, partial thromboplastin time, and platelet count.**

      4. **Management** should consist of **analgesia only.** Symptoms improve within 3 to 4 days.

This chapter is a revision of the third edition chapter by Lois F. O'Grady.

B. Ruptured cyst
  1. **History.** The patient may have **known fibrocystic disease, may complain of trauma,** or both.
  2. **Physical examination**
      a. **Localized moderate to severe tenderness and some swelling** may be present.
      b. **Fibrocystic disease may be found in the other breast.**
  3. **Investigative procedures.** Further investigation is **not helpful.** Although a mammogram would show the cystic disease, it is not usually needed.
  4. **Management.** With **analgesia,** all symptoms should be gone within 1 week.
C. Fat necrosis
  1. **History. Sudden onset of inflammation and pain occurs without a history of trauma. This is benign, but may mimic cancer clinically.**
  2. **Physical examination. Local pain, erythema, and swelling** may be present.
  3. **Investigative procedures**
      a. The **mammogram** is characteristic.
      b. A **biopsy** to exclude malignancy may be needed.
  4. **Management**
      a. **Analgesia** may be needed.
      b. **If symptoms persist** longer than 1 week, a **biopsy** should be done.
D. Infection and abscess
  1. **History.** Most patients with breast infection or abscess are lactating or have an obvious cause of infection (e.g., bite). **If there is no history of a bite, penetrating trauma, or lactation, be very, very suspicious of underlying cancer.**
  2. **Physical examination.** Local or diffuse **pain** (usually more severe than that discussed in foregoing sections A., B., or C.), **swelling, marked erythema, fever,** or a combination of these symptoms may be present.
  3. **Investigative procedures.** A **complete blood cell count** (CBC) **with a differential leukocyte count and a culture of the abscess** should be done.
  4. **Management.** Because of the loose connective tissue in the breast, **infection can spread rapidly** and dissect along duct systems deep into the breast.
      a. **Minor infection, very localized, in a reliable patient. Local warm, moist compresses and oral antistaphylococcal** (the most common organism) **antibiotics** should be used. If the patient is **not distinctly better in 48 hours, open drainage** is required. Breast-feeding need not be stopped as this will help clear the infection. Alternatively, a woman may pump her breasts and discard the milk.
      b. **Severe infection, abscess, or deep infection. Nursing should be discontinued** and the **wound drained and cultured. Antibiotics** should be given IV for 2 to 3 days, then PO.
      c. **If the patient is not nursing and has no history of penetrating trauma, the chance of an underlying malignancy is so high that a biopsy is mandatory at the time of the incision and drainage.**
E. Mondor's disease (thrombophlebitis) is generally the result of trauma or surgery.
  1. **History.** The patient presents with a painful, localized area of the breast. She may have a positive history for a recent surgical event or may or may not recall having direct trauma to the area.
  2. **Physical examination** reveals a superficial phlebitis of the veins on the breast or chest wall. Skin retraction may be present as well.

3. **Investigative procedures.** This problem is generally recognized by inspection and palpation. In the event that there is skin retraction or more than a superficial palpable lesion, a **mammogram** should be ordered.
4. **Management** is centered on symptom relief.
   a. Analgesics either over-the-counter or prescription are useful.
   b. Warm, moist compresses at least qid for at least 10 minutes will provide comfort.
F. **Differential diagnosis.** The differentiation of hematoma, ruptured cyst, and fat necrosis may be impossible. Finding a bruise or other cysts in the breast is helpful. However, very often the exact cause is never found, and **therapy is expectant with analgesia** used for comfort.
   1. This should become **asymptomatic with 1 week to 10 days.**
   2. If **symptoms and signs persist, a mammogram or biopsy** should be considered.

III. **Diseases of the major ducts** are grouped by anatomic consideration and by the fact that the **primary presenting symptom is nipple discharge** in a nonlactating woman **or a change in character of the milk** in a lactating woman. When nursing is discontinued, prolactin levels return to normal in 2 to 4 weeks. All signs of lactation should be gone within 6 to 8 weeks.

   Some degree of nipple discharge is not unusual in healthy women. Up to 30% of women may have occasional clear or opalescent (milky) fluid spontaneously draining from the breast or produced by palpation. This is more often noted **just before the menses** when the breasts are enlarged. In many of these women, breast manipulation or suckling is an important part of their sexual activity. The amount of fluid is small and is unchanged over the years.

   In recent years, there has been an **increased incidence of galactorrhea in women who jog or run.** Two causes are cited for this increase: **friction between nipple and clothes,** which stimulates prolactin and **release of endorphins** from the hypothalamus, which, in turn, stimulates prolactin.

   There are **drugs that are associated with galactorrhea,** all by a common pathway of **increased prolactin.** They can be divided into the following three groups:

   Estrogens and drugs that increase estrogen
   Digitalis
   Marijuana
   Heroin
   Dopamine receptor blockers
   Phenothiazines
   Haloperidol
   Metoclopramide
   Isoniazid
   Central nervous system dopamine depleters
   Tricyclic antidepressants
   Reserpine
   Methyldopa
   Cimetidine
   Benzodiazepines

   A careful **history of sexual and athletic activity** must be obtained. It is important to determine that the fluid comes from many different ducts; that it has not changed in character; and that it goes away within a month when exercise, breast manipulation, or drug ingestion is halted on a trial basis. If the galactorrhea fits all these criteria, the activity that produces it may be resumed.

   A. **Galactorrhea** (other than foregoing)
      1. **History** reveals the following:
         a. **Recent onset of large or increased amounts of milk** being discharged spontaneously or on mild palpation.
         b. **No history of recent childbirth.**
         c. **No history of excessive breast stimulation.**
         d. **Milk from multiple ducts** of (usually) both nipples.

2. **Physical examination.** Galactorrhea is **present on palpation.**
3. **Investigative procedures.** As a screening test, determination of the **serum prolactin** level would be advisable. If elevated, there is reason for further evaluation, initially by checking the normality of **follicle-stimulating hormone** (FSH), **luteinizing hormone** (LH), **estradiol interrelationships,** and serum thyrotropin (thyroid-stimulating hormone [TSH]). **Evaluation of the hypophyseal-pituitary-ovarian axis** is often required and should be done by a qualified endocrinologist (medical or gynecologic).

B. **Galactocele**
   1. **History.** A galactocele appears as a **sudden development of a mass in the breast of a nursing woman.** It is usually **nontender.**
   2. **Physical examination** reveals a **localized area of swelling** that may be firm, soft, or cystic.
   3. **Investigative procedures. None are necessary,** except as in management.
   4. **Management.** A 10- to 20-ml syringe with a 22-gauge needle is used to **aspirate the milk.** If the mass **does not resolve or if it recurs** within 2 months, a **biopsy** should be considered.

C. **Duct ectasia (comedomastitis).** After many years of nursing, some or all of the major ducts become permanently distended and fluid collects and becomes inspissated (like cheese), which may result in a **chronic inflammatory reaction.**
   1. **History.** A multiparous woman in her 40s or older notes a **thick, white or discolored, cheesy material draining from the nipple(s).** There may be a history of local subareolar infection.
   2. **Physical examination**
      a. **Ropy induration** is found just under the areola, radiating outward a few centimeters.
      b. It is easy to **express thick cheesy fluid.** This symptom **may be segmental,** affecting only a few major ducts.
   3. **Investigative procedures. None are indicated.** A mammogram shows classic findings if one is obtained.
   4. **Management**
      a. **None is required if the lesion is not bothersome.**
      b. However, mammary duct ectasia is **often associated with repeated infections** around or under the areola. If so, **local excision** of the major duct system under the areola is indicated.

D. **Papilloma** is a **benign tumor (with a slight potential for malignant degeneration)** originating in the cells lining one of the major ducts. The finding of a **bloody discharge demands prompt investigation** to exclude the presence of cancer. All pathologic discharges require further evaluation by excision to rule out the possibility of cancer.
   1. **History.** Discharge of **clear, bloody, or discolored** (brown-green from old blood) **fluid** occurs **from a single duct opening on one breast.** The bloody discharge often frightens both the patient and the physician.
   2. **Physical examination.** On **milking the breast,** the fluid can be seen coming **from a single duct** on the nipple.
   3. **Investigative procedures**
      a. There is no need to send the fluid for cytologic diagnosis because this test has a low sensitivity and the results do not affect management (5).
      b. A **mammogram** may show the **classic finding of small ball-like lesions in a major duct,** but the lesions must measure 1 cm or more to be evident.
   4. **Management.** Treatment consists of **insertion of a polyethylene catheter or fine wire** into the draining duct, followed by **surgical exploration** of the duct and **removal** of the papilloma and duct.

IV. **Diseases of the lobule and lobular ducts** are grouped together for three reasons: (a) because of their **anatomic relationship,** (b) because they present a

common clinical picture of mastodynia and mass, and (c) because they are the **result of an endocrine imbalance in the breast.** There appears to be a relative excess of estrogen over progesterone. Some clinicians believe that a shortened luteal phase of the menstrual cycle causes deficiency of progesterone. The imbalance can also lead to an increase in prolactin. **Therapy is directed toward reversal of these hormonal imbalances.**

A. **Fibroadenoma** is the **most common benign tumor of the breast.** It occurs in young women, often teenagers. It is the result of **focal area(s) of increased sensitivity to estrogen.**

   1. **History.** The young patient accidentally discovers a **mass that is usually painless** but may be cyclically tender. One third of fibroadenomas spontaneously regress especially those less than 1 cm in size in adolescent and young adult women or those that occur during pregnancy. Fibroadenomas are not premalignant **nor** do they convert to cancer.

   2. **Physical examination.** The mass is small or large, **sharply circumscribed,** freely **movable, rubbery** in consistency, and usually **located in the upper quadrant.**

   3. **Investigative procedures. Aspiration of fluid** should be attempted. A fine-needle biopsy (FNA), core needle biopsy, or excisional biopsy may be diagnostic. An ultrasound can also confirm the diagnosis.

   4. **Management. Surgical excision** is diagnostic and curative and may be considered for cosmetic reasons or to allay anxiety. However, removal is not necessary.

B. **Mastodynia and fibrocystic disease. Mastodynia,** or **mastalgia,** simply means **painful breasts.** The majority of these patients are more concerned about the possibility of cancer than the pain itself. Classically, the pain is one of aching discomfort and **may radiate** to the neck, arm, back, or side. It usually is worse **2 to 4 days before menses** but can occur up to **2 weeks prior.** It can be unilateral **or** bilateral in its presentation. It can be associated with change in the size of the breast premenstrually, sometimes by one to two bra cup sizes. It can be associated with underlying fibrocystic disease. This association is so strong that to many doctors mastodynia has come to mean fibrocystic disease. However, we must remember that an **occasional patient with breast cancer presents** with a **painful mass** (see section V.F.). Fibrocystic disease is actually a misnomer because these changes are present to some degree in most women and do not represent true disease (5). However, fibrocystic disease is the commonly used terminology and for consistency, is used here.

There are a number of conditions that can cause pain in the chest wall with mastalgia. Some of these include, but are not limited to angina, cervical radiculopathy, costochondritis, arthritis, myalgia, neuralgia, pleurisy, rib fracture, and other trauma. It is important to keep the differential in mind while performing the physical examination and determining what investigative procedures are warranted.

These patients represent a **spectrum of symptoms and signs.** Some have such mild discomfort that it is apparent only on close questioning, and some are so incapacitated they cannot bear the touch of clothes, let alone a child or lover. In some the breasts feel normal; in others, the breast is dense, lumpy, and bumpy. The clinical approach must be gentle, understanding, and reassuring. It must be based on **knowledge of the disease process, which is caused by exaggeration and distortion of the normal cyclic menstrual changes secondary to estrogen-progesterone imbalance.** Symptoms improve after menopause, but may recur with estrogen replacement therapy. There is a **definite familial incidence.**

Classically, **fibrocystic disease** has been divided into **three types: fibrosis, adenosis,** and **cystic disease.** Most fibrocystic breasts contain varying mixtures of all three, although one may predominate. There is so much overlap, and the signs and symptoms are so similar that, clinically, they can be considered together.

The presence of fibrocystic disease increases the risk of breast cancer **only if there are findings of atypical hyperplasia.** If **atypical hyperplasia** is found, the **risk** is **five times** that of the general population. A positive family history of cancer increases the risk even further. There is **no increased risk of breast cancer** in women whose **biopsies show nonproliferative changes.**

1. **History.** The patient may complain of **mild to moderate pain and tenderness in the breasts premenstrually,** and may note lumpiness in the breast. It is most common in women between the ages of 35 and 45.

2. **Physical examination**
   a. **Multifocal, bilateral nodularity and thickening** may be present.
   b. **Individual cysts may be soft or hard** depending on the amount of fluid.

3. **Investigative procedures.** Fibrocystic disease becomes a prominent problem in the same age group at risk for breast cancer. Therefore, **the investigation becomes directed at excluding cancer as well as diagnosing the fibrocystic disease.**
   a. **Often the history and physical examination are enough** to make the diagnosis, and no other procedures are necessary **until a suspicious new mass arises.**
   b. **Mammograms** may be diagnostic, and since the disease peaks at the age when first mammograms should be done (see section V.C.), it is a reasonable tool to use. One must remember that mammography has a 15% error rate overall that is increased in women younger than the age of 35 and in the presence of dense nodular breast. Mammography should be done before aspiration or biopsy.
   c. **Aspiration.** When a patient develops a new mass or nodule in the breast, needle aspiration is an excellent first step. It can be done in the office. Many clinicians do not even use local anesthesia since the procedure involves only a single stick with a small needle.
      (1) After a thorough skin cleansing, the operator puts on gloves and **stabilizes the nodule firmly between two fingers and against the chest wall,** much like stabilizing an artery for a puncture.
      (2) A 21- or 22-gauge needle attached to a 10-mL **syringe is introduced into the nodule with a sharp penetrating motion** (again, like piercing an artery).
      (3) The stabilizing hand may then be moved to aid in **withdrawal of fluid.**
      (4) **If clear or milky fluid is drained and the mass goes away and stays away for 3 months,** two things have been accomplished:
         (a) **A diagnosis of cystic disease of the breast has been made.**
         (b) **Cancer has been ruled out.**
      (5) **If no fluid is obtained, excisional biopsy** is indicated.
      (6) **If the mass recurs, biopsy** is indicated.

4. **Management.** The treatment of fibrocystic disease depends on an **understanding of the hormonal imbalance** that produces it, **knowledge of the severity of the disease** in an individual patient, and an appreciation of the basic tenet to **alter the physiology as little as possible** to achieve a goal and avoid side effects.
   a. Many patients have **disease mild enough** to need only **reassurance or mild analgesia** premenstrually. They may also benefit from a more supportive bra and mild, warm, moist compresses.
   b. Those whose disease is a little more severe may benefit from **mild diuresis in the week before menses,** which counteracts the salt and water retention of hormones, relieves pressure in the breast, and decreases pain.

c. Other treatment modalities include dietary and vitamin supplementation.

   (1) **Obese women produce increased amounts of endogenous estrogen.** Women who are more than 30-lb (13.6-kg) overweight benefit from **weight reduction.**

   (2) Many clinicians believe that **removing caffeine and theophylline** from the diet ameliorates the disease, although the association has not been proven as yet. It is certainly worth a 4- to 6-month **trial of elimination of coffee, tea, cola drinks, and chocolate** from the diet. There is no clear understanding of how the methylxanthines cause increased symptoms, but they are regulators of cyclic adenosine monophosphate (AMP), which may be the mediator.

d. **Thiamine,** 50 to 100 mg/day, is proposed by some clinicians. It is involved in the **detoxification of estrogen,** so theoretically it would make sense that it would decrease available endogenous estrogen. Unfortunately, there are **no good clinical trials to validate the claims of benefit.**

e. **Vitamin E,** 400 units a day, has been advocated by many providers for fibrocystic disease however, conclusive proof of its benefit has not been established.

f. Women who wish to use herbal methods may try evening primrose oil 1,000 mg. qd.

g. **Hormones.** Since the disease is caused by a relative increase of estrogen to progesterone (or increase in the breasts' sensitivity to normal endogenous levels of estrogen) and a resultant increased activity of prolactin, **any decrease in estrogen or increase in progesterone will help.** There are several ways to accomplish this regulation.

   (1) **Cyclic hormones.** The **low-estrogen, high-progesterone oral contraceptives** have been very helpful.

      (a) After 3 to 4 months, a **significant number of patients note improvement** in symptoms. There are reports in the literature of improvement in the physical and mammographic findings.

      (b) **Side effects are well known and minor.**

      (c) The oral contraceptives **do not cause breast cancer.**

   (2) **Progesterone.** Increasing progesterone during the week before the menstrual period will accomplish the same results as in (1). **Side effects** of progesterone are well known and minor. Of the two following methods, one method may be more convenient, the other more sensuous, and either will work.

      (a) Medroxyprogesterone (Provera) can be given in **doses of 5 to 10 mg/day PO** for 10 days before the onset of menses.

      (b) In Europe, **progesterone-rich cream is massaged into the breasts daily for the week before the period,** with about 5 mg progesterone being absorbed.

   (3) Patients with **subclinical hypothyroidism** have increased amounts of thyroid-releasing hormone (TRH) as well as increased amounts of TSH. Increased TRH causes increased prolactin secretion. In these patients, **thyroid function tests are normal but TSH levels are increased.** If TSH is elevated, a **3- to 4-month trial of thyroid replacement** (0.15 to 0.20 mg/day levothyroxine [Synthroid] or its equivalent) may be helpful.

   (4) **Androgen.** It is possible to counteract estrogen effects using androgens, but the **side effects are severe.**

      (a) Danazol is currently the only Food and Drug Administration (FDA) approved therapy for severe mastalgia. It is 80% effective. It **decreases both prolactin secretion and estrogen secretion.** The drug is given in doses of 200 mg bid. Once the desired effect is obtained, 50 to 100 mg/day may be used as maintenance.

   (b) The side effects may include **weight gain** (4–6 lb), **amenorrhea,** and hot flashes, which occur in most patients. Acne and masculinization have also been reported to occur.

   (c) The results are dramatic. Symptomatic relief may occur in 1 to 2 weeks. Within 4 to 6 months, there is a **marked decrease in symptoms and signs of disease and a dramatic improvement in mammographic evidence of disease.** The drug can be discontinued after 6 to 8 months of use since **improvement persists for months to years.**

   (d) The drug has **not been in use long enough to know whether there is a long-term effect on incidence of cancer** in these patients.

   (e) Because of the side effects and the altered physiology, this drug should be **reserved for only the most severely affected patients.**

(5) **Tamoxifen** is an **antiestrogen used widely in the treatment of breast cancer.**

   (a) This drug **counteracts estrogen.** Studies have shown benefit in fibrocystic disease similar to that of danazol.

   (b) The dosage is 10 mg PO bid for 3 to 4 months, and may be repeated as necessary.

   (c) The side effects include amenorrhea, hot flashes, and a slightly increased risk of thromboembolic disease, but the incidence of side effects is significantly lower than for danazol.

   (d) There should be no concern about endometrial cancer since the duration of treatment is short.

(6) **Prolactin suppression. Bromocriptine** is a drug that inhibits prolactin. It is a long-acting dopaminergic drug. Although effective, it has **severe side effects** of nausea, vomiting, and postural hypotension and **cannot be recommended for routine use.**

h. **Surgery**

(1) Mastodynia and fibrocystic disease cannot be treated by **subcutaneous mastectomy with or without implants.** However, there are occasional patients whose disease is so severe, who require so many biopsies for new masses, and whose risk of malignancy is so high because of the atypical hyperplasia, that drastic measures are worth considering. Such a step should be **undertaken only after consultation with medical or surgical oncologists and after much soul-searching by the patient and her physician(s).**

(2) Since menopause results in amelioration of symptoms, an **oophrectomy could also be considered as a drastic measure.** Symptoms would remit over several months, but the risk of malignancy, if atypical hyperplasia is present in the breast, would not decrease for years, if ever.

V. **Breast cancer.** Although benign breast disease takes its toll in discomfort, worry, and cost, breast cancer takes its toll in lives. It is the **most common cancer** of women in the United States. There were predicted to be 182,000 new cases in the year 2000 with 40,800 deaths from breast cancer. It affects 12% of women, one in nine women by the age of 95, and over 50% are cured. **Of those who are cured of their disease, most (if not all) are cured by the initial therapy.** Once breast cancer recurs, only a rare exceptional patient is rendered free of disease. Therefore, the number who are cured by the primary therapy must be increased, whether it be surgery, radiation, or a combination. This number can be increased by **discovering tumors when they are small and before they have spread to the axillary nodes,** which is the initial manifestation of metastatic disease. We can accomplish this by **identification of patients at high risk, patient education, and improved use of detection methods.**

A. **Risk.** Although the cause of breast cancer in humans is unknown, several things that increase the risk of disease are known. However, only 25% of breast cancer occurs in defined risk groups and only 5% of breast cancer is genetic. Although it does occur in women under the age of 30, it is uncommon. There is a sharp rise in incidence in women older than the age of 50.

1. **Major risk factors**
   a. **History of breast cancer.** Depending on the type of cancer, the chance of developing cancer in the opposite breast varies from 10% to 50%, with an overall incidence of 20%.
   b. **Family history.** The gene that is related to familial breast cancer may be inherited from either parent. The closer the relative with cancer and the more aggressive her cancer, the greater the risk. A mother or sister with breast cancer is a distinct threat and increases the risk two to three times. A patient whose mother had bilateral cancers before menopause may have a 40% chance of developing the disease.
   c. **The presence of fibrocystic disease with atypical hyperplastic changes increases the risk to 16% to 33%.**

2. **Minor risk factors**
   a. **Prolonged reproductive life.** A patient who had early menarche and late menopause is at increased risk.
   b. **Nulliparity.**
   c. **Late age at first birth (older than 25!).** For an early pregnancy to exert a protective effect, it must be a term pregnancy.
   d. **Prolonged use of postmenopausal estrogen therapy** is more of a risk if the patient has any of the major risk factors. This risk should not deter use of postmenopausal estrogen since the beneficial effects of estrogen usually outweigh the risk.
   e. There is **no firm proof as yet that diet, increased fat intake in particular, is a risk factor.** However, many clinicians believe it is. Excessive alcohol consumption before the age of 30 is being evaluated as a risk factor, but studies have been inconsistent.

B. **Patient education**
1. All women should be **aware of the risk** of breast cancer **and its common clinical sign of a painless mass or a bloody nipple discharge.**
2. All women should be taught **breast self-examination** (BSE). Some studies show that the most effective teacher of BSE is the physician, next is the nonphysician practitioner, third is the office nurse, and last (but still effective!) is the nonmedical instructor. All cancers are not detected by mammogram; hence, **BSE is an important screening tool.**
   a. **The American Cancer Society** (ACS) **has programs of instruction in BSE,** which are a major community resource.
   b. BSE is best taught as **part of the routine physical examination,** after the practitioner has examined the breast thoroughly and can attest to its normality. It should be **reinforced on a regular basis.**
   c. **Ideal technique.** BSE should be done **just after the menstrual period,** when breasts are smallest and least tender.
      (1) The patient should inspect the breast **in front of a mirror looking for lumps, dimples, and retraction of the skin.**
      (2) Then, the patient should lie on a bed. **A small pillow or folded towel should be placed under the left shoulder, and the left arm is placed over the head.** This position arches the chest wall and spreads the breast out.

(3) The patient takes the **flat part of the fingers of the right hand and massages the left breast tissue between the fingers and the chest wall.** The breast is imagined as a clock. **The patient should palpate** at each hour around the outer edge of the breast. **The patient repeats around the inner circle of the breast and under the nipple-areola area.** The patient is feeling for nodules not present on the last month's examination.

(4) The process is repeated for the right breast.

(5) The process is repeated while standing **in the shower or sitting in the bathtub,** while the hands and breasts are soapy and slippery.

    d. Adequate technique. The ideal technique (see section c.) takes only a few minutes, but that may be too much for some patients. Rather than skip the process, they may lie flat in bed, raise one arm, and perform the technique described in foregoing section c.(3).

C. Screening techniques all involve **some kind of image of the breast.** At the present time, thermography and ultrasound have not been developed to the point that they are accurate or reliable for general use. Thermography may have as much as a 30% positive or negative error.

Currently, the **only reliable screening method is mammography.** New techniques of film screen mammography have the dose of radiation down to 50 mrad (compare 0.1–0.5 rad per chest x-ray study). This dosage is safe enough that **fear of inducing cancer by radiation exposure has been eliminated almost entirely.** In discussing mammography, one must differentiate carefully its **two uses.**

1. **Screening is looking for cancer in a normal-appearing breast.** The technique of mammography is reliable, with a false-negative rate of 15%.

2. **Diagnosis.** A mammogram is **done when a lump is found in the breast.** In this instance, the decision track of evaluating the lump is made regardless of the mammographic findings. The test is used to screen the rest of the breast and the opposite one. In a young patient with dense breasts and fibrocystic disease, the error rate may be as high as 30% (5).

D. History. Despite the widespread use of screening mammography, **the large majority of breast cancer is found by the women themselves.** The typical story is that of a painless lump found while bathing. Much less often, there is **history of skin change or dimpling, nipple retraction, or bloody nipple discharge.**

1. The history to be elicited includes **menstrual and reproductive history, hormonal uses, family history of cancer, history of mastalgia, and prior masses.**

2. Of course, a **general review of systems should be obtained** for pain and change in function.

E. Physical examination. The **classic finding** is that of a 2- to 5-cm, firm but not rock-hard, mass in the upper outer quadrant. The **actual examination findings may vary** from an area of soft ill-defined thickening to actual skin erosion and ulceration. Thorough examination includes the following:

1. **Examination of the mass itself with notation of skin or muscle fixation.**

2. **A careful examination of supraclavicular and axillary nodes, bilaterally.**

3. **Examination of the skin on the chest wall** for cutaneous lesions, often best felt by running the flat of the hand across the skin.

4. **Liver size.**

5. **Above all, the patient should be listened to. If she feels a mass and the clinician does not, SHE IS RIGHT!**

F. **Investigative procedures depend on the degree of suspicion of malignancy. If suspicion is low** and the plan is for observation and re-examination in 1 month, then **no further investigation** is needed. **If the suspicion of malignancy is high,** the following procedures should be done:

   1. **Mammography should be done to assess the mass and the rest of the breast. A negative mammogram should not fool the clinician.** The error rate should be thought of. **Some institutions set a minimum age of 30 for mammography.** About 0.5% of breast cancers occur under the age of 30. Ultrasonography can be helpful. If suspicion is high, a personal request to the radiologist (or through an oncologist) can usually circumvent the administrative block. If not, the clinician should **not be deterred: The mass should be biopsied even without the mammogram.**

   2. **No scans need be done until the diagnosis of malignancy is established, and then only if an advanced stage is diagnosed.**

   3. If the practitioner feels competent, **needle aspiration should be attempted** (see section IV.B.4.c.). **Otherwise, a surgical referral** should be made.

G. **Comment.** It is essential to have **special concern for the patient at this time. Her anxiety is high, as is that of her friends and family. Reassurance is critical.** Only one in eight breast biopsies is positive for malignancy.

VI. **Protocols**

A. **Screening for breast disease. Many groups, including the ACS, the American Medical Association (AMA), and the National Cancer Institute (NCI), have issued guidelines for screening.**

   1. The recommendations for which there is general agreement include the following:

     a. **BSE for all women older than 20.**

     b. **Physical examination every 3 years** between the ages of 20 and 40 and yearly thereafter.

     c. **Mammography** yearly in women older than the age of 50.

   2. **Areas of controversy are:**

     a. **Women between the ages of 40 and 50** Many groups, including the ACS continue to recommend mammograms every 1 to 2 years for women between the ages of 40 to 50. Other groups, including the NCI, no longer endorse this recommendation. The studies in this age group have failed to conclusively show any reduction in mortality from screening. Conversely, they have also failed to show that there is no benefit. The recommendations should be individualized based on the patient's risk.

     b. **Baseline mammography. Most groups no longer recommend baseline mammograms for women from 35 to 40. However, some groups continue to recommend it.**

     c. The ACS points out that these **recommendations emphasize the role of the personal physician** in determining mammography. This may be so, but they also **place the personal physician right in the middle of a major controversy without guidelines.**

B. **Approach to the patient with a new mass in the breast**

   1. **A thorough history and physical examination** must be done.

   2. If the mass is **not suspicious** (soft discrete mass but similar to the rest of breast), the practitioner may **watch the mass through one menstrual cycle.**

   3. **If the mass persists**

     a. **Fine-needle aspiration** must be done. If fluid is obtained and the mass disappears and does not recur in 3 months, it may be assumed to have been a benign cyst. The fluid need not be sent for pathologic workup because it is seldom of help.

  b. If there is a **residual mass** after the aspiration or if the mass is **solid** (no fluid obtained), a **biopsy** must be done. Fine-needle biopsy is acceptable if cytopathology expertise is available. Otherwise, core needle or excisional biopsy is recommended.
  c. Rapidly recurring cysts require excisional biopsy.
  d. The mammogram should be ordered if not current.

References

1. Belchetz PE. Hormonal treatment of postmenopausal women. *N Engl J Med* 1994;330:1062.
2. Donegan WL. Evaluation of a palpable breast mass. *N Engl J Med* 1992;327:937.
3. DuPont MD, Page DL. Risk factors for breast cancer in women with proliferative breast disease. *N Engl J Med* 1985;312:146.
4. Hughes LE, Mansel RE, Webster DJT, eds. *Benign disorders and diseases of the breast.* London: Bailliere Tindall, 1989.
5. O'Grady LF, Lindfors KK, Rippon MB, et al., eds. *A practical approach to breast disease.* Boston: Little, Brown, 1995.
6. Vorherr H. Fibrocystic breast disease: pathobiology, pathomorphology, clinical picture, and management. *Am J Obstet Gynecol* 1986;154:161.
7. Greenlee RT, Murray T, Bolden S, et al. Cancer statistics, 2000. *CA Cancer Clin* 200;50;7–33.
8. Stomper PC, Gelman RS, Meyer JE, et al. New England Mammography Survey 1988: public misconceptions of breast cancer incidence. *Breast Disease* 1990;9.
9. Love SM, Gelman RS, Silen W. Sounding board. Fibrocystic "disease" of the breast—a nondisease? *N Engl J Med* 1982;307:1010–1014.
10. Mansel RE, Hughes LE. Breast pain and nodularity. In: Hughes LE, Mansel RE, Webster DJT, eds. *Benign disorders of the breast: concepts of clinical management.* London: WB Saunders, 2000:95–121.
11. Pye JK, Mansel RE, Hughes LE. Clinical experience of drug treatments for mastalgia. *Lancet* 1985;2:373–377.
12. Rohan TE, Cook MG, McMichael. Methylxanthines and benign proliferative epithelial disorders of the breast in women. *Int J Epidemiol* 1989;18:626–633.
13. Allen SS, Froberg DC. The effect of increased caffeine consumption on benign proliferative breast disease: a randomized clinical trial. *Surgery* 1986;101:720–730.
14. London RS, Sundaram GS, Murphy L, et al. The effect of vitamin E on mammary dysplasia: a double-blind study. *Obstetrics Gynecology* 1985;65:104–106.
15. Holland PA, Gately CA. Drug therapy of mastalgia: what are the options? *Drugs* 1994;48:709–716.
16. Jackson VP. The current role of ultrasonography in breast imaging. *Radiol Clin North Am* 1995;33:1661–1170.
17. Hughes LE. Cysts of the breast. In: Hughes LE, Mansel RE, Webster DJT, eds. *Benign disorders and diseases of the breast: concepts and clinical management.* London: WB Saunders, 200:123–135.
18. Watt-Boolson S, Ryegaard R, Blichert-Toft M. Primary periareolar abscess in the nonlactating breast: risk of recurrence. *Am J Surg* 1987;153:571–573.
19. Leitch AM, Dodd GD, Costanza M, et al. American Cancer society guidelines for the early detection of breast cancer: update 1997. *CA Cancer J Clin* 1997;47:150–153.
20. Sattin RW, Rubin GL, Webster LA, et al. Family history and the risk of breast cancer. *JAMA* 1985;253:1908–1913.
21. Dupont WD, Page DL. Breast cancer risk with proliferative disease, age at first birth, and a family history of breast cancer. *Am J Epidemiol* 1987:125:769–779.
22. Chu KC, Smart CR, Tarone RE. Analysis of breast cancer mortality and stage distribution by age for the health insurance plan clinical trial. *J Natl Cancer Inst* 1988;80:1125–1132.

10. PREMENSTRUAL SYNDROME

Janet M. Walker

Premenstrual syndrome (PMS) is a diverse constellation of cyclic physical and emotional symptoms, occurring monthly during the luteal phase of the menstrual cycle (ovulation to menstruation). This phase is followed by a symptom-free period of at least 1 week, beginning after the onset of menses. Of all the symptoms, the emotional and behavioral symptoms are the most devastating. In an attempt to define and treat the psychological symptoms, the American Psychiatric Association has described premenstrual dysphoric disorder (PMDD). PMDD requires the presence of at least one of 4 core symptoms (irritability, dysphoria, labile mood, tension) and at least 5 of 11 other symptoms. Symptoms must markedly impair functioning and interfere with normal activities.

I. **Incidence.** It has been reported that 70% to 90% of the female population will admit to recurrent menstrual problems. Between 20% and 40% report some degree of temporary mental and physical dysfunction and 2% to 5% may be incapacitated.

   PMS is cross-cultural and affects women of all races, socioeconomic status, and professions. There may be an **increased incidence** with **age** and **major life stresses.** Demographic data are contradictory concerning genetic contribution, effects of number of pregnancies, and educational level. Women with severe PMS may have a lifetime increased incidence of affective disorders.

II. **Etiology.** Evidence supports the **association** of PMS with **abnormal neurotransmitter response to normal ovarian function.** Recent research has confirmed that women with PMS have **normal levels** of both **estrogen** and **progesterone,** are **not vitamin** or **mineral deficient,** have **normal prolactin** and **thyroid levels,** and are **euglycemic.** Of the possible mediators of ovarian steroid action in the central nervous system, serotonin, gamma-amino butyric acid (GABA) receptors, and beta-endorphins are the best studied.

   A. **Serotonin.** The association of serotonin with **mood** and **appetite disturbances** is **well documented,** and the sex steroidal hormones do modulate serotonergic activity. Women with PMS have significantly **lower serotonin levels** during the **luteal phase,** as measured in peripheral blood, compared with normal controls. This may be due to impaired postsynaptic serotonergic response in PMS patients. Compounds that increase serotonin levels have been shown to decrease symptoms of PMS.

   B. **Beta-endorphin** levels **may be lower** in PMS patients during both the periovulatory and premenstrual phases of the menstrual cycle. Substances that increase beta-endorphins improve PMS symptoms.

   C. The **GABA receptors,** associated with control of anxiety, are stimulated by progesterone, which **may** be a **mechanism** in the modulation of **anxiety** in PMS.

III. **History.** PMS is a **polysymptomatic disorder** and the syndrome may last anywhere from 3 to 21 days. Symptoms do not all begin on the same day nor will women have the same symptoms each month or throughout their lives. The following is a partial list of symptoms:

   A. **Behavioral symptoms:** depression, irritability, tension, lethargy, mood swings, anger, uncontrolled crying, aggression, panic attacks, anxiety, social withdrawal, change in memory or concentration, change in libido, poor impulse control.

   B. **Physical symptoms**
      1. Neurologic: migraines and other headaches, syncope, vertigo.
      2. Metabolic: breast tenderness, edema.
      3. Cardiovascular: palpitations, ectopic beats, paroxysmal tachycardia.

      4. Gastrointestinal: nausea, abdominal bloating, flatulence, constipation, diarrhea.
      5. Urinary: oliguria, urethritis, cystitis, enuresis, urinary retention.
      6. Dermatologic: acne, urticaria.
      7. Musculoskeletal: pain and swelling of the joints and muscles.
  C. Chronic medical problems, such as diabetes and asthma, as well as psychological disorders may worsen premenstrually, a condition termed **premenstrual magnification.**

IV. Physical examination. A complete physical examination including a pelvic examination is necessary to rule out other causes such as ovarian cysts, fibroids, pelvic inflammatory disease, endometriosis, and thyroid disease. It is also important to perform a **complete mental status examination to rule out psychopathology.** There are no characteristic physical findings of PMS.

V. Investigative procedures. The **diagnosis** of PMS **depends** on the temporal **relationship** of **psychological** and **somatic symptoms with menstruation** rather than the presence of symptoms alone. It is the recurring symptoms during the luteal phase followed by a symptom-free time that defines PMS. A thorough medical, sexual, and psychological history as well as physical examination and laboratory studies are necessary to identify PMS and to rule out other disorders.

  A. Menstrual chart. Evaluation should include a detailed diary of symptoms charted against the menstrual cycle (Fig. 10.1).
      1. The **chart** should show the **length** of the menstrual cycle, **duration** of bleeding, and **regularity or irregularity** of menstruation. By definition, PMS occurs only during ovulatory cycles.
      2. **Each symptom** along **with** its **severity** can be charted each day. The patient should be sure to **include eating patterns** if they vary with the cycle.
      3. A **full three cycles** are optimal for evaluation.
      4. **Posthysterectomy** patients **may** still **experience** PMS if they **retained** their **ovaries,** so their 3-month chart will show the same characteristic pattern.
  B. Laboratory tests should be ordered as indicated by history and/or examination to rule out other disease as a source of the patient's symptoms.

VI. Management. Since PMS represents an abnormal response to the physiologic ovulatory cycle, management can be directed to:
- Altering the cycle.
- Changing the body's response to the cycle.
- Treating the symptoms themselves.

  A. Self-help steps
      1. Education is one of the most important components in the management of PMS.
        a. Knowledge of the menstrual cycle, as well as female anatomy and physiology can aid in understanding this disorder.
        b. It is also helpful to read the available literature on PMS.
        c. Keeping a menstrual chart helps a woman achieve awareness of her menstrual cycle as well as her premenstrual symptoms.
      2. Exercise. Regular aerobic exercise at least three or four times per week, continuing through the premenstrual phase, may reduce symptoms of PMS. This is especially true of the physical symptoms including breast tenderness, fluid retention, and abdominal cramping. Exercise has been shown to reduce stress and anxiety, increasing one's sense of well-being.
      3. Stress management. Women should be encouraged to reduce the demands that they make on themselves and on others. Relaxation, visualization, and hypnosis are some other important methods of stress reduction. Supportive psychotherapy and reflexology may also be beneficial (15).
      4. Diet and nutrition improves one's overall feeling of health and may be helpful with PMS. **Recommended dietary changes** include **increasing**

Patient Name _____   MR# _____

Rating Scale: 0 — No symptoms
1 — Mild symptoms, does not interfere with daily activities
2 — Moderate, some interference with daily activities
3 — Severe, significant interference with work, home, or interpersonal relationships

DAY OF CYCLE	1	2	3	4	5	6	7	8	9	10	11	12	13	14	15	16	17	18	19	20	21	22	23	24	25	26	27	28	29	30	31	32	33	34	35
DATE																																			
WEIGHT																																			
MENSES																																			
SYMPTOMS																																			
MEDICATIONS																																			
NOTES																																			

FIG. 10.1. Sample menstrual chart with rating scale. The patient should record information for each day of her menstrual cycle and for three consecutive cycles to facilitate the diagnosis of premenstrual syndrome.

complex carbohydrates and **green vegetables** and **decreasing** simple **sugars, fats,** and **processed foods.** Unfortunately, specific studies of the effect of diet on PMS have not demonstrated a benefit, with the exception of **eliminating caffeine,** which helps **reduce breast tenderness** and **low salt/low fat diet,** which improves fluid retention.

B. **Food supplements**

1. **Vitamin B6.** Pyridoxine is a coenzyme in the biosynthesis of serotonin and dopamine, probable mediators of PMS. Some studies have shown a benefit with vitamin B6 in doses well above the recommended daily allowance (RDA), starting at 25 mg twice daily and increasing to 100 mg per day. Higher doses to 300 mg have been studied but carry a significant **risk** of **peripheral neuropathy.**

2. **Vitamin E** in doses of 400 to 600 IU/day has, in some studies, alleviated the symptom of breast tenderness associated with PMS.

3. **Calcium** improves symptoms of water retention, abdominal cramps, and mood changes in doses of 1,000 mg/day. One study has also shown improvement with food cravings.

4. **Magnesium** supplementation, 300 to 500 mg daily during the luteal phase, has been shown to improve symptoms of mood changes and fluid retention in small randomized crossover trials.

5. There are now many PMS formulae that **combine vitamins** and **mineral supplements.** Of these only a few, Lurline PMS tablets and Optivite have been studied and shown to have some efficacy.

6. The use of **cis-linoleic acid (evening primrose oil),** 1,500 mg bid, is an old remedy for depression and anxiety symptoms of PMS. Randomized, double-blind trials have been unable to substantiate its efficacy.

C. **Drug therapy.** Drug therapy can be tailored to alleviate specific symptoms or to obliterate the menstrual cycle itself.

1. **Oral contraceptive pills (OCPs)** are often used as a first-line treatment for premenstrual symptoms but few studies have substantiated efficacy except with some physical symptoms such as cramps and bloating.

   a. Monophasic preparations may be more effective than triphasic combinations.

   b. Patients should be warned that psychological symptoms could worsen when taking OCPs.

2. In the past, **progesterone** was widely used for PMS, but well designed studies do **not demonstrate** efficacy. The general popularity of using progesterone for PMS may be due to its mildly sedative properties.

   a. Synthetic progestins (medroxyprogesterone acetate, norethindrone) are used as contraceptives or to regulate menstrual flow.

   b. In some women, medroxyprogesterone acetate (Depo-Provera) eliminates the menstrual cycle and can in this way improve some of the physical symptoms of PMS.

   c. Progestins should be used with caution in women with PMS because they can exacerbate psychological symptoms, especially anxiety and depression.

3. **Gonadotropin releasing hormone (GnRH) agonists** obliterate the menstrual cycle and are therefore very effective in controlling symptoms of PMS. Randomized trials have demonstrated significant improvement in PMS symptoms; however, **psychological symptoms** are **not** as **consistently improved** as physical symptoms.

   a. These medications are expensive and **must be used with add-back estrogen and progesterone to reduce menopausal side effects such as osteoporosis.**

   b. Use of GnRH agonists without add-back hormonal replacement must be limited to less than 6 months.

      (1) Leuprolide acetate, 3.75 mg IM monthly **OR** 11.25 mg q 3 months **OR**

      (2) Goserelin, 3.6 mg SQ implant monthly, **OR**

      (3) Nafarelin, 200 g bid intranasally, are the most commonly used preparations.

  4. Selective serotonin reuptake inhibitors (SSRIs) are highly effective in the treatment of severe PMS. Multiple controlled double-blind studies have shown efficacy, with resolution of symptoms nearly immediately and in smaller doses than is normally used for depression.

    a. Fluoxetine has been studied in the most detail and is effective in doses as small as 5 mg and up to 20 mg po qd. Efficacy has been shown with a daily dose throughout the month and also with treatment only during the luteal phase of the menstrual cycle (i.e., with symptoms). Although generally well tolerated, side effects include insomnia, anxiety, gastrointestinal disturbances, and sexual dysfunction.

    b. Paroxetine, 5 to 30 mg/day, and sertraline, 25 to 150 mg/day, have not been as extensively studied as fluoxetine for PMS but are **probably equally** as **effective.**

  5. Clomipramine, a **tricyclic antidepressant** with serotonin and noradrenaline reuptake inhibiting properties, has been successfully used to treat severe psychological symptoms of PMS.

    a. Effective doses are 25 to 75 mg PO qd during the luteal phase of the menstrual cycle.

    b. Side effects including fatigue, weight gain, nausea, seizures, and dry mouth may limit its usefulness.

  6. Anxiolytics

    a. Buspirone may be useful in patients with **predominant** symptoms of **anxiety** and it is neither sedating nor habit forming. The **initial** dosage is 5 mg tid, gradually increasing to cessation of symptoms with a **maximum** dose of 60 mg/day.

    b. Alprazolam controls anxiety and irritability if given during the symptomatic period.

      (1) However, its use is associated with sedation, tolerance, and dependence and it should be used cautiously.

      (2) Dosage is 0.25 mg tid, increasing to a total daily dose of 4 mg. At the beginning of menses, the dose should be decreased by 25% each day.

  7. Diuretics. Abdominal bloating and water retention are some of the most common symptoms of PMS. Despite this, actual weight gain and change in total body water have not been well demonstrated in studies. In this light, diuretics should be used **with caution.** Spironolactone, 25 mg tid or qid, during the luteal phase of the menstrual cycle may be effective for abdominal bloating and also may improve irritability, depression, and food cravings.

  8. Danazol, a synthetic androgen, is effective in suppressing symptoms of PMS. However, its side effects, including weight gain and virilization may be unacceptable to patients.

D. Surgery. Bilateral oophorectomy is rarely indicated in PMS treatment and should be reserved only for patients with severe PMS and after failure of all conservative measures. Complete resolution should be demonstrated with GnRH agonist suppression prior to undertaking surgery. Consideration should also be made of the number of years left until menopause.

References

1. Backstrom T. Neuroendocrinology of premenstrual syndrome. *Clin Obstet Gynecol* 1992;35:612.
2. Barnard ND, et al. Diet and sex-hormone binding globulin, dysmenorrhea, and premenstrual symptoms. *Obstet Gynecol* 2000;95:245–250.
3. Chuong CJ. Periovulatory B-endorphin levels in premenstrual syndrome. *Obstet Gynecol* 1994;83:755.
4. Collins A, et al. Essential fatty acids in the treatment of premenstrual syndrome. *Obstet Gynecol* 1993;81:93–98.

5. Dennerstein L, et al. Menstrual cycle hormonal profiles of women with and without premenstrual syndrome. *J Psychosom Obstet Gynecol* 1993;14:259.
6. *Diagnostic and statistical manual of mental disorders,* 4th ed. Washington, DC: American Psychiatric Association, 1994.
7. Facchinetti F, et al. Oral magnesium successfully relieves premenstrual mood changes. *Obstet Gynecol* 1991;78:177–181.
8. Freeman E, et al. Ineffectiveness of progesterone suppository treatment for premenstrual syndrome. *JAMA* 1990;264:349–353.
9. Halbreich U, Smoller JW. Intermittent luteal phase sertraline treatment of dysphoric premenstrual syndrome. *J Clin Psychiatry* 1997;58:399–402.
10. Halbreich U, Tworek H. Altered serotonergic activity in women with dysphoric premenstrual syndromes. *Int J Psychiatry Med* 1993;23:1.
11. Helvacioglu A, et al. Premenstrual syndrome and related hormonal changes: long-acting gonadotropin releasing hormone agonist treatment. *J Reprod Med* 1993; 38:864.
12. Johnson S. Premenstrual syndrome therapy. *Clin Obstet Gynecol* 1998;41:405–421.
13. Korzedwa M, Steiner M. Assessment and treatment of premenstrual syndromes. *Primary Care Update OB/GYN* 1999;6(5):153–162.
14. Kouri E, Halbreich V. State and trait serotonergic abnormalities in women with dysphoric premenstrual syndromes. *Psychopharmacology Bull* 1997;33:767–770.
15. Ling F, et al., eds. *Premenstrual syndrome and PMDD: scope, diagnosis, and treatment.* APGO Educational Series on Women's Health Issues, 1998:1–24.
16. London RS, Bradley L, Chiamore NY. Effect of a nutritional supplement on premenstrual symptomatology in women with premenstrual syndrome: a double-blind longitudinal study. *J Am Coll Nutr* 1991;10:494–499.
17. Mortola J. Applications of gonadotropin-releasing hormone analogues in the treatment of premenstrual syndrome. *Clin Obstet Gynecol* 1993;36:753.
18. Penland JG, Johnson PE. Dietary calcium and manganese effects on menstrual cycle symptoms. *Am J Obstet Gynecol* 1993;168:1417.
19. Romano S, et al. The role of fluoxetine in the treatment of premenstrual dysphoric disorder. *Clin Therapeutics* 1999;21(4):615–637.
20. Schmidt PJ, et al. Thyroid function on women with premenstrual syndrome. *J Clin Endocrinol Metab* 1993;76:671.
21. Steiner M, et al. Intermittent fluoxetine dosing in the treatment of women with premenstrual dysphoria. *Psychopharmacol Bull* 1997;33:585.
22. Steiner M, et al. Fluoxetine in the treatment of premenstrual dysphoria. *N Engl J Med* 1995;323:1529–1534.
23. Stewart A. Clinical and biochemical effects of nutritional supplementation on the premenstrual syndrome. *Reprod Med* 1987;32:435–441.
24. Sunblad C, et al. A naturalistic study of paroxetine in premenstrual syndrome: efficacy and side-effects during ten cycles of treatment. *Neuropsychopharmacol* 1997;7:201–206.
25. Sunblad C, et al. Clomipramine administered during the luteal phase reduces the symptoms of premenstrual syndrome: a placebo-controlled trial. *Neuropsychopharmacol* 1993;9:133.
26. Thys-Jacobs S, et al. Calcium carbonate and the premenstrual syndrome: effects on premenstrual and menstrual symptoms. Premenstrual Syndrome Study Group. *Am J Obstet Gynecol* 1998;179:444–452.
27. Wood SH, et al. Treatment of premenstrual syndrome with fluoxetine: a double-blind, placebo-controlled, crossover study. *Obstet Gynecol* 1992;80:339.
28. Wyatt KM, et al. Efficacy of vitamin B6 in the treatment of premenstrual syndrome: systematic review. *BMJ* 1999;318:1375–1381.
29. Yonkers KA, et al. Paroxetine as a treatment for premenstrual dysphoric disorder. *J Clin Psychopharmacol* 1996;16:3–8.
30. Yonkers DA, et al. Symptomatic improvement of PMDD with sertraline treatment: a randomized controlled trial. *JAMA* 1997;278:983–988.

11. AMENORRHEA

Condessa M. Curley

Disorders of menstruation are among the most common reasons women seek medical attention. **Amenorrhea** is the absence or cessation of menstrual bleeding. The etiology of amenorrhea can be **physiologic** as occurs during childhood, pregnancy, lactation, and after menopause **or** it can be a manifestation of a **variety of pathophysiologic disorders.** Amenorrhea has been categorized as primary or secondary.

- **Primary amenorrhea** is the failure of menarche by age 16, regardless of the presence or absence of secondary sex characteristics (2,7,17,19,30).
- **Secondary amenorrhea** is the failure of menstruation for 6 months in a woman with previous periodic menses or the absence of menses for 12 months in a woman with a history of prior oligomenorrhea (bleeding at intervals of greater than 40 days that is usually irregular) (2,7,17,19,30).

Primary and secondary amenorrhea are useful terms to describe the timing of menstrual cycle interruption but offer minimal information on the underlying etiology, management, or prognosis of menstrual cycle interruptions. Strict adherence to the criteria discussed previously may result in inappropriate management of individual cases. Therefore any patient fulfilling the following criteria should be evaluated as having the clinical symptom of amenorrhea.

1. A woman who has been menstruating **and** has an absence of periods for a length of time equivalent to a total of at least three of the previous cycle intervals or 6 months of amenorrhea (27).
2. No menses by age 14 in the absence of growth or development of secondary sex characteristics (27).
3. No menses by age 16 regardless of the presence of normal growth and development with the appearance of secondary sex characteristics (27).

Amenorrhea is a symptom, **not** a diagnosis. Establishing the etiology of amenorrhea is essential for safe and effective management. A basic understanding of the normal menstrual cycle, puberty, and hormonal changes are key for the recognition and treatment of menstrual dysfunction.

I. Physiology of menstruation and normal growth and development
   A. **Physiology.** The evaluation and treatment of patients with amenorrhea can, for the most part, be readily performed in an outpatient setting. A clear understanding of normal growth and development, as well as the physiology of the normal menstrual cycle, is a prerequisite to **rapid** and **accurate diagnosis** while minimizing expense to the patient. From the onset of menarche, the regular cyclic occurrence of uterine bleeding takes place with ovulation and an absence of conception. Regular cyclic menstruation signifies a complex series of events including an interplay between the ovaries, hypothalamus (median eminence, particularly the arcuate nucleus), anterior pituitary, and uterine endometrium. The developing follicle and subsequent corpus luteum feed back steroid signals **(estrogen and progesterone)** through the bloodstream to the central nervous system (CNS) (hypothalamus). The **hypothalamus monitors and translates these hormone levels** into messages to the anterior pituitary, which raises or lowers the levels of gonadotropic hormones (follicle-stimulating hormone [FSH] and luteinizing hormone [LH]). This system has both positive and negative feedback components. FSH and LH stimulate follicular growth and ovulation. The endometrium passively responds with growth (proliferation), maturation

This is a revision of the third edition chapter by Frederick W. Hanson.

(secretion), and regular shedding (menstruation) to the steroid signals from the developing follicle and corpus luteum.

Typical **intermenstrual intervals** ranging from 24 to 35 days are thought to be indicative of ovulatory function. The age at menarche is associated with race, nutritional status, body fat, and maternal age at menarche. Improved nutrition and living conditions have produced a gradual but progressive fall in the mean age of menarche over the past century. The mean age of menarche in United States is **12.7 years** (29). The normal menstrual cycle varies from 21 to 45 days and remains fairly constant for a given individual. Normal menstrual flow lasts 2 to 7 days with an average blood loss of 30 to 40 mL (23). **Regular bleeding implies** an intact hypothalamic-pituitary-ovarian system, as well as responsiveness of the endometrium and patency of the outflow tract.

B. **Normal growth and development.** Puberty is a complex **sequence** of **maturational changes** consisting of development of **secondary sex characteristics,** adolescent **growth spurts, fertility onset, psychological changes,** and **sex steroid secretions.** In the female, puberty usually begins between ages 9 and 13 years and is completed within 1½ to 6 years, with menarche usually occurring within 2 years of the onset of breast development (23,26,30). Breast development is the first sign of normal sexual development, followed by the appearance of pubic and axillary hair. Puberty and its preceding events may be divided into the following stages:

1. **Growth spurt.** Girls reach peak height velocity prior to menarche. The mean female growth from the growth spurt to cessation is 25 cm. Its hormonal control is due to a combination of growth hormone and sex steroids. The three stages of growth spurt are minimum growth velocity, peak height velocity, and decreased velocity.

   a. **Bone age** is **one indicator** of **physiologic maturation and** a **better indicator** of onset of **secondary sexual development** than chronologic age **in cases of delayed puberty.** It is also useful in predicting ultimate adult height. **Retarded bone age suggests hypothyroidism,** whereas **advanced bone age suggests** a diagnosis such as **constitutional or organic brain disease.**

   b. **An increase in body mass is the earliest change at puberty.** Attempts have been made to relate weight and body fat content to onset of menarche.

2. **Thelarche (breast development).** The beginning of breast development at puberty and cornification of the vaginal mucosa are primarily under the control of ovarian estrogen, which is influenced by FSH.

3. **Pubarche or adrenarche (sexual hair development).** Both **pubic** and **axillary hair development** is stimulated primarily by adrenal androgens, although there may also be an ovarian contribution. The appearance of pubic hair usually precedes the development of axillary hair.

4. **Menarche**

C. **Hormonal changes**

1. **Gonadotropins.** Fetal levels of gonadotropins rise until midgestation, then fall until term, rise and fall during the first 2 years of life, and then remain low until puberty. At puberty, there is an **enhanced release of LH due to gonadotropin-releasing hormone (GnRH), a sleep release (diurnal variation) of LH** (disappears in adulthood), and an **increased episodic or pulsatile release pattern of FSH and LH.**

2. **Estrogen.** The rising levels of plasma gonadotropins stimulate the ovary to produce increasing amounts of estradiol. **Estradiol** is the major ovarian secretory product, although **estrone, androstenedione, testosterone** and other steroids are produced. **Estradiol** is responsible for the development of secondary sex characteristics (growth and development of breasts and reproductive organs, fat redistribution [hips and breasts]) and bone maturation. The uterine endometrium is affected by wide fluctuations in estradiol and undergoes cyclic proliferation and regression, until

a point is reached when substantial growth occurs so that withdrawal of estrogen results in the first menstruation (menarche). The first ovulation usually does not take place until 6 to 9 months after menarche because the positive feedback mechanism of **estrogen** is not fully developed (19,27).

   a. Estrogen levels are high at birth, then drop until puberty.

   b. Estradiol rises steadily through the stages of puberty.

   c. Estrone plateaus in midpuberty.

3. **Adrenal hormones.** The **adrenal gland** is also implicated in puberty. Circulating levels of aromatizable androgens such as dehydroepiandrosterone and androstenedione, mostly of adrenal origin, begin to increase in the bloodstream at about 7 to 8 years of life and reach their maximum value by ages 13 to 14 (7). This phenomenon is called **adrenarche.** Adrenal androgens are responsible to a large extent for the growth of pubic and axillary hair and are not believed to play a decisive role in determining the start of **puberty.**

D. **Hypothalamic-pituitary-ovarian axis.** The CNS, through the hypothalamus, orchestrates the release of neurotransmitters and neuropeptides, which influence the amount and frequency of pulsatile GnRH into the pituitary portal system. *Gonadarche* is the **maturation of the hypothalamic-pituitary-ovarian axis** and develops in two stages: **negative-feedback** (active in midfetal life) and **positive-feedback** (active in midpuberty).

   1. GnRH stimulates the pituitary to release LH and FSH.

   2. LH stimulates the ovary (theca cells) to make androgens, which are converted into estrogens by the follicular granulosa cells.

   3. The main estrogen is estradiol.

   4. Estradiol and FSH promote growth and maturation of the follicle.

   5. At the middle of the menstrual cycle, an LH surge induces ovulation and conversion of the follicle to a corpus luteum.

   6. The corpus luteum secretes both progesterone and estradiol.

   7. Estradiol acts to exert a positive feedback control on LH, which then peaks, leading to ovulation.

   8. Progesterone and estradiol act together to inhibit gonadotropin.

   9. The adrenal gland is responsible for most of the circulating levels of aromatizable androgens such as dehydroepiandrosterone and androstenedione which begins to increase in the bloodstream at approximately 7 to 8 years of age and reach maximum value by 13 to 14. This phenomenon is called adrenarche.

      a. Adrenal androgens are responsible, to a large extent, for the growth of pubic and axillary hair.

      b. It is believed that these androgens do not play a decisive role in determining the onset of puberty.

E. **The determinants of the onset of puberty are genetic inheritance and environmental factors** such as health, nutrition, light, geography, and altitude. Whether a metabolic signal, such as body weight or composition, triggers the CNS onset of puberty is open to question.

II. **Primary amenorrhea.** Primary amenorrhea is the failure of menarche by age 16 **regardless** of the presence or absence of secondary sex characteristics.

A. **Prevalence.** Although a rare disorder, the most common cause of primary amenorrhea involves gonadal failure, congenital absence of the uterus and vagina, and constitutional delay. The prevalence is 0.3% (17).

B. **Etiology.** Errors in the fetus and errors in development of the gonads, müllerian and wolffian system, and the urogenital sinus are the most frequent causes of primary amenorrhea. Nearly all individuals **without** secondary sex characteristics have a genetic basis for primary amenorrhea (19,27).

C. **History.** A detailed history is essential. The questions asked should be directed toward the following subjects:

   1. **Family history.**

      a. Mother and sister(s) history of menarche, menopause, menstrual dysfunction, and infertility.

   b. **Genetic abnormalities.**
   c. **Autoimmune disorders.**
   d. **Congenital abnormalities.**
   e. **Endocrinopathies.**
   f. **Genetic disorders.**
  2. **Birth.**
   a. Appearance of **external genitalia and ambiguity** suggest the possibility of early maternal drug ingestion or adrenogenital syndrome.
   b. **Anomalies such as nonpatency of the vagina** suggest the possibility of müllerian tract abnormalities.
  3. **Growth and development,** including appearance and timing of secondary sex characteristics.
  4. **Medications** can increase prolactin levels and **may cause amenorrhea.** These include antipsychotics (e.g., phenothiazines, haloperidol, pimozide, and clozapine), tricyclic antidepressants, monoamine oxidase inhibitors, and antihypertensives (e.g., calcium channel blockers, methyldopa, and reserpine).
  5. **Nutritional and dietary factors.**
  6. **Systemic diseases.**
  7. **Hospitalizations and surgeries.**
  8. **Emotional difficulties.**
  9. **Prior diagnostic studies and results.**
  10. **The possibility of pregnancy should be considered.**
 C. **Physical examination** is an extremely important part of the evaluation of primary amenorrhea. It should serve as a **highly suggestive indicator of the etiology** of the amenorrhea. It should not, however, cause the physician to deviate from a compulsive and thorough workup and thereby omit steps that would have detected a different etiology. Screening for abnormal anatomy or development is the primary purpose of the physical examination. The physical and pelvic examination serves to confirm the history, which should suggest the most likely etiology of primary amenorrhea. Evaluation of an adolescent requires familiarity with the Tanner staging system, in particular stages II and III (7). The pelvic examination assists in narrowing the differential diagnosis to gonadal factors, end-organ causes, or dysregulation of the hypothalamic-pituitary-ovarian axis.
  1. Beyond the usual features covered in a thorough physical examination, **particular attention should be paid** to the following features:
   a. **Stature** (<60 in. suggests gonadal dysgenesis).
   b. **Secondary sex characteristics.**
    · (1) **Breasts** (e.g., development, galactorrhea).
    (2) **Hair distribution** (pubic and axillary hair, bitemporal baldness).
    (3) **Body habitus** (female vs. male).
    (4) **Inguinal or labial masses** (e.g., hernias, ectopic gonads, or uterus).
    (5) **Cutaneous lesions** such as extra pigmented nevi (gonadal dysgenesis), acanthosis nigricans (sclerocystic ovary syndrome).
    (6) **Musculoskeletal anomalies** (increased muscle mass, male carrying angle).
    (7) **Pelvic examination** (external and internal genitalia including adnexa).
  2. **Abnormalities of the external genitalia** may vary from anomalous development (labioscrotal fusion) to nonpatency of the vagina (testicular feminization or imperforate hymen).
   a. **Nonpatency of the vagina** may be due to something as simple as an imperforate hymen or transverse vaginal septum or as complex as müllerian dysgenesis or testicular feminization.
   b. Inadequate estrogen stimulation (Turner's syndrome) may have resulted in **infantile external genitalia.**

    c. Intrauterine exposure to maternal sources of androgen or incomplete forms of testicular dysgenesis may result in **varying degrees of defeminization, virilization, or ambiguous external genitalia.**

  3. The **presence of a uterus,** although it may not be palpable because of lack of estrogen stimulation (premenarcheal or gonadal dysgenesis), is always **confirmed by visualization of a cervix.**

  4. **Absence of menarche** with the **normal appearance and** progression of **secondary sex characteristics** is suggestive of an **abnormality** of the müllerian tract (i.e., congenital absence of the uterus), hypothalamus (stress), anterior pituitary (tumor), **or** ovaries (premature failure).

  5. **Total absence of secondary sex characteristics** suggests a **genetic basis** or the rare **gonadotropin or releasing factor deficiencies** as the basis for the observed abnormalities.

  6. The presence of **breasts without pubic and axillary hair** suggests testicular feminization.

  7. If there is **hair and absence of breasts,** male pseudohermaphroditism is suspected.

  8. The forgoing examples are not intended to be a complete list of problems.

E. **Investigative procedures.** The most common causes of primary amenorrhea can be classified according to pathophysiologic disorders of the Hypothalamic-pituitary-ovary axis, uterus and vagina, and the ovaries. Fig. 11.1 represents an investigative protocol (similar to those found in many of the standard texts listed in the reference section at the end of the chapter). **Rigid adherence to such a protocol** will usually result in efficient and rapid diagnosis, minimize expense, and identify those patients requiring referral to specialized centers.

Steps I and IV of the algorithm in Fig. 11.1 will provide a focus for the diagnostic work-up of primary amenorrhea. In the majority of cases laboratory and other diagnostic tests will be confirmatory. The following is a brief description or explanation of each step in the algorithm:

  1. **Urine pregnancy.** If early pregnancy is possible, this should be ruled out by urine pregnancy test.

  2. **Pelvic ultrasound** to identify the presence of ovaries and uterus.

  3. **Serum prolactin** level is **elevated** with prolactinomas of the pituitary gland. Thyrotropin-releasing hormone also stimulates the release of prolactin. Serum prolactin and thyroid-stimulating hormone (TSH) levels should therefore be obtained at the same time.

    a. **Elevated prolactin** as well as **TSH** levels require **pituitary tumors be ruled out.** Magnetic resonance imaging (MRI) of the **anterior pituitary** is indicated along with a referral to an appropriate specialist if indicated.

    b. **Medications** must also be considered. Drugs that increase prolactin are antipsychotics (phenothiazines, haloperidol, pimozide, and clozapine), tricyclic antidepressants, monoamine oxidase inhibitors, and antihypertensives (calcium channel blockers, methyldopa, and reserpine) (17).

  4. **TSH.** Hypothyroidism must also be ruled out. Patients with primary hypothyroidism and hyperprolactinemia can present with either primary or secondary amenorrhea. TSH measurement is warranted because the treatment yields prompt return of ovulatory cycles and the disappearance of galactorrhea (17,19,27).

  5. **Progesterone challenge.** The purpose of the progesterone challenge is to assess the level of endogenous estrogen and the competence of the outflow tract.

    a. A 10-mg dose of medroxyprogesterone acetate is given for 5 days.

    b. Withdrawal bleeding usually occurs 2 to 7 days after the last dose (2,13,16,17,27).

    c. If the patient bleeds, any amount beyond a few spots, a diagnosis of **anovulation** is reliably diagnosed and the presence of a functional

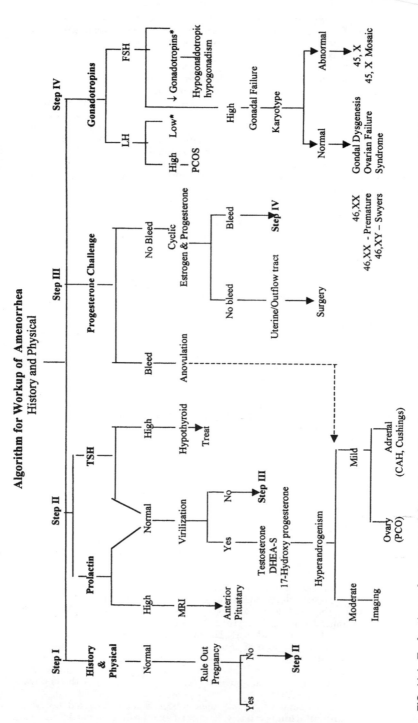

FIG. 11.1. Evaluation and treatment of the patient with primary amenorrhea. TSH, thyroid-stimulating hormone; MRI, magnetic resonance imaging; FSH, follicle-stimulating hormone.

outflow tract with reactive endometrium is confirmed. **Withdrawal bleeding** demonstrates the **presence** of estrogen and minimal function of the ovary, pituitary, and CNS. No further evaluation is necessary (13,16,17,27).

   d. A positive withdrawal bleeding response to progesterone, in the absence of galactorrhea, and a normal prolactin level together **rule out** the presence of a significant tumor (17,27).

   e. **Negative withdrawal** response despite evidence of adequate levels of endogenous estrogen can be found in anovulatory state such as **polycystic ovaries** and **specific adrenal enzyme deficiency** (13,16,27).

6. The **estrogen and progesterone withdrawal** test is obtained if the progesterone withdrawal test is negative. A **negative test** implies **inadequate follicular estrogen priming of the endometrium** (17,27).

   a. Conjugated estrogen (Premarin) 1.25 mg PO is given for 25 days with medroxyprogesterone acetate added during the last 10 days.

   b. Ethinyl estradiol, 10 µg/day, may be substituted for the conjugated estrogen.

   c. Withdrawal bleeding indicates that the uterus is capable of responding, given the appropriate hormonal stimuli; therefore, the uterus is eliminated as a cause of amenorrhea.

7. **Gonadotropins (LH and FSH). Elevated gonadotropins and a low estrogen** level indicate the ovarian follicle is not responding to gonadotropin stimulation, therefore not providing negative feedback to the pituitary and hypothalamus. This is most commonly reflected in ovarian failure. Ovarian failure is considered premature when it occurs in women less than 40 years.

   a. **A single measurement of FSH greater than 50 miU/mL is a reliable indicator of ovarian failure** (27).

   b. Twenty percent to 40% of women with premature ovarian failure have associated autoimmune disorders (8,17,23); therefore, one should consider obtaining the following blood tests to rule out autoimmune disease: thyroid antibody, TSH, free T4, complete blood count (CBC), rheumatoid factor, antinuclear antibody, morning cortisol, calcium, and phosphorus (17,27).

8. **Chromosome evaluation.** All patients under the age of 30 diagnosed with ovarian failure on the basis of elevated gonadotropins must have a **karyotype determination.**

   a. Thirty percent of patients with X chromosome anomalies will not develop signs of virilization; therefore, normal adult appearing women with elevated gonadotropin levels must be karyotyped.

   b. The presence of any testicular component carries a significant chance of a malignant tumor formation (gonadoblastoma, dysgerminoma, yolk sac tumor, and choriocarcinoma).

   c. A karyotype determination positive for 45,X and mosaicism with an X chromosome as well as the presence of a Y chromosome, therefore, require excision of the gonadal tissue (7,19,27).

F. **Management.** Appropriate management of patients with amenorrhea depends upon the correct diagnosis and presenting symptom and whether or not pregnancy is desired. The treatment modalities can consist of hormone replacement, surgery, ovulation induction, and counseling.

   1. **Hormone replacement** is directed at controlling uterine bleeding and creating a normal cyclic hormonal pattern, preventing osteoporosis, and resulting in development of secondary sex characteristics.

      a. When reliable **contraception** is needed, the use of a **low-dose oral contraceptive pill** in the usual cyclic fashion is appropriate.

      b. **All anovulatory** patients require therapeutic management. **Minimal** therapy **requires** the monthly administration of a progestational agent, i.e., 10mg medroxyprogesterone daily for the first 10 days of the month.

   c. **If a uterus is present, the addition of progesterone to the estrogen is required** to prevent unopposed estrogen stimulation **and** its potential adverse sequelae (cancer of the endometrium and possibly breast). This is done in a fashion similar to that described earlier for the combined estrogen and progesterone withdrawal test (see section II.E.6).
   d. **When development of secondary sex characteristics is the initial goal,** one method of treatment is as follows:
      (1) Conjugated estrogen is given daily with dosage increases at approximately 3-month intervals (e.g., 0.30 mg, 0.625 mg, 1.25 mg).
      (2) Once vaginal bleeding occurs, progesterone is added each month in combination with estrogen to the last 10 days of medication, and the patient takes no medication the last week. This leaves the last week of each month for withdrawal bleeding if a uterus is present.
   e. Hormonal treatment **is** indicated for the entire life of the patient to **prevent the development of osteoporosis.**
2. **Ovulation induction requires a gynecology fertility consult and/ or referral.** Therapy is rendered **according** to the **etiology** of the amenorrhea.
   a. Drug therapy for a negative progestin challenge is clomiphene citrate. Patients showing some ovarian stimulation by clomiphene can be treated with a combination of clomiphene and human menopausal gonadotropin (HMG). Ovulation induction with HMG must be carefully monitored with serial ultrasound and estradiol determinations to avoid hyperstimulation, which is associated with ovarian enlargement and ascites (1,2).
      (1) Clomiphene citrate may be started at 50 mg orally daily for 5 days and increased to a maximum of 250 mg orally daily in 50 mg increments until ovulation is induced.
      (2) Ovulation occurs 5 to 10 days after the last dose.
      (3) Patients with elevated androgens who do not respond to clomiphene citrate may respond to combined treatment with corticosteroids and clomiphene (1,13,16).
   b. Bromocriptine is used to treat amenorrhea-galactorrhea.
      (1) Bromocriptine 2.5 mg orally is given twice daily and generally titrated until serum prolactin is within normal limits.
      (2) Once ovulation has been documented by basal body temperature, bromocriptine can be discontinued then resumed after menses or continued until pregnancy occurs (1,2,27).
3. **Surgery.** The need for surgical intervention for diagnosis should be **infrequent,** and patients are best **referred to specialized centers** for specific diagnoses and removal of gonads when indicated.
   a. Patients who will require corrective surgery for ambiguous genitalia, vaginal agenesis, correctable uterine anomalies, or a combination of these are also best referred.
   b. Generally speaking, the **prognosis for fertility is poor,** and these patients should be carefully and tactfully counseled.
   c. **Surgical wedge resection** of the ovary in patients with polycystic ovary disease will often lead to ovulation. This is usually reserved for patients who have failed clomiphene citrate and refuse HMG (27).
4. **Counseling.** Every patient deserves counseling which includes an adequate explanation of the physiologic or pathophysiologic event that the patient is experiencing, all available treatments, and associated risk factors.
   a. **Phenotypic appearance is far more important** than either gonadal or chromosomal identification. Tactless divulgence of the latter information is unnecessary and can be devastating to the individual.
   b. **The potential for normal sexual activity,** albeit in the face of decreased fertility potential, **is to be stressed** to these individuals.

III. Secondary amenorrhea. Secondary amenorrhea is the **cessation** of menstrual periods for at least 6 months once menarche has occurred. This is a somewhat arbitrary and artificial distinction from primary amenorrhea. **Since** considerable overlap exists, such as ovarian dysgenesis and premature gonadal failure demonstrating early cyclic gonadal function prior to the subsequent onset of amenorrhea, it is extremely important to consistently **rule out pregnancy** as a **cause** for secondary **amenorrhea.**

The evaluation of secondary amenorrhea is organized around the disruption of the menstrual cycle at the levels of the hypothalamus, pituitary, and ovary.

  A. Incidence: The overall incidence of secondary amenorrhea is 1% to 3%, but in selected subgroups it is even higher. Two percent to 5% of women of reproductive age who are not pregnant or lactating experience some form of secondary amenorrhea (26,30). **Endurance athletes, ballet dancers, and college women may have rates as high as 60%, 44%, and 5%, respectively** (9,17,22).

  B. Etiology: The most **common physiologic etiologies** of secondary amenorrhea are **pregnancy, breast-feeding,** and **postmenopause. Nonphysiologic causes** of secondary amenorrhea maybe due to **chronic anovulation, hypothyroidism, hyperprolactinemia,** and **weight loss or anorexia.** Chronic anovulation leaves the practitioner with the task of defining the biologic cause for anovulation (prolactinoma, Cushing's syndrome, malnutrition, altered steroid production, or adrenal tumors). Endometrial suppression by medications is also a common cause of secondary amenorrhea (13,19,27).

   1. The **most common physiologic causes** of secondary amenorrhea are **pregnancy** and **menopause.**
   2. Pathologic causes of amenorrhea can be divided into categories by **levels of gonadal steroid production.**
      a. Intrauterine synechiae and hysterectomy are examples of **normal steroid production.**
      b. Primary ovarian failure on a **congenital** (e.g., gonadal dysgenesis) or **acquired** (e.g., autoimmune disease, postoperative irradiation, postinfection) basis is a common example of decreased gonadal steroid production with high gonadotropin production.
      c. Normal pituitary gonadotropins are seen with secondary ovarian failure. More common examples are **pituitary prolactinomas, injury or tumors of the pituitary gland and hypothalamus,** and **hypothalamic-pituitary dysfunction** secondary to extrinsic factors such as psychogenic disorders, acute diseases, endocrine disease, or anorexia nervosa.
      d. Increased ovarian steroid production, with estrogen- or androgen-secreting tumors or the polycystic ovary syndrome, can result in secondary amenorrhea.
   3. The availability of an assay for prolactin has led to the diagnosis of the **galactorrhea-amenorrhea syndrome,** including prolactinomas, hypothyroidism, and drug-induced symptoms (e.g., phenothiazines, reserpine, alpha-methyldopa), as a **major diagnostic etiology of secondary amenorrhea.**

  C. History taking is similar to primary amenorrhea and, for that matter, any gynecologic problem. There are, however, **additional** factors that are more important when considering secondary amenorrhea.
   1. Menstrual history.
      a. Menarche.
      b. Menstrual interval and flow.
      c. Prior episodes of oligomenorrhea or amenorrhea.
   2. Obstetric history.
      a. Date of last delivery.
      b. Complications such as hemorrhage (Sheehan's syndrome), dilations and curettages (D & Cs), or postpartum infection (Asherman's syndrome).
      c. Cesarean sections.

3. **Surgical history.**
   a. **Salpingectomy** for ectopic pregnancy (often accompanied by oophorectomy).
   b. **Ovarian cystectomies or wedge resections** (e.g., polycystic ovaries or endometriosis).
   c. **Myomectomy.**
   d. **Hysterectomy.**
4. **Systemic diseases. Any generalized illness,** including other endocrine diseases (e.g., those involving the thyroid, adrenal glands, and pancreas), may result in cessation of reproductive function.
5. **Nutritional status. Obesity as well as starvation** (i.e., anorexia nervosa) can result in aberrations of steroid production and metabolism and ovulatory dysfunction. Health professionals caring for female athletes as well as young women must inquire about weight loss, excessive dieting, eating disorders, and a history of stress fractures.
6. **CNS.** Head injury, intrinsic lesions of the pituitary or hypothalamus, or treatment (e.g., irradiation, surgery) of CNS lesions can interfere with hypothalamic-pituitary-ovarian function.
7. **Drugs.** Many drugs can affect menstrual function either directly via an effect on the endometrium (progesterone) or indirectly via effects at the hypothalamic-pituitary level (e.g., oral contraceptives, dopamine-blocking agents), which in turn may result in cessation or irregularity of ovulation. It is important to elicit a history of the following:
   a. **Oral contraceptive use.**
   b. **Psychiatric drugs.**
   c. **Hypertensive medication.**
   d. **Hormone replacement.**
   e. **Fertility-stimulating agents.**
   f. **Cancer chemotherapy.**
8. **Extrinsic factors** such as stress, obesity, and intercurrent illness can result in amenorrhea.
9. **Hormone deficiency symptoms.** Menopause-like symptoms of estrogen deficiency, such as hot flashes and vaginal dryness may suggest premature gonadal failure.
10. **Hormone excess symptoms.** There are several relatively uncommon ovarian tumors that can provide signs of excessive feminization or the more obvious defeminization or virilization.
    a. **Androgen excess** is seen with gonadoblastomas, dysgerminomas, and lipoid or hilar cell tumors.
    b. The most common cause of secondary amenorrhea with **excess estrogen secretion** is the **polycystic ovary syndrome.**
    c. Symptoms of defeminization are **loss of feminine fat distribution,** certain degrees of **hirsutism,** and **acne.**
    d. **Virilization** is characterized by **male muscle mass and body habitus, clitoromegaly, bitemporal baldness, and deepening of the voice.**
D. **Physical examination.** The same general principles apply as those for primary amenorrhea (see section II.D). More emphasis is to be applied in searching for the following:
   1. Signs of **pregnancy.**
   2. **Estrogen deficiency.**
   3. **Defeminization.**
   4. **Galactorrhea.**
   5. **Virilization.**
   6. **Abnormalities on pelvic examination,** particularly with the presence of adnexal masses and abnormalities of the external genitalia (e.g., clitoromegaly).
E. **Investigative procedures.** Steps I, II, and III of the algorithm reflect the standard work-up for secondary amenorrhea (Fig. 11.1).
   1. Confirmation of the diagnosis of a uterine cause of secondary amenorrhea is usually made by **hysterography or hysteroscopy** to confirm intrauterine adhesions or synechiae (1,8,15,26).

2. The laboratory evaluation of hyperandrogenic anovulation is controversial. The standard evaluation varies. The evaluation may include
measurement of levels of free or total **testosterone** or both, 8 AM
17 α-hydroxyprogesterone during the follicular phase, **dehydroepiandrosterone sulfate (DHEA-S),** and prolactin if galactorrhea
is present. Initial laboratory tests should be obtained in the fasting
state (13,17,19,26,27).

   a. **Testosterone, androstenedione, dehydroepiandrosterone
(DHEA), and DHEA-S levels** are also obtained with hirsutism,
virilization, or both. **Elevated androgen levels are abnormal.**

     (1) **Mildly elevated levels of testosterone** suggest a more
benign ovarian disease process such as the polycystic ovary
syndrome.

     (2) **Mildly elevated DHEA-S levels** suggest adrenal hyperplasia.

     (3) **Markedly elevated levels of testosterone or DHEA-S** sug-
gest tumors. These patients are best referred to centers for
**differential suppression studies and specific long-term
treatment.** Surgical exploration may be required for removal
of steroid-secreting tumors.

   b. **17 α-hydroxyprogesterone.** This is to screen for nonclassical
late-onset adrenal hyperplasia resulting from a heterozygous state
21-hydroxylase deficiency. Therapy for this disorder is specific, glucocorticoids (13,17,27). Identification of women with late-onset adrenal
hyperplasia may have implications for preconception counseling.

3. LH increases cause ovarian stroma and theca cells of women with hyperandrogenism to secrete more androstenedione and testosterone. Ovarian
androgen overproduction may be the result of chronic exposure of the
ovary to excessive LH as seen in polycystic ovary syndrome (1,13,19).
Women with polycystic ovary syndrome have three times the risk of
hypertension and six times the risk of type 2 diabetes mellitus, therefore, they need to be evaluated for these diseases (8,25).

4. MRI is indicated when:

     (1) A CNS hypothalamic cause is suspected from an anatomic
lesion.

     (2) Elevated prolactin levels, nipple discharge, and neurologic
findings are present to rule out tumors of the pituitary gland.

F. **Management** of secondary amenorrhea is similar to that of primary amenorrhea. Accurate diagnosis is the key to management. In many cases, the **options for management depend on the patient's desires for fertility.**
With treatment options involving essentially equal success rates, **conservative nonoperative management is always preferable to surgery.
The main treatment options are as follows:**

1. **Hormone replacement is necessary in all cases of ovarian failure** (see Chapter 25). It is also important that the patient clearly understands that fertility is impossible.

2. **Ovulation induction** is used when fertility is desired (see Chapter 23).

3. **Hirsutism management depends on the source of elevated androgens and end-organ sensitivity.** Suppression of the adrenal gland or
ovary (or both), tumor removal, ovulation induction in the case of polycystic ovary syndrome, or end-organ suppression with spironolactone
may be required (see Chapter 21). Any potential offending drugs should
be discontinued, **such as** testosterone, danazol, anabolic steroids, and
synthetic progestins.

4. **Surgery** is used for steroid-secreting tumors, prolactinomas, intrauterine
synechiae, wedge resection of ovaries, and endometrial biopsy. Direct
lysis of adhesions through the operative hysteroscope may result in restoration of menses in 90% of patients (17,25). A wedge resection of the
ovaries for those with polycystic ovary syndrome and endometrial biopsy
along with surgical removal of tumors may relieve obstructions (26).

5. Cosmetic: waxing, depilatories, electrolysis, and shaving. Eflornithine
has been formulated for topical use to decrease facial hair. The topical

eflornithine (Vaniqua 13.9%) applied bid is the latest drug on the market that may be considered to limit the symptom of excessive facial hair growth in hirsute patients.

6. Management of galactorrhea-amenorrhea syndromes depends on the patient's desire to conceive and the size of the prolactinoma (26). **Observation, medical management** (bromocriptine), **transsphenoidal surgery,** and **irradiation** are the possible treatment modalities.

IV. **Athletic (hypoestrogenic) amenorrhea.** The female athlete triad was first described 1970s and refers to an interrelationship of eating disorder, osteoporosis, and amenorrhea. Athletic amenorrhea is the second component of the female athlete triad (3,5,9,14,18,22,23,28,31). This discussion will be limited to that component.

A. **Incidence.** The incidence of athletic amenorrhea among endurance athletes, ballet dancers, and college women may be as high as 60%, 44%, and 5%, respectively (3,9,22,26,28,30).

B. **Prevalence.** Women deny or underreport symptoms of primary and secondary amenorrhea, therefore, the true prevalence is unknown.

C. **Etiology.** The cause of hypothalamic-induced amenorrhea is unknown. It may be related to (a) psychosocial stressors, (b) training intensity, and (c) reduced caloric intake. Excessive exercise in women is believed to affect the hypothalamic-pituitary-gonadal axis leading to a reduction of estrogen and progesterone release from the ovaries (8,14,18,28). A combination of these two factors is thought to change the body composition, in particular a reduction in body fat. The **Critical Weight Concept of Frisch** suggests that the onset and regularity of menstrual function necessitate maintaining weight and body fat above a critical level. Losing 10% to 15% of normal weight for height represents about one third of body fat loss, which may result in abnormal menstrual function (9,12,27).

D. **History.** A complete history with special emphasis on (a) menstrual history and irregularities of the patient as well as family history, (b) psychological stressors, (c) intensive athletic training in childhood, and (d) a heightened body awareness may be key factors that cause a delay in the onset of puberty and menstruation (3,5,14,18,20,28,31).

E. **Physical examination.** Assessment of symptoms of anorexia nervosa, reduced bone mineral density, stress fractures, delayed epiphyseal closure, and complete physical examination as described previously for both primary and secondary amenorrhea (3,27,28) should be done.

F. **Management.** The management of amenorrheic athletes can be difficult. If the athlete has been amenorrheic for 6 months or more, she should be medically assessed. Health care professionals, parents, and coaches who work with female athletes should be diligent in monitoring for signs and symptoms of this triad. Recognition and prevention are key. Athletes who complain of any eating disorder, menstrual irregularity, and stress fractures are considered high risk (3,28,31).

1. If the cessation of menses correlates with the timing of intensive athletic training then exercise is the most likely cause and should be stopped or decreased until the return of menses (28).

2. If there is **no** clear-cut association with exercise, an in-depth medical and gynecologic work-up is indicated. Treatment options include:
   a. Nutritional assessment with correction of dietary calcium deficits.
   b. Increase in caloric intake.
   c. Reduction of training intensity.
   d. Measurement of bone mineral density (BMD).
   e. Estrogen replacement in the form of oral contraception (3,28,31).

Patient Education
What Is Amenorrhea?
Amenorrhea is the absence of menstrual bleeding and is a symptom, not a diagnosis. It requires a complete medical work-up to establish its cause. It is classified as both

primary and secondary. **Primary** amenorrhea is when **no** period has occurred by age 14 and there are no secondary sex characteristics (such as breast development, pubic hair) **or** by age 16 with normal development. **Secondary** amenorrhea is the failure to menstruate for 6 months in a woman who has had previous regular periods **or** in a woman with a history of irregular periods who does not have a period for 12 months.

What Are Common Causes of Amenorrhea?
Many women will experience the absence of a period sometime during their life, such as with pregnancy, breast-feeding and postmenopause. However there are some causes that are congenital (born with) problems or lifestyle problems. **Primary amenorrhea** is usually caused by congenital problems such as an obstruction in the uterus, vagina, or ovary or by a hormonal imbalance. **Secondary amenorrhea** may be from very strenuous exercise (athlete), anorexia nervosa, weight loss, psychological or emotional stress, illness, medications (psychotropics, antihypertensives, oral contraceptives), tumors of the pituitary and hypothalamus, and disorders of the ovaries and adrenal gland as well as multiple metabolic and endocrine disorders. **The most common cause of secondary amenorrhea is pregnancy.**

What Are Common Signs and Symptoms?
Common signs and symptoms are related to hormonal imbalances that affect the body. These symptoms occur with menstrual irregularities and might include vaginal dryness, thinning of the vaginal mucosa, pain with intercourse (dyspareunia), decreased cervical mucus, mood swings, and irritability. Elevated levels of certain hormones such as testosterone may produce truncal obesity (increased waist to hip ratio), acne, male pattern baldness, or enlargement of the clitoris.

How Is It Diagnosed?
A detailed history is needed and will include menstrual and reproductive history, general medical and surgical history, and family history. A complete physical examination including a breast and pelvic examination will be necessary. Various laboratory tests and imaging tests may be needed. However, the history and physical will establish most of the diagnosis and tests may be used only to confirm the diagnosis.

How Is Amenorrhea Treated?
The treatment depends upon the cause and may include surgery, hormone replacement, and/or drug therapy.

What Is the Female Athlete Triad and How Does It Relate to Amenorrhea?
Some highly competitive female athletes have been known to develop multiple problems known as **the female athlete triad.** This triad refers to an interrelationship of eating disorders, osteoporosis, and amenorrhea. Parents, health care professionals, and coaches who work with female athletes should monitor female athletes for signs and symptoms of this triad. Athletes who complain of any eating disorder, menstrual irregularity, and/or stress fractures are considered to be at high risk. Recognition of early symptoms and prevention are key.

What Is the Treatment for Athletic-associated Amenorrhea?
If the athlete has been without a period for 6 months or more, a medical and gynecologic evaluation is indicated. If menses ceased after the onset of intensive training, then exercise is the most likely cause and should be reduced or stopped until menses returns. If there is no clear-cut association with exercise then an in-depth medical and gynecologic assessment is needed. Treatment includes nutritional assessment, especially for calcium intake; an increase in caloric intake; reduce training intensity; possible hormone replacement in the form of oral contraception pill; and close follow-up with the primary care provider.

References
1. *Managing the anovulatory state: medical induction of ovulation.* ACOG Technical Bulletin, 1994; No. 197.

2. Aloi JA. Evaluation of amenorrhea. *Compr Ther* 1995;21:575–578.
3. Anderson SJ, et al. Medical concerns in the female athlete. *Pediatrics* 2000;106: 610–613.
4. Baird DT. Amenorrhea. *Lancet* 1997;350:275–279.
5. Benson JE, et al. Nutritional aspects of amenorrhea in the female athlete triad. *Int J Sport Nutr* 1996;2:134–145.
6. Carr BR, Bradshaw KD. Disorders of the ovary and female reproductive tract. In: Fauci AS, ed. *Harrison's principles of internal medicine*, 14th ed. New York: McGraw-Hill, 1998:2098–2110.
7. Carr BR. Disorders of the ovaries and female reproductive tract. In: Wilson JD, Foster DW, et al. *Williams' textbook of endocrinology*, 9th ed. Philadelphia: WB Saunders, 1998:782–794.
8. Crosigani PG, Vegetti W. A practical guide to the diagnosis and management of amenorrhea. *Drugs* 1996;52:673–671.
9. DeSouza MJ, Metzger DA. Reproductive dysfunction in amenorrheic athletes and anorexic patients: a review. *Med Sci Sports Exerc* 1991;23:995–1007.
10. Doody KM, Carr BR. Amenorrhea. In: Chihal HJ, London SN, eds. Menstrual cycle disorders. *Obstetrics and Gynecology Clinics of North America* 1990;17:361–389.
11. Felmar E. Menstrual disorders. In: Taylor RB, ed. *Family medicine principles and practice*, 5th ed. New York: Springer-Verlag, 1998:900–906.
12. Frisch RE. Body fat, menarche, and reproductive ability. *Semin Reprod Endocrinol* 1985;3:45–54.
13. Galle PC, MacRae M. Amenorrhea and chronic anovulation. *Postgrad Med* 1992; 92:255–260.
14. Gidwani GP. The athlete and menstruation. *Adolesc Med* 1991;2:227–246.
15. Hammond CB, Riddick DH. Menstruation and disorders of menstrual function. In: Danforth DN, ed. *Obstetrics and gynecology*, 8th ed. Philadelphia: Lippincott Williams & Wilkins, 1999:501–607.
16. *Hyperandrogenic chronic anovulation.* ACOG Technical Bulletin. February, 1995; 202:1–7.
17. Kiningham RB, Apgar BS, et al. Evaluation of amenorrhea. *Am Fam Physician* 1996;53:1185–1194.
18. Marshall LA. Clinical evaluation of amenorrhea in active and athletic women. *Clin Sports Med* 1994;13:371–387.
19. McIver B, Romansiki SA, et al. Evaluation and management of amenorrhea. *Mayo Clin Proc* 1997;72:1161–1169.
20. Nattiv A, et al. The female athlete triad: the inter-relatedness of disordered eating, amenorrhea, and osteoporosis. *Clin Sports Med* 1994;13:405–418.
21. Neddlman RD. Growth and development. In: Behrman RE, Webb KH, eds. *Nelson textbook of pediatrics*, 15th ed. Philadelphia: WB Saunders, 1996:57–59.
22. Needless CF. Resumption of menses in anorexia nervosa. *Arch Pediatr Adolesc Med* 1997;151:634–635.
23. Plectcher JR, Slap GB. Menstrual disorders amenorrhea. Adolescent gynecology, part I: Common disorders. *Pediatr Clin North Am* 1999;46:505–543.
24. Practice Recertification 1998;20:58–74.
25. Reid RL. Amenorrhea. In: Copeland LJ, ed. *Textbook of gynecology*, 2nd ed. Philadelphia: WB Saunders, 2000:541–569.
26. Sanford CE, Miller KE. Evaluation and treatment of secondary amenorrhea. Family. Practice Recertification 1998;20:58–74.
27. Speroff L, Glass R, et al. Amenorrhea. In: Speroff L, ed. *Clinical gynecologic endocrinology and infertility*, 5th ed. Baltimore: Williams & Wilkins, 1994:401–456.
28. Thein LA. The female athlete. *J Orthop Sports Phys Ther* 1996;23:134–148.
29. US Department of Health and Human Services. Centers for Disease Control and Prevention. National Center for Health Statistics. *Vital and health statistics. Fertility, family planning and women's health: new data from the 1995 national survey of family growth* 1997;23:29.
30. Warren PM. Clinical review 77. Evaluation of secondary amenorrhea. *J Clin Endocrinol Metab* 1996;81:437–442.
31. Wolman RL. ABC of sports medicine: osteoporosis and exercise. *BMJ* 1994;309: 400–403.

12. ABNORMAL UTERINE BLEEDING

Gary S. Leiserowitz and Clara K. Paik

Abnormal uterine bleeding is the most common presenting gynecologic complaint. Although often assumed to be uterine in origin by both patient and physician, **abnormal bleeding can occur from other sites.** A systematic approach to the problem will identify the source and lead to an explanation for the abnormal bleeding.

I. **Normal menstruation.** The normal menstrual cycle involves a series of complex hormonal events integrating hypothalamic, pituitary, ovarian, and uterine functions. The local hormonal milieu achieved during ovarian follicular maturation and ovulation induces secretory changes in the endometrium to facilitate implantation of the fertilized ovum. Normal menstrual bleeding occurs in the absence of endometrial implantation of the fertilized ovum. The menstrual flow represents sloughing of the endometrial lining and is the direct result of the withdrawal of hormonal stimulation in the absence of early pregnancy.
   A. **Normal volume of menstrual blood loss** is less than 80 mL, with an average volume loss of 30 mL (1).
   B. **Normal interval between menstrual cycles** is considered to be 28 days (±7 days) (7).
   C. **Duration of flow** ranges between 2 and 7 days for normal menses.
II. **Overview of abnormal bleeding.** The ten different abnormal bleeding patterns are described in Table 12.1. The appropriate management of patients with abnormal bleeding is dependent upon an accurate diagnosis. It is important to remember that not all bleeding originates from the uterus, or even the genital tract; therefore, a thorough investigation of potential bleeding sites is mandatory. Considerations in the **differential diagnosis of abnormal bleeding** are shown in Table 12.2.
   A. **General etiologies** for abnormal bleeding fall into four categories (12):
      1. **Dysfunctional bleeding, with no evidence of organic lesions.**
      2. **Pregnancy and its complications.**
      3. **Organic pelvic lesions, benign or malignant.**
      4. **Extragenital problems (coagulopathies, endocrinopathies, iatrogenic).**
   B. **Age-dependent causes** of abnormal bleeding should be considered during the investigation. This way of approaching the problem directs the evaluation toward the most probable etiologies in each age category. This chapter focuses on the potential diagnostic considerations in the prepubertal, perimenarcheal, reproductive, and postmenopausal age groups and discusses their management.
III. **Dysfunctional uterine bleeding** (DUB) results from a loss of coordinated cyclic hormonal changes and excludes organic lesions (e.g., neoplasms, polyps, leiomyomas). The age of the patient will determine the likelihood that DUB is the primary cause.
   A. **Age categories**
      1. **Menarche to 20 years.** Majority of these patients will have abnormal bleeding secondary to anovulatory DUB.
      2. **Age 20 to 40 years.** Less than 20% of abnormal bleeding is due to anovulatory DUB. More common etiologies include pregnancy and its complications, pelvic inflammatory disease, intrauterine devices, oral contraceptives (OCPs), neoplasia, thyroid disease, endometriosis, and adenomyosis.

This is a revision of the third edition chapter by Gary S. Leiserowitz and Richard Graves.

Table 12.1. Abnormal uterine bleeding patterns

Amenorrhea: absent menstrual flow for >90 days

Hypermenorrhea: excessive uterine bleeding occurring during a regular menstrual duration

Hypomenorrhea: decrease in the amount of menstrual flow, often with a decrease in duration

Menometrorrhagia: prolongation of the menstrual flow associated with irregular intermenstrual bleeding

Menorrhagia: excessive bleeding at the time of menstrual period, either in number of days, amount of blood loss, or both

Metrorrhagia: bleeding occurring irregularly between menstrual cycles

Oligomenorrhea: episodes of menstrual bleeding occurring at intervals of >35 days

Polymenorrhea: episodes of menstrual bleeding occurring at intervals of <22 days

Postmenopausal bleeding: bleeding that occurs >1 year after the normal menopausal cessation of menses

Premenstrual spotting: a variant of metrorrhagia occurring frequently and limited to the few days immediately preceding the menstrual flow

---

3. **Age greater than 40 years.** Anovulation again becomes a prominent cause of abnormal bleeding until menopause. However, **neoplasia must be ruled out prior to attributing the bleeding to DUB.**

B. **Etiologies.** DUB is usually associated with anovulatory cycles but it can also be seen in ovulatory cycles. The differentiation between anovulatory and ovulatory DUB is based on bleeding patterns and predisposing factors. These differences are elaborated in the following paragraphs:

1. **Anovulatory DUB** is often seen in the **adolescent and perimenopausal age** groups. In these age groups, 90% of DUB is anovulatory (3). In regular ovulatory cycles, estrogen causes endometrial proliferation. Progesterone provides stromal support and acts as an antiestrogen to prevent excessive proliferation, thereby controlling endometrial height. Endometrial shedding occurs following cyclic withdrawal of estrogen and progesterone. In an anovulatory cycle, the prolonged effect of estrogen on the endometrium results in abnormal proliferation and hyperplasia. Once the endometrial height is greater than the stromal support, irregular menstrual shedding occurs, which can lead to excessive and prolonged bleeding.

2. **Ovulatory DUB** can result in **midcycle bleeding or abnormal menstrual cycles.** Midcycle bleeding occurs when estrogen levels are reduced at ovulation (i.e., estrogen withdrawal bleeding) (3). Abnormal intervals between cycles can manifest as polymenorrhea or oligomenorrhea. Corpus luteum insufficiency (or luteal phase defect) can result from inadequate progesterone production or a shortened period of progesterone secretion, which usually leads to unexpected early menses.

IV. **Prepubertal bleeding** or bleeding that occurs **prior to the age of 9 years is abnormal.** The average age of menarche in the United States is 12 years (12). A complete history and physical examination are essential for diagnosis.

A. **History.** In addition to questions concerning the character of the bleeding, the following should be elucidated:

1. The possibility of maternal diethylstilbestrol (DES) use during pregnancy.

2. Ingestion of steroid-containing substances (e.g., OCPs).

3. A family history of blood dyscrasias or sexual precocity.

Table 12.2. Differential diagnosis of abnormal bleeding

I. Dysfunctional uterine bleeding
    A. Anovulatory
        1. Perimenarcheal (immature hypothalamic-pituitary-ovarian axis)
        2. Perimenopausal (aging or insensitive ovarian follicles)
        3. Polycystic ovarian syndrome (PCO)
        4. Obesity
        5. Endocrinopathies (other than PCO, such as thyroid or adrenal dysfunction)
        6. Drugs
           a. Nonsteroidal hypothalamic depressants (e.g., morphine, phenothiazines)
           b. Sex steroids (e.g., oral contraceptives, testosterone)
        7. Stress
    B. Ovulatory
        1. Dysfunctional corpus luteum leads to unexpected early menses
        2. Midcycle bleeding
II. Organic lesions
    A. Pregnancy-associated causes
        1. Normal first-trimester implantation spotting
        2. Spontaneous or induced abortion
        3. Ectopic pregnancy
        4. Gestational trophoblastic disease
        5. Postabortion or postpartum endometritis
    B. Anatomic uterine lesions
        1. Leiomyomas
        2. Adenomyosis or endometriosis
        3. Polyps
        4. Endometrial hyperplasia
        5. Cancer
        6. Infection
           a. Sexually transmitted disease
           b. Tuberculosis
        7. Mechanical causes
           a. Intrauterine device
           b. Perforation
    C. Anatomic nonuterine lesions
        1. Ovarian lesions
           a. Adnexal torsion (limiting ovarian blood supply and resulting in the loss of hormonal support for the endometrium)
           b. Functional neoplasms (benign or malignant) secreting estrogens or androgens
        2. Fallopian tube lesions
           a. Cancer
           b. Salpingitis
         3. Cervical and vaginal lesions
           a. Neoplasms
              (1) Cancer
              (2) Adenosis
           b. Infections
              (1) Sexually transmitted diseases
              (2) Nonspecific polymicrobial diseases
           c. Atrophic vaginitis
           d. Trauma
              (1) Sexual assault
              (2) Foreign bodies
              (3) Postcoital bleeding
              (4) Self-mutilation

continued

Table 12.2. (*continued*).

---

   4. Urinary tract
   a. Infection
   b. Stones
   c. Cancer
   5. Gastrointestinal tract
   a. Hemorrhoids
   b. Fissures
   c. Inflammatory bowel disease
   d. Neoplasms
D. Systemic abnormalities
   1. Exogenous hormone administration
   a. Oral contraceptives
   b. Sex steroids
   c. Corticosteroids
   2. Coagulopathies
   a. Von Willebrand's disease (most common)
   b. Thrombocytopenia
   c. Hepatic failure
   3. Endocrinopathies
   a. Thyroid disorders (hypothyroidism and hyperthyroidism)
   b. Adrenal disorders (hyperplasia and neoplasia)
   c. Diabetes mellitus
   d. Hypothalamic-pituitary disorders (hyperprolactinemia, neoplasia, failure)
   4. Malnutrition (obesity or inadequate nutrition)

B. Physical examination
  1. The physical examination should be done with a proper **pediatric-sized speculum**, a **long otoscope**, or a **long nasal speculum**.
  2. Materials for culturing and biopsy should be readily available for use as indicated.
  3. The recto-vaginal-abdominal examination can often detect vaginal masses or foreign bodies.
  4. The extremely small child **may require** vaginoscopy and cystoscopy **under anesthesia** to ensure completeness of the evaluation.
  5. The status of secondary sexual characteristics such as breast development and pubic hair should be noted to look for signs of sexual precocity.
  6. If the physical examination is not helpful in establishing the cause of bleeding, one must consider whether the child actually bled.
C. Etiologies of vaginal bleeding usually are easily recognized in this age group. Management strategies for the following diagnoses are discussed in their context.
  1. Vulvovaginitis is the most common cause of pediatric gynecologic complaints (2). The offending organisms are usually bacterial, monilial, and occasionally protozoan. Superinfection associated with a vaginal foreign body is a common finding.
    a. The **clinical presentation** includes pruritus, burning, erythema, discharge, and occasionally a small amount of bleeding.
    b. Poor hygiene is often the cause but other etiologies include irritation from soap, cosmetics, clothing, and sand.
    c. The vaginitis can result from a sexually transmitted infection which would require careful and sensitive questioning of the child, her parents and/or caregivers.
    d. The **diagnosis** is established by gentle examination, looking for evidence of a foreign body.

   e. Any discharge should be sent for routine cultures as well as cultures for gonorrhea and chlamydia.
   f. If a **sexually transmitted disease** is strongly suspected, then **throat** and **anal cultures**, as well as the Venereal Disease Research Laboratories (**VDRL**) test and **HIV** test, should be done.
   g. **Treatment** is specific to the etiology. Antibiotics are necessary for identified bacterial infections, and the dose should be calculated for the age and weight of the child. Instruction in hygiene is valuable to avoid repeat infections.
2. **Trauma to the perineum** is another common cause of bleeding in children. Since a child's vulva lacks subcutaneous fat, it is less able to withstand trauma compared with an adult's vulva.
   a. **Sexual molestation** of the child is a potential cause of perineal or vaginal lacerations. Any suspicion should be pursued in a discreet investigation.
   b. **Treatment** of large lacerations should be carried out in the operating room under anesthesia to allow better exposure and to minimize further trauma to the child. Examination under anesthesia is also necessary to rule out intraabdominal perforation or rectal entry. Large hematomas should be observed for further enlargement. Retroperitoneal bleeds with unilateral back pain can follow development of a large hematoma. A continuing fall in hematocrit is an indication for laparotomy.
3. **Prolapse of the urethra** can also cause bleeding. It usually occurs in girls aged 6 to 9 years and is more common in blacks than whites.
   a. **Predisposing factors** are congenital weakness, mucosal redundancy, increased intraabdominal pressure, and external trauma.
   b. **Presenting symptoms** include bleeding, pain, and dysuria.
   c. **Examination** will reveal tender, grayish or dark-red tissue outside the urethral meatus.
   d. **Management** is initiated with the use of estrogen cream, which is often effective and may eliminate the need for surgery. If unsuccessful, then ligation, cautery, or surgical excision of the prolapsed tissue is indicated. Manual repositioning of the prolapsed tissue and sitz baths are no longer recommended for conservative therapy since recurrence is common.
4. **Genital neoplasms** are distinctly **uncommon in** the **prepubertal age** group.
   a. **Benign growths** include vaginal and cervical polyps, vaginal adenosis, and vaginal and vulvar hemangiomas (10). Biopsy of the latter can lead to massive hemorrhage.
   b. **Malignant tumors** include sarcoma botryoides, adenocarcinoma of the cervix or vagina (especially in DES progeny), and ovarian tumors. Ovarian tumors, such as granulosa-theca cell tumors and other sex-cord stromal tumors, as well as dysgerminomas, can cause vaginal bleeding and incomplete isosexual precocity as a result of estrogen production (10).
   c. **Diagnosis** usually requires biopsy. Ultrasound is useful in looking for ovarian or other pelvic tumors.
   d. **Management** of malignant tumors requires referral to a gynecologic oncologist. Vaginal bleeding associated with sexual precocity also may require evaluation by a pediatric or gynecologic endocrinologist.
V. **Perimenarcheal bleeding.** Anovulatory DUB is the most common cause of abnormal bleeding in this age group, usually representing an immature hypothalamic-pituitary-ovarian axis. Following menarche at an average of 12 to 13 years, 80% of menstrual cycles are anovulatory in the first year. Regular ovulatory menstrual cycles are usually not established until the second year, with some irregularity persisting up to 5 years. It is well to remember that

coagulation defects, especially Von Willebrand's disease, can cause 20% of excessive abnormal uterine bleeding in this age group (13). If a patient has severe anemia (hemoglobin <10 g/dL) because of menorrhagia, the risk of a coagulopathy increases to 45% (13).

A. **History.** A history of irregular, heavy menses is classic for anovulatory DUB in this age group. In general, patients should be queried about onset of menses, duration and amount of flow, dysmenorrhea, sexual activity, and excessive bleeding resulting from minor surgical procedures (often dental procedures). A history of DES exposure leads to a search for vaginal or cervical adenosis or adenocarcinoma (see DES, Chapter 17).

B. **Physical examination.** The adolescent should be examined carefully and with sensitivity. DUB is often the precipitating event that leads to the first pelvic examination.
   1. **Abnormalities of the genital tract** should be noted.
   2. **Signs of pregnancy** should be sought.
   3. In most adolescents with abnormal bleeding, **the examination will be normal.**
   4. **In the virginal patient,** clinical judgment will decide the extent of the pelvic examination.

C. **Investigative procedures**
   1. **A complete blood cell count** (CBC) is often all that is needed to document the presence of anemia or thrombocytopenia. If anemia is present, the red cell indices should be noted since not all anemia is due to excessive menstruation.
   2. **Prothrombin (PT), partial thromboplastin (PTT), and bleeding time tests should be done if a coagulopathy is suspected.**
   3. **Thyroid function tests** should be done for evaluating thyroid dysfunction.
   4. **A pregnancy test** should be considered if sexual activity is suspected. Teenagers will often deny sexual activity.
   5. **A Papanicolaou (Pap) smear** is indicated in the sexually active adolescent.
   6. **Cultures for gonorrhea and chlamydial infections** should be done in the sexually active teenager.
   7. **Gonadotropin levels** are rarely necessary to investigate abnormal bleeding in this age group.
   8. **Ultrasound** is usually unnecessary unless a palpable mass is present.
   9. **Uterine curettage** is rarely necessary unless an organic etiology is suspected or the patient fails hormonal treatment. **Pregnancy must first be ruled out.**
   10. **Diagnostic hysteroscopy** may be a better choice to investigate the uterine cavity.

D. **Management.** Hormonal treatment will usually be effective if anovulatory DUB is the etiology of the bleeding. The lack of response to hormonal treatment should make the clinician suspicious of another cause for the abnormal bleeding. Other determined etiologies should be addressed specifically (e.g., pregnancy, pelvic inflammatory disease [see Pelvic Inflammatory Disease, Chapter 5]).
   1. **OCPs are the treatment of choice, especially if the teenager is sexually active.**
      a. Any OCP can be used in a dose of 1 tablet qid for 5 to 7 days. This is **followed by** use of a low-dose estrogen pill daily for 21 days.
      b. This regimen is then followed by 7 days of withdrawal that usually leads to a heavy menses. The patient and her family should be warned to expect this heavy period since this may be interpreted as failure of therapy.
      c. After several cycles of the pill, each succeeding period will become lighter. The pill can then be discontinued, and the patient can be followed for the onset of regular menses.

    d. The pill can also be continued in the sexually active patient, in those with a history of severe anemia, or in patients who are anxious about recurrence of heavy bleeding.

  2. Progestational agents

    a. Medroxyprogesterone (Provera), 10 mg qd, or **norethindrone,** 5 to 10 mg qd to bid, can be used. Patients must understand that this regimen does not provide contraception.

    b. This is continued for several days and then withdrawal bleeding is allowed. Since the withdrawal bleeding will be heavy, the patient must be warned that this does **not** represent treatment failure.

    c. OCPs can then be used cyclically.

    d. Alternatively, medroxyprogesterone, 10 mg qd for 10 days at the beginning of each month may be used to induce regular withdrawal bleeding.

  3. Profuse, persistent bleeding associated with anemia or hemodynamic changes is treated differently.

    a. Blood transfusion is indicated for severe anemia or unstable hemodynamics.

    b. Intravenous conjugated estrogens (Premarin), 25 mg IV, can be given every 4 hours for up to three doses to stop acute bleeding (11). Failure to control bleeding with this regimen mandates further investigation and usually requires curettage. After the acute bleeding stops with this regimen, OCPs or progesterone, as described earlier, should be started immediately to continue to control the bleeding.

VI. Reproductive age. The potential etiologies are noted in Table 12.2. DUB is less common in this age group. Pregnancy and its complications must be ruled out. Other common causes are noted in section III.A.2.

  A. History

    1. A **detailed menstrual history,** including the last menstrual period, age at menarche, frequency, duration, and amount of menstrual flow, must be obtained from all patients with abnormal bleeding.

    2. The **abnormal bleeding episode(s)** should be described in detail and related chronologically to the patient's menstrual pattern.

    3. Coexisting as well as precipitating factors, such as medical illnesses, medications, stress situations, changes in weight, dietary alterations, pain, dyspareunia, and any other relevant symptomatology, should be carefully sought.

    4. A **comprehensive medical history** should be obtained, looking for systemic causes for abnormal uterine bleeding. The possibility of a cagulopathy should be considered.

    5. Bleeding from other orifices should be considered as a possibility.

    6. Endocrinopathies, such as thyroid or adrenal diseases, should be noted. The combination of hirsutism, obesity, and oligomenorrhea suggests polycystic ovarian syndrome.

  B. Physical examination

    1. A **general physical examination** should be performed.

    2. Signs of anemia and chronic systemic diseases are sought.

    3. Obesity and hirsutism are noted if present.

    4. Pain or masses should be noted.

    5. A **thorough pelvic examination,** beginning with careful inspection of the external genitalia, urethral meatus, perineum, and perianal area is performed. The vaginal walls and cervix are inspected for the presence of gross lesions and retained foreign objects.

      a. Bimanual examination will document the shape and contour of the uterus and adnexa, as well as the presence of any tenderness or masses.

      b. Rectovaginal examination will evaluate the presence of lesions in the cul-de-sac or primary rectal lesions.

C. Investigative procedures
  1. **Cultures for gonorrhea and chlamydial infection** should be taken.
  2. **Cervical cytologic studies** are done to screen for cervical dysplasia or cancer.
      a. **Gross lesions of the cervix, vagina, and external genitalia** are biopsied for pathologic identification unless obvious.
      b. **All lesions suspicious for malignancy** must be biopsied.
      c. **Patients with abnormal Pap smears** showing dysplasia should be referred for colposcopy.
  3. **Stool occult blood** screening should be done to evaluate potential gastrointestinal sources for the bleeding.
  4. A **CBC** is useful to document anemia and/or thrombocytopenia.
  5. **PT, PTT, and a bleeding time** should be obtained if a coagulopathy is suspected.
  6. **Thyroid function tests** and **prolactin levels** are done to rule out endocrinopathies.
  7. **Urinalysis** is done to look for hematuria which can be caused by urinary tract infection, stones, or tumor.
  8. A **pregnancy test** is necessary to rule out pregnancy and its complications, such as abortion or ectopic gestation. Current urine pregnancy tests are sensitive; however, if doubt persists after a negative urine pregnancy test, a serum assay for the beta-subunit of human chorionic gonadotropin (hCG) will settle the issue.
  9. **Pelvic ultrasound** should be done for any palpable mass.
D. Management is dependent upon the determined etiology of the bleeding. Treatment issues pertaining to specific causes of abnormal bleeding, such as pelvic inflammatory disease (see Pelvic Inflammatory Disease, Chapter 5), leiomyomas or neoplasms (see Enlarged Uterus, Chapter 13; Adnexal Masses, Chapter 20), and pregnancy complications, are not covered in this chapter.
  1. **Ovulatory DUB** is usually due to midcycle bleeding or abnormal corpus luteum function.
      a. **Midcycle bleeding** occurs at the time of ovulation when the level of estrogen drops. It commonly manifests only as spotting and is usually not bothersome. In those patients who have bleeding and require treatment, oral estrogen therapy is used. **Conjugated estrogens (Premarin), 1.25 to 2.5 mg, or ethinyl estradiol, 20 µg, is given daily from 3 days before to 2 days after ovulation.**
      b. **Abnormal corpus luteum function** is usually diagnosed in association with infertility. It is suspected by menstrual cycles that have a shortened interval (<24 days). It is **diagnosed with an endometrial biopsy** that shows endometrial maturation 1 to 2 days out-of-phase in the secretory period. Its treatment is controversial.
          (1) If the patient desires pregnancy, then vaginal progesterone suppositories are sometimes used to augment the endogenously produced progesterone.
          (2) **Clomiphene citrate (Clomid)** is often used instead (see Infertility, Chapter 23).
          (3) OCPs can be used if contraception is desired.
          (4) If neither fertility nor contraception is important, then it is not necessary to treat the patient unless the irregular menstruation is bothersome, in which case, OCPs will serve well.
  2. **Anovulatory DUB** that occurs during reproductive years is often due to **polycystic ovarian syndrome or obesity.** These women often have prolonged amenorrhea or oligomenorrhea followed by menorrhagia. On the other hand, women who experience significant stress, perform strenuous exercise (marathon runners), or lose excessive weight (e.g., anorexics) have amenorrhea or oligomenorrhea with hypomenorrhea. This latter pattern results from hypothalamic hypogonadism (see Amenorrhea, Chapter 11).

    a. **Anovulatory cycles associated with amenorrhea or oligomenorrhea,** due to resulting from polycystic ovarian syndrome or obesity, lead to excessive estrogen exposure on the endometrium. The absence of a corpus luteum means that progesterone is not produced to balance the estrogen-stimulated proliferation. This persistently estrogen-stimulated endometrium is at risk to develop hyperplasia or cancer.

    b. **Endometrial biopsy** is indicated in patients older than 30 years with 12 months or more of anovulatory DUB and in occasional patients older than 20 years with frequent, prolonged, or excessive periods (1,3). This is necessary to identify those patients at risk for endometrial hyperplasia, atypical hyperplasia, or rarely cancer. Most often, biopsy will show evidence of hyperplasia.

    c. **Infertility** is a common problem in this group because anovulation results in no ovum being available for fertilization in the cycle.

    d. **Hirsutism** is also common. It results from chronic exposure to excessive ovarian production of androgens, primarily androstenedione (11).

    e. **Treatment** depends on the patient's desire for fertility.

        (1) **If pregnancy is desired,** then ovulation induction is indicated (see Infertility, Chapter 23).

        (2) **To regulate menses** when pregnancy is not desired, supplemental progesterone or OCP is used.

            (a) The patient can be treated with medroxyprogesterone (Provera), 10 mg qd, for 10 days each month, followed by withdrawal bleeding.

            (b) Occasionally, sporadic ovulation occurs in these patients, and thus, they are at risk for pregnancy.

            (c) If the patient desires to avoid pregnancy, then low-dose estrogen OCPs can be used instead. The OCPs have the added advantage of helping to control hirsutism (11).

3. **Functional ovarian cysts** are often responsible for abnormal periods. They are either follicular cysts or persistent corpus luteum cysts. They are referred to as functional cysts because they produce hormones.

    a. **They are often palpable** and can reach 6 cm in diameter.

    b. **Any adnexal mass of 6 cm or more** requires further investigation (see Adnexal Masses, Chapter 20).

    c. **Use of OCPs** may be successful in suppressing the cysts.

    d. **Failure to resolve within 1 to 2 months,** with or without use of OCPs, requires further evaluation to rule out a neoplasm.

4. **Functional ovarian tumors** are neoplastic growths that do not resolve spontaneously and are not suppressible with OCPs. They also produce hormones, usually either estrogen or androgens. These include granulosa cell and theca cell tumors, arrhenoblastomas, and some malignant ovarian tumors. The management is primarily surgical.

5. **Menorrhagia or intermenstrual bleeding** is a common menstrual disorder. It is one of the most common causes of iron deficiency anemia (3). When not associated with DUB, it often represents anatomic abnormalities. The differential diagnosis includes uterine fibroids, endometrial polyps, endometriosis, adenomyosis, chronic pelvic inflammatory disease, ovarian abnormalities, massive obesity, coagulopathies, severe hypothyroidism, and endometrial hyperplasia or carcinoma. Pregnancy and its complications must be ruled out. Some evaluation of the uterine cavity is indicated by endometrial biopsy, formal dilation and curettage (D & C), or hysteroscopy.

    a. **Diagnostic hysteroscopy** has become popular in the evaluation of abnormal uterine bleeding because of its ability to visualize the uterine cavity directly. There is literature to suggest that it is more accurate in defining the exact pathology compared to endometrial biopsy since hysteroscopy can visualize the entire cavity, whereas endometrial sampling recovers only 1% of the endometrial volume (6).

    b. Hysteroscopic surgery is commonly performed for the treatment of uterine bleeding disorders. In skilled hands, submucous leiomyomas and endometrial polyps can easily be removed using a resectoscope (7).

        (1) If no specific pathologic process can be found and the patient has persistent menorrhagia, then endometrial ablation can be used to destroy the endometrium, with resultant cessation or decrease of menses.

        (2) Current methods for endometrial destruction involve laser ablation, use of the resectoscope, "roller-ball" cautery, or the thermal balloon. Roller-ball cautery is still the most common method used (7).

        (3) Endometrial atypia, pregnancy, or cancer must be ruled out prior to endometrial ablation.

        (4) The endometrium should be hormonally prepared with medroxyprogesterone (Provera or Depo-Provera), danazol, gonadotropin-releasing hormone (GnRH) agonists, or OCPs. The specifics for hormonal preparation are beyond the scope of this book.

    c. Nonsteroidal antiinflammatory agents are sometimes effective in controlling menorrhagia. Agents that have been used include **mefenamic acid (Ponstel),** 500 mg tid, and **naproxen (Naprosyn),** 500 mg as an initial dose followed by 250 mg tid. Gastrointestinal side effects are diminished if taken with food (7).

    d. Hysterectomy has been used to control menorrhagia as a last resort when medical therapy and uterine curettage fail.

VII. Perimenopausal bleeding. The causes of bleeding in this age group include those mentioned for the reproductive-age group (discussed in section VI.). Anovulatory DUB again becomes a common cause of abnormal bleeding. This occurs as a result of the greatly diminished number of follicles remaining in the ovary and the growing refractoriness of the residual follicles to gonadotropin stimulation (1). As a consequence, follicle-stimulating hormone (FSH) levels are elevated and circulating estradiol levels are lower, compared with the reproductive years. As the follicles fail to ovulate, corpus luteum function ceases. Unopposed estrogen leads to endometrial proliferation, hyperplasia, and sometimes endometrial cancer. The irregular menstrual shedding is responsible for the abnormal bleeding.

    A. Evaluation of the perimenopausal woman with abnormal bleeding is the same as in the reproductive-aged woman.

        1. Pregnancy is an unusual cause but should be ruled out if the sexually active woman is not using birth control.

        2. A menstrual history should be taken, as well as a description of the abnormal bleeding episodes.

        3. A careful pelvic examination is mandatory, looking for evidence of neoplasia or other anatomic causes for the bleeding.

        4. A Pap smear must be done.

        5. A CBC should be obtained to determine whether anemia is present if bleeding has been excessive.

        6. Endometrial sampling is necessary to rule out endometrial hyperplasia (with or without atypia) or endometrial cancer.

        7. An ultrasound should be obtained to rule out fibroids.

    B. Treatment of anovulatory DUB in the perimenopausal woman involves use of **progesterone** to counterbalance the effects of unopposed estrogen on the endometrium. If the endometrial sampling shows simple proliferation or simple, adenomatous, or cystic hyperplasia without atypia, then the condition should respond to progestin therapy.

1. **Medroxyprogesterone,** 10 mg qd for 10 to 14 days each month, is used until menopause occurs.
2. **If the initial pathologic workup revealed endometrial hyperplasia,** then repeat endometrial sampling is done in 3 to 6 months to demonstrate the reversal of the endometrial hyperplasia. Preferably, the timing should be after completion of 10 days of progesterone therapy and prior to the next menses to show the secretory effects on the endometrium.
3. **The presence of atypical hyperplasia or cancer** requires hysterectomy for definitive treatment since these conditions will not resolve with progestin therapy.

VIII. **Postmenopausal bleeding** is defined as any amount of bleeding that occurs after a 12-month cessation of regular menstrual flow. The irregular, acyclic bleeding that characterizes the perimenopausal period can make it difficult to determine when menopause has begun. Bleeding that occurs 1 year after cessation of flow or that begins after the onset of vasomotor changes demands investigation. Those at risk for endometrial cancer, such as obese, hypertensive, or diabetic patients or those receiving unopposed estrogen therapy, should have investigation as soon as possible.

A. **History.** A complete description of the bleeding episode as well as a thorough medical history must be obtained.
1. **Any history of systemic diseases,** particularly diabetes mellitus, hypertension, liver disease, or obesity, should be noted.
2. **Use of medications,** especially that of estrogen or progesterone, is especially relevant.

B. **Physical examination** includes a general examination, with careful attention to the abdominal and pelvic examination.

C. **Investigative procedures**
1. **Routine pap smear.**
2. **Cultures for gonorrhea and chlamydia.** These infections may be considered but are an unusual cause of bleeding in the postmenopausal woman.
3. **CBC.**
4. **Stool occult blood testing.**
5. **Urinalysis** for hematuria.
6. **Pelvic ultrasound.** Any palpable mass requires this procedure.
7. **Endometrial sampling** by endometrial biopsy or D & C. **An endocervical curettage** or cytobrush sampling should also be done to rule out endocervical disease.
   a. If a diagnosis is made by endometrial biopsy, then a formal D & C is not necessary.
   b. Lesions can still be missed in the uterine cavity with the four-quadrant technique.
   c. If the pathologic findings on endometrial biopsy are not consistent with the clinical impression, then a formal D & C or hysteroscopy should be performed.
8. **Diagnostic hysteroscopy** (see section VI.D.5.a.).

D. **Etiology**
1. The **benign causes** of postmenopausal bleeding are most common.
   a. **Atrophic vaginitis** is due to lack of estrogen stimulation. The vaginal wall becomes thin and atrophic, with loss of rugae (folds). It is susceptible to bleeding resulting from the slightest trauma.
   b. **Atrophic endometrium** also results from estrogen deficiency. The endometrium becomes thin, with simple tubular glands and occasionally, cystically dilated glands. The stroma is dense, cellular, and compact (4). The thin endometrium is susceptible to bleeding, usually manifesting as spotting. Endometrial sampling will demonstrate atrophy. Unfortunately, endometrial cancer can be present in limited foci with surrounding atrophic endometrium. Persistent postmenopausal bleeding in a patient with atrophic endometrium

should have further evaluation by formal D & C or hysteroscopy or both.

    c. Endometrial or endocervical polyps occasionally contribute to vaginal spotting.

        (1) Cervical polyps are almost invariably benign. They can be removed by twisting off with a ring forceps.

        (2) Endometrial polyps can be missed, even with the most careful curettage. Often they are discovered only at hysteroscopy or after hysterectomy.

    d. Endometrial hyperplasia is caused by excess endogenous estrogen (as seen in obesity and diabetes) or unopposed estrogen therapy.

  2. The **malignant causes** should be ruled out systematically. Malignancy is more likely the longer the interval since cessation of menses.

    a. Endometrial adenocarcinoma is seen in about 20% of postmenopausal women who present with bleeding (4). Atypical endometrial hyperplasia is considered a precursor and can be documented with endometrial sampling.

    b. Cervical cancer can be found on routine screening with a **Pap smear. Gross cervical lesions should be biopsied even if the Pap smear is negative.**

    c. Ovarian cancer occasionally produces hormones (estrogen or androgens) that can lead to postmenopausal bleeding.

    d. Fallopian tube cancer classically presents with a **watery vaginal discharge** and a **pelvic mass,** but more commonly, **scant vaginal bleeding** occurs. **If endometrial sampling fails** to yield a diagnosis, ultrasound should be done.

    e. Gastrointestinal and urinary tract cancers also cause bleeding, and bleeding from the rectum or urethra can be misinterpreted as vaginal bleeding.

E. Management of postmenopausal bleeding is primarily directed at determining the etiology of the bleeding and then providing appropriate treatment.

  1. Atrophic changes of either the vulva or vagina can readily be treated with exogenous estrogen replacement.

    a. Conjugated estrogens, 0.625 mg/day, is sufficient to reverse atrophy of the vagina. Alternatively, estrogen cream will suffice to treat atrophic vaginitis on a short-term basis.

    b. Progesterone is needed to counterbalance the effects of estrogen on the endometrium. This can be accomplished by cyclic regimens or continuous, combined hormone replacement therapies.

        (1) Medroxyprogesterone, 5 to 10 mg qd is given for 10 to 14 days each month. This is sufficient to reverse the effects of estrogen on the endometrium.

        (2) Continuous, combined estrogen and progesterone regimens reduce the doses of progesterone needed. **Conjugated estrogens, 0.625 mg, and medroxyprogesterone, 2.5 to 5 mg,** are each given daily. Irregular spotting is common for the first 3 to 6 months. **A baseline endometrial biopsy is recommended prior to starting therapy** to ensure that the baseline endometrium is benign.

  2. Adenomatous hyperplasia in the postmenopausal woman is abnormal and represents either unopposed exogenous estrogen therapy or excess endogenous estrogen production.

    a. The diabetic, hypertensive, or obese patient is at risk for endogenous estrogen production.

    b. Hysterectomy and bilateral salpingo-oophorectomy is indicated for definitive treatment.

    c. In those patients who are not candidates for surgery, high-dose progesterone therapy (e.g., Megace) can be considered as an alternative.

    d. Repeat endometrial sampling is mandatory to document that the lesion has not progressed to cancer.

    3. **Endometrial cancer and other malignancies** in their early stages are amenable to therapy by surgery, radiation, or chemotherapy. These malignancies are best managed in consultation with a gynecologic oncologist.

References

1. Bayer SR, DeCherney AH. Clinical manifestations and treatment of dysfunctional uterine bleeding. *JAMA* 1993;269:1823.
2. Droegemuller W. Pediatric gynecology. In: Herbst AL, Mishell DR Jr, Stenchever MA, et al., eds. *Comprehensive gynecology,* 3rd ed. St. Louis: Mosby-Year Book, 1997.
3. Field CS. Dysfunctional uterine bleeding. *Primary Care* 1988;15:561.
4. Fortier KJ. Postmenopausal bleeding and the endometrium. *Clin Obstet Gynecol* 1986;29:440.
5. Kustin J, Rebar RW. Menstrual disorders in the adolescent age group. *Primary Care* 1987;14:139.
6. Loffer FL. Hysteroscopy with selective endometrial sampling compared with D&C for abnormal uterine bleeding: the value of a negative hysteroscopic view. *Obstet Gynecol* 1989;73:16.
7. Mishell DR. Abnormal uterine bleeding. In Herbst AL, Mishell Jr DR, Stenchever MA, et al., eds. *Comprehensive gynecology,* 3rd ed. St. Louis: Mosby-Year Book, 1997.
8. Richards-Kustan CJ, Kase NG. Diagnosis and management of perimenopausal bleeding. *Obstet Gynecol Clin North Am* 1987;14:169.
9. Sandler B, Kase NG. Normal and abnormal menstruation. In Kase NG, Weingold AB, Gershenson DM, eds. *Principles and practice of clinical gynecology.* New York: Churchill Livingstone, 1990.
10. Sanfilippo JS, Wakim NG. Bleeding and vulvovaginitis in the pediatric age group. *Clin Obstet Gynecol* 1987;30:653.
11. Speroff L, Glass RH, Kase NG. Dysfunctional uterine bleeding. In: Speroff L, Glass RH, Kase NG, eds. *Clinical gynecologic endocrinology and infertility,* 6th ed. Philadelphia: Lippincott Williams & Wilkins, 1999.
12. Weingold AB. Abnormal bleeding. In: Kase NG, Weingold AB, Gershenson DM, eds. *Principles and practice of clinical gynecology.* New York: Churchill Livingstone, 1990.
13. Zimmermann R. Dysfunctional uterine bleeding. *Obstet Gynecol Clin North Am* 1988;15:107.

13. THE ENLARGED UTERUS

Jeanne A. Conry

The enlarged uterus may present in a variety of ways. During a routine bimanual examination, an **enlarged uterus** may be found **unexpectedly.** It is **most common during the reproductive years.** There are no unique problems in the prepubertal or postmenopausal aged groups, with the exception of hematometra at the beginning of menarche.

Historically, an enlarged uterus may be suspected in association with **symptoms such as abnormal bleeding, pelvic pain, dysmenorrhea, missed menstrual periods, and difficulty with urination or defecation.** The **uterus should be examined for size, shape, consistency, mobility, position, and tenderness.** The actual size of the uterus should be compared with normal dimensions.

The uterus is pear-shaped. The nulliparous uterus is approximately 8 cm long, 5 cm wide, and 2.5 cm in the anteroposterior diameter and weighs 40 to 50 g. The uterus of a multiparous woman is approximately 9 cm long, 6 cm wide, and 3.5 cm in the anteroposterior diameter and can weigh up to 80 g. The **prepubertal** and **postmenopausal** uteri are much **smaller.** On **transabdominal ultrasound,** the approximate size of the uterus in a normal adult woman is $8 \times 4 \times 4$ cm. It will appear smaller in the postmenopausal and larger in the multiparous patient.

At times, the origin of the pelvic mass may not be clear, and other **diagnostic methods,** such as transabdominal or transvaginal ultrasound, CT scanning, pyelogram, MRI, and barium enema are useful for diagnosis. In some cases, the diagnosis remains uncertain and the patient will require a **diagnostic laparoscopy, exploratory laparotomy, or hysteroscopy.**

I. **Hematometra.** The uterus is distended with blood secondary to partial or complete obstruction of the lower genital tract. The obstruction of the uterus, cervix, or vagina may be congenital or acquired.
   A. **History**
      1. The **adolescent menarchal** patient may present with **amenorrhea, cyclic lower abdominal cramping pain** of increasing severity, and a gradually enlarging **pelvic mass** if the drainage of the uterus is blocked at the level of the vagina or hymen.
      2. **Urinary frequency or even urinary retention** may be reported because of the mass effect of the enlarged uterus.
      3. **Hematometra** in a postmenopausal woman may be asymptomatic or associated with lower abdominal pain as well. The etiology may range from a malignant process to a blockage of the withdrawal bleeding during estrogen and progesterone therapy.
      4. Hematometra can develop secondarily in response to cervical stenosis, following a LEEP, cryotherapy, laser ablation, or cone biopsy.
   B. **Physical examination**
      1. **Secondary sex characteristics** consistent with menarche are found.
      2. **If the hymen is imperforate,** there may be a tense bulging hymnal membrane.
      3. **If the blockage is higher, a transverse vaginal septum** may be seen on pelvic examination.
      4. With **congenital absence of the vagina,** the external genitalia are normal, and there is a 1- to 2-cm dimple above the hymen.
      5. **Rectovaginal examination** will reveal a **large boggy pelvic mass.**
      6. If the cervix is visible, it can be probed with a small dilator. Old dark blood will escape. If pus is found, a diagnosis of pyometra is made.

C. **Investigative procedures**
   1. **Ultrasonography** may be useful in demonstrating cystic enlargement of the uterine cavity and the presence or absence of pelvic structures.
   2. A **pyelogram** should be ordered if a congenital defect is suspected as the cause of the hematocolpometra since anomalies of the vagina may be associated with urinary tract defects.
   3. In complicated cases in which **duplication of the vagina, cervix, or uterus is suspected, laparoscopy** may aid in diagnosis.
D. **Management**
   1. The **imperforate hymen** can be opened by a cruciate incision using scalpel, cautery, or laser, preferably before puberty.
   2. A **complete vaginal septum** can be sharply excised or removed.

II. **Pregnancy.** The **diagnosis of a normal or abnormal pregnancy must be considered** in any woman of reproductive age when an enlarged uterus is found.
A. **History**
   1. The patient usually (but not always) reports a **missed menstrual period or abnormal menses.**
   2. The normal symptoms of pregnancy may be present or may be exaggerated in the case of **molar pregnancy.**
B. **Physical examination**
   1. **In a normal pregnancy**
      a. **The uterine size** is consistent with the last menstrual period.
      b. **The uterus is soft, smooth, and symmetric.**
      c. **Heart tones** may be heard with Doppler ultrasound at 12-weeks gestation.
      d. **Fetal cardiac activity** is apparent by 6-weeks gestation on vaginal probe ultrasound.
   2. With **a missed abortion,** the uterus may be smaller than expected and can be confirmed by vaginal probe ultrasound.
   3. **In a molar pregnancy**
      a. The **uterus may be larger.**
      b. **Heart tones are absent.**
C. **Investigative procedures**
   1. A **pregnancy test,** especially the quantitative measurement of the serum beta-subunit of human chorionic gonadotropin (hCG), will be helpful.
   2. **Ultrasonography** may distinguish viable pregnancies from missed abortions and molar pregnancies.
D. **Management**
   1. **Viable pregnancies** are managed as the patient desires.
   2. **Appropriate counseling and follow-up** must be given to the patient who originally denies that her abdominal mass could be a pregnancy.
   3. **Abnormal pregnancies** may be evacuated **or** managed expectantly, depending on clinical indications and patient preference.
   4. **Molar pregnancies** must be evacuated and monitored.

III. Adenomyosis is a benign condition characterized by the presence of endometrial glands and stroma within the myometrium. The uterus may be enlarged to two to three times normal size. Adenomyosis is found in 20% of hysterectomy specimens (15).
A. **History.** Although often an incidental finding at the time of hysterectomy, the typical patient is a parous woman older than 30 years who presents with a history of menorrhagia and secondary dysmenorrhea.
   1. Both the **quantity and duration of flow** may be increased.
   2. Often there is **progressive dysmenorrhea** occurring just before and during the menstrual period. Adenomyosis causes dysmenorrhea because of menstrual flow occurring within the myometrium (5).
   3. Approximately 30% of patients will be completely asymptomatic.
B. **Physical examination**
   1. There may be **diffuse globular enlargement of the uterus.** This uterine enlargement may be two to three times normal size.

2. There may be **soft and tender areas in the uterus** just before or during menstruation.

C. **Investigative procedures**
1. **Ultrasonography** may be helpful to distinguish adenomyosis from leiomyomas.
2. **Hysteroscopy** is useful in identifying the entrance of the diverticula into the mucosal layer (3).
3. **MRI** provided a correct diagnosis in 88% of the pathologically proven cases of adenomyosis (2). The distinction between fibroids and adenomyosis is of clinical importance because of the alternative treatments available (19). However, this is a very expensive test and not cost-effective for diagnosis.
4. An **endometrial biopsy, dilation and curettage (D & C), or hysteroscopy are done in all cases of abnormal bleeding during the later reproductive years** to rule out an endometrial malignancy.

D. **Management**
1. **Hysterectomy is the definitive treatment for adenomyosis and the only way to establish the diagnosis** with certainty. The decision to proceed with this step depends on reproductive goals and symptomatology.
2. The **decision to remove the ovaries** should be based on the patient's age and the presence or absence of ovarian lesions.
3. **Endometrial ablation** is a technique that is used to control abnormal bleeding without a hysterectomy by destroying the endometrial lining.
4. **Medical management** of biopsy-proven adenomyosis with continuous gonadotropin-releasing hormone (GnRH) analogues (such as depot leuprolide 3.75–7.5 mg IM per month) results in amenorrhea and relief of severe dysmenorrhea. It may prove useful for temporary management of adenomyosis (12). Add-back replacement with hormone therapy is advised if GnRH is continued beyond 6 months.

IV. **Leiomyomas** (also called **myomas** or **fibroids**) are benign tumors of the uterus and are composed mainly of smooth muscle with some fibrous connective tissue elements. Leiomyomas are the most common pelvic tumors and one third of the hysterectomies performed annually are for fibroids (22). Approximately 20% to 25% of women older than 35 years have a uterine myoma. Leiomyomas are usually asymptomatic, more common in black women than in white women, rare before puberty, and usually shrink after menopause. They are estrogen-dependent and may grow during estrogen replacement therapy (peri- and postmenopausal) or during pregnancy. They are single or, more commonly, multiple tumors in the uterine corpus (i.e., intramural, subserosal, or submucosal). They can be pedunculated and, on occasion, involve the cervix, round ligament, or broad ligament.

A. **History**
1. **Abnormal bleeding** is the most common symptom associated with leiomyomas. Initially, there may be an increase only in menstrual flow. However, patients may have any type of abnormal bleeding, including continuous bleeding and severe hemorrhage. Other sources of abnormal bleeding should also be considered in the work-up of leiomyomas. **Fibroids will usually cause menorrhagia rather than metrorrhagia.**
2. **Pain is not characteristic** of leiomyomas, although it can be present in up to one third of patients.
   a. It generally occurs with the menstrual cycle and may be caused by a submucous or pedunculated leiomyoma stimulating uterine contractions.
   b. Acute pain with leiomyomas is **associated with torsion** of a pedunculated leiomyoma **or degeneration** of a large myoma.
3. As leiomyomas enlarge, they may cause a feeling of **pelvic heaviness or produce pressure symptoms** by compressing nearby organs.

       a. Constipation may occur as well as decreased bladder capacity or urinary retention.

       b. Occasionally, there may be **compression of one or both ureters.**

    4. Infertility may be a presenting complaint with leiomyomas. Although large leiomyomas are compatible with pregnancy, they may on occasion be a factor in infertility, according to one large study (20). When leiomyomas are the presumed cause of infertility, 17% of patients become pregnant after myomectomy (16). Preconception counseling regarding fibroids should address an 18% risk of spontaneous abortion, a 15% risk of painful myomas, 20% to 30% preterm labor rate, and the risk of malpresentations and malformations (16).

B. Physical examination. On bimanual examination, the **uterus is distorted by one or more smooth, spherical, firm masses.** The uterine size is estimated in weeks, corresponding to the pregnant uterus of the same size. It is often not obvious whether the pelvic mass is of uterine origin.

C. Investigative procedures

    1. A blood count may show findings consistent with **iron-deficiency anemia,** even in the face of iron supplementation.

    2. A fetus can coexist with a leiomyomatous uterus, hence before other studies are done, **pregnancy should be ruled out.**

    3. An endometrial biopsy, D & C, or hysteroscopy should be done for abnormal bleeding to rule out other endometrial anomalies in women who are at risk.

    4. Ultrasonography may aid in the definition of a mass but it cannot always differentiate between a uterine and ovarian mass.

    5. Occasionally, an **intravenous pyelogram** may be useful in the case of a large uterus, because it may show urethral deviation or compression. Calcifications in leiomyomas may be seen on the x-ray films.

    6. If there is any question of whether the pelvic tumor is **ovarian, rather than uterine** in origin, **laparoscopy or laparotomy** should be performed to rule out an ovarian malignancy.

    7. Hysteroscopy may aid in the diagnosis and treatment of **submucous fibroids.**

D. Management of leiomyomas depends on the patient's symptoms, age, parity, desire for future pregnancies, and the size of the leiomyomatous uterus.

    1. Surgical intervention has been recommended routinely when a uterus reaches a 12- to 14-week size, although no prospective studies have established the degree of risk for not intervening. Size alone is not an adequate indication for treatment (14).

       a. Normally, the treatment would be a **hysterectomy.**

       b. Myomectomy may be done to preserve fertility by performing laparoscopy, hysteroscopy, or exploratory laparotomy. The 10-year recurrence risk is 27% (4).

    2. Leiomyomas are removed when they cause pain, abnormal bleeding that is uncontrolled by hormone management, pressure, compromise to pelvic organs, or a rapid change in size.

       a. Hysterectomy is the procedure of choice **if** fertility is not a consideration.

       b. For **infertility** with no other origin, **myomectomy may improve** fertility.

       c. If bleeding is the only symptom and uterine pathology has been ruled out, **endometrial ablation with fibroid resection** may be indicated.

    3. Asymptomatic leiomyomas may be followed by annual examinations.

       a. After menopause, the leiomyomas usually **shrink and they should never grow.**

       b. Rapid growth, or any growth after menopause, is cause for hysterectomy to rule out sarcoma.

    c. **Estrogens** should be used cautiously before and after the menopause since they **may cause leiomyomas to grow.**
    d. **Medical therapy** can be used to control bleeding or to shrink fibroids (14). **Progestins,** such as medroxyprogesterone acetate (Provera), 10 mg PO for 10 to 13 days each month, can control excessive bleeding and are useful especially for perimenopausal women. The **GnRH analogues** induce pseudomenopause, resulting in decreased tumor volume. Although their use in long-term management is limited, presurgical treatment and temporary symptomatic relief prove useful. Most studies have shown that myomas return to their previous size within 6 months of treatment (17). In a study of perimenopausal women treated for 6 months with GnRH agonists, about 30% did not experience a regrowth of fibroids.
    e. **Radiologic uterine artery embolization** is becoming an alternative to hysterectomy in the treatment of fibroids (13). Reports have shown up to a 60% reduction in uterine volume within 2 to 4 months of treatment. Presently, the procedure is **not** recommended for women who desire future fertility.

V. Uterine cancers. Of all the causes of the enlarged uterus, uterine cancers are the most serious and **are always considered in the differential diagnosis.**

    Endometrial carcinoma is now the most frequent pelvic genital cancer in women. Carcinoma of the endometrium occurs during the reproductive and postmenopausal years, with a median age of 61. Risk factors include obesity, nulliparity, unopposed estrogen, tamoxifen therapy, and late menopause. Diabetes mellitus and hypertension can be associated with endometrial cancer.

    Uterine sarcomas are rare and usually fatal. The most common symptoms are a **rapidly enlarging uterus and vaginal bleeding.** However, in a literature review, less than 3% of patients with leiomyosarcoma had a history of a rapidly growing uterus (1). Endometrial stromal sarcomas are usually composed of endometrial glands and stroma. Leiomyosarcomas develop from the myometrium. The rarely occurring angiosarcomas and fibrosarcomas arise from supporting tissues. The mean age for patients with leiomyosarcoma is in the mid-50s. Patients with mixed mesodermal or endometrial and stromal sarcomas are usually in their mid-40s.

    A. History
        1. **Painless vaginal bleeding** is the hallmark of endometrial carcinoma. Postmenopausal bleeding or abnormal perimenopausal bleeding should always be assumed to be an underlying malignancy until proven otherwise.
        2. Patients may complain of **pelvic pain caused by uterine contractions** if the cervix is blocked off and there is blood, pus, or tumor trapped in the uterus. Pain usually occurs as a late symptom in the disease process.
        3. The **symptoms of uterine sarcoma** are not distinctive and are **similar to myomas.**
            a. **Abnormal bleeding may be absent.**
            b. **Serosanguinous vaginal discharge** may occur.
            c. The patient may notice a **rapidly growing uterus** and have pain from pressure on surrounding organs.
            d. The patient may also have **symptoms of generalized disease,** such as weight loss and weakness.
    B. Physical examination
        1. **The uterus is often symmetrically enlarged.** The patient should be questioned carefully concerning a history of uterine enlargement.
        2. **A necrotic mass** may be protruding from the os, and a biopsy specimen should be taken.
        3. **If the uterine cancer is advanced,** there may be induration or fixation of the tissue surrounding the uterus.

C. **Investigative procedures**
  1. Sampling of the endometrium by **endometrial biopsy or fractional D & C** is the definitive procedure for diagnosis of endometrial carcinoma and also may make the diagnosis of uterine sarcoma.
  2. **Routine laboratory evaluation** should include blood count, urinalysis, liver function tests, and creatinine.
  3. **Ultrasonography, CT scan, or MRI** of the pelvis may be useful to clarify the uterine or ovarian origin of the tumor and also to demonstrate tumor spread.
  4. The **pyelogram** can be used to evaluate the ureters.
  5. A **chest x-ray** film should be obtained to rule out pulmonary metastasis.
  6. **In spite of adequate history, physical examination, and investigative procedures,** the diagnosis of uterine sarcoma may not be appropriately made (8). There may be confusion with leiomyomas, adenomyosis, and ovarian pathologic processes.
     a. **Therefore, when any question exists concerning the diagnosis of an enlarged uterus, laparoscopy or laparotomy must be used as a diagnostic procedure.**
     b. Since the diagnoses of uterine sarcoma and adenomyosis are often made only after study of the removed uterus, **hysterectomy may be necessary** to make the proper diagnosis.
D. **Management**
  1. **Endometrial carcinoma** may be treated in several ways:
     a. **Abdominal hysterectomy** with removal of the tubes and ovaries is the treatment of choice.
     b. **Pelvic and paraaortic lymph node dissection** is used in selected cases.
     c. If extensive disease within the uterus is found or if metastases outside the uterus is noted, appropriate **radiation, progestins, or chemotherapy** are employed.
  2. **Uterine sarcoma**
     a. **Abdominal hysterectomy with removal of the tubes and ovaries** is by far the most effective therapy for uterine sarcomas.
     b. **Bilateral pelvic lymphadenectomy** may be especially helpful in low-grade lesions.
     c. **Radiation** when used **in combination with surgery** may improve survival slightly, but the efficacy of this therapy is questionable.
     d. **Adjuvant chemotherapy** is being used selectively in the hope of improving outcome.

References
1. Allen-Davis JT, Schlaff WD. Dysfunctional uterine bleeding, polyps, and fibroids. *Infertility Reprod Med Clin North Am* 1995;6:401.
2. Ascher SA, et al. Adenomyosis: prospective comparison of MRI and transvaginal sonography. *J Radiol* 1994;190:803.
3. Baggish MS, et al. *Diagnostic and operative hysteroscopy: a text and atlas*. Chicago: Year Book Medical, 1989.
4. Candiani GB, et al. Risks of recurrence after myomectomy. *Br J Obstet Gynaecol* 1991;98:385.
5. Dawood MY. Dysmenorrhea. *Infertility Reprod Med Clin of North Am* 1995.
6. DiSaia PJ, Creasman WT. Adenocarcinoma of the uterus. In: DiSaia PJ, Creasman WT, eds. *Clinical gynecologic oncology*. St. Louis: Mosby, 1997.
7. DiSaia PJ, Creasman WT. Sarcoma of the uterus. In: DiSaia PJ, Creasman WT, eds. *Clinical gynecologic oncology*. St. Louis: Mosby, 1997.
8. Dover RW, et al. Sarcoma and the conservative management of uterine fibroids: a cause for concern. *Aust NZ J Obstet Gynecol* 2000;40:308.
9. Droegemueller W. Anatomy. In: Droegemueller W, et al., eds. *Comprehensive gynecology*. St. Louis: Mosby, 1987.

10. Droegemueller W. Benign gynecologic lesions. In: Droegemueller W, et al., eds. *Comprehensive gynecology*. St. Louis: Mosby, 1987.
11. Gompel C, Silverberg SG. The corpus uteri. In: Gompel C, Silverberg SG, eds. *Pathology in gynecology and obstetrics*. Philadelphia: Lippincott-Raven, 1994.
12. Grow DR, Valle RF. Treatment of adenomyosis with long-term GnRH analogues: a case report. *Obstet Gynecol* 1991;78:538.
13. Hurst BS, et al. Uterine artery embolization for symptomatic myomas. *Fertility and Sterility* 2000;74:855.
14. Hutchins FL. Uterine fibroids: current concepts in management. *Female Patient* 1990;15(10):29.
15. Lacey CG. Benign disorders of the uterine corpus. In Pernoll ML, Benson RC, eds. *Current obstetric and gynecology diagnosis and treatment*. Norwalk, CT: Appleton & Lange, 1987.
16. Lanouette JM, Diamond MP. Pregnancy in women with myoma uteri. *Infertility Reprod Med Clin North Am* 1996;7:19.
17. Lemay, A. and R. Maheux. GnRH agonists in the management of uterine leiomyoma. *Infertility Reprod Med Clin North Am* 1996;7:33.
18. Merrill JA, Creasman WT. Lesions of the corpus uteri. In: Danforth DN, Scott JR, eds. *Danforth's obstetrics and gynecology*, 7th ed. Philadelphia: Harper & Row, 1996.
19. Murase E, et al. Uterine leiomyomas: histopathologic features, MR imaging findings, differential diagnosis, and treatment. *Radiographics* 1999;19:1179.
20. Neuwirth RS. Leiomyomas of the uterus. In: Sciarra JJ, ed. *Gynecology and obstetrics*. Philadelphia: Lippincott, 1987.
21. Sarti DA. Gynecologic application of ultrasound. In: Sarti DA, ed. *Atlas of obstetric and gynecology ultrasound*. Boston: GK Hall, 1984.
22. Sullivan MW, Guzick DS. The natural history of uterine myomas. *Infertility Reprod Med Clin North Am* 1996;7:1.
23. Thompson HE. Diagnostic ultrasound in gynecology. In Sciarra JJ, ed. *Gynecology and obstetrics*. Philadelphia: Lippincott, 1988.

14. DYSMENORRHEA

Patti Tilton

The word **dysmenorrhea** means **painful menstruation.** It also refers to a syndrome or **symptom complex that may encompass nausea, vomiting, headache, nervousness, fatigue, diarrhea, syncope, lower abdominal cramping, bloating, breast tenderness, mood changes, backache, and dizziness.** These symptoms often appear just before (24–48 hours) or at the onset of menstruation and are maximal during the first 48 hours afterward. Pelvic pain associated with the menses may be a result of physiologic events such as ovulation, premenstrual syndrome, or primary or secondary dysmenorrhea. These conditions can include similar symptoms; however, each is believed to have a different pathophysiology.

Dysmenorrhea is one of the most common gynecologic disorders. Estimates of incidence among menstruating women vary from 3% to 90%, depending on the population studied and the criteria used to define dysmenorrhea. It is perhaps the **greatest single cause of lost work and school days among young women.** Therefore, correct diagnosis and treatment can have a significant effect on individual well-being and economic loss.

Parous women usually have less dysmenorrhea than nulliparous women do. Some studies have shown that obesity increases the severity of dysmenorrhea. Older women in higher socioeconomic groups are at increased risk of having dysmenorrhea, especially if they are single. Women who start menstruating at a younger age and who have heavy bleeding during their periods are more prone to have dysmenorrhea. In families where mothers and sisters have dysmenorrhea, there is an increased risk that the remaining sisters will also have it.

Dysmenorrhea is usually divided into two categories, primary and secondary.

   I. **Primary dysmenorrhea.** In primary dysmenorrhea (intrinsic, essential, idiopathic), there is **no macroscopic clinically detectable pelvic pathologic process.** It usually begins with the onset of ovulatory cycles from 6 to 12 months to 2 years after menarche and generally becomes more severe with time, peaking at ages 23 to 27, then decreasing in severity. Primary dysmenorrhea is believed to be **caused by factors intrinsic to uterine physiology** and is often associated with the symptom complex mentioned previously. It has been postulated that **two types of primary dysmenorrhea** may exist. **Spasmodic dysmenorrhea** is pain that begins with the onset of menstruation and is experienced as severe cramping and general discomfort in the lower abdomen and back. **Congestive dysmenorrhea** usually occurs prior to the onset of menstruation and is also characterized by general discomfort in the lower abdomen as well as in other areas of the body.

   The pain of primary dysmenorrhea is usually a **lower midline, dull abdominal ache or cramping** that generally occurs with ovulatory menstruation. It tends to be **spasmodic and cyclic** and may radiate to the back or inner aspects of the thighs. Discomfort may begin 2 days before, at, or after the onset of menstruation. Pain can be severe on the first day and usually lasts no more than 48 hours. It may be accompanied by increased menstrual flow and the symptom complex mentioned previously. There is usually a progressive increase in severity of pain over the years, followed by a decrease after age 27 or pregnancy. A few women may experience pain at menarche if they are having ovulatory cycles.

   A. **Etiology.** Several theories have been postulated to explain the cause of primary dysmenorrhea.

     1. **Increased uterine prostaglandin** (PGE$_2$ and PGF$_{2\alpha}$) **production and release.** Prostaglandins are 20-carbon molecules derived from arachidonic acid through the action of several enzymes that are collectively termed **prostaglandin synthetase.** Currently, evidence indicates that

139

in many women with primary dysmenorrhea, there is an increased production and release of endometrial prostaglandins during menstruation, giving rise to increased abnormal uterine activity resulting in ischemia. Prostaglandins may also sensitize the nerve endings to other pain-producing substances.

2. **Behavioral and psychologic factors have never been convincingly demonstrated as causes** of primary dysmenorrhea. It should be considered a physiologic phenomenon in the majority of women. However, based on a number of studies, it is accepted that there is a small association between dysmenorrhea and psychologic factors. **Dysmenorrhea has been associated with severe depression and increased suicide rates.**

3. **Cervical factors.** Hysterographic studies have found a significant narrowing of the cervical canal in some dysmenorrheic women. However, these studies were not performed when pain was present. In addition, true narrowing would constitute secondary dysmenorrhea.

4. **Neuronal factors.** Recent investigations have demonstrated the **presence of short adrenergic nerves in the uterus** that seem to disappear almost completely during pregnancy (in guinea pigs) and regenerate only partially after pregnancy.

5. **Hormonal factors.** Classically, women who are anovulatory do not have menstrual pain with bleeding.
   a. The clinical efficacy of progesterone and the combination oral contraceptives in some patients suggest that **estrogens and progesterones are somehow involved in the pathophysiology of dysmenorrhea.**
   b. **Vasopressin or oxytocin may be involved in increasing uterine tone** with resulting dysmenorrhea. A decreased concentration of oxytocin results in uterine contractions, mainly stimulated by vasopressin, that are dysrhythmic and painful.

6. **Constitutional factors. Conditions causing general debilitation,** such as anemia, fatigue, tuberculosis, and diabetes, may be associated with an increased incidence of primary dysmenorrhea. However, these women are also more likely to become amenorrheic.

B. **History**
   1. A **gynecologic history** should include:
      a. **Age.**
      b. **Gravidity.**
      c. **Parity.**
      d. **First day of the last menstrual period.**
      e. **Age at onset of menses.**
      f. **Length and regularity** of cycles.
      g. **Duration of flow.**
   2. **Documentation of previously known or suspected pelvic problems** such as infection, endometriosis, pelvic masses, undiagnosed pelvic pain, dyspareunia, infertility, or other pelvic disease is important.
   3. An **obstetric history including complications,** along with bowel, urinary tract, musculoskeletal, or vascular **disease** and abdominal, pelvic, or vaginal **surgery, injury, or procedure** should be noted.
   4. The **history of the pain** must include the following:
      a. **Severity.**
      b. **Duration.**
      c. **Character.**
      d. **Location.**
      e. **Radiation.**
      f. **Its relationship to:**
         (1) **Menarche.**
         (2) **Menses.**
         (3) **Mittelschmerz.**

(4) **Coitus.**
(5) **Bowel movements and voiding.**
(6) **Any associated symptoms.**
5. The provider needs to know the other factors that may influence dysmenorrhea, such as **family history of painful menses,** and should be aware of the **cultural, educational, and social milieu** in which the patient deals with her pain. The influence of the pain on the women's personal, partner, family, and career expectations must be established.
6. **Previous therapy** and its effectiveness are also pertinent.
C. **Physical examination. A complete gynecologic examination, including abdominal and rectal examinations,** should be performed with special attention directed toward reproducing the pain and detecting endometriosis, pelvic masses, or uterine enlargement.
   1. **A retroflexed uterus** was once considered to be a significant cause of dysmenorrhea. However, approximately 25% of women normally have retroflexed uteri, and many of these have no pain with menstruation. The retroflexion **should not be corrected unless it is fixed by endometriosis.**
   2. **A pelvic examination with negative findings strongly supports the diagnosis of primary dysmenorrhea.**
D. **Investigative procedures. No investigative procedures are necessary.** The diagnosis of primary dysmenorrhea is suggested by appropriate history, absence of positive findings on pelvic examination, and a therapeutic response to either ovulation-blocking agents or prostaglandin synthetase inhibitors.
   1. **Any positive pelvic finding requires further evaluation** (see section II.).
   2. **Individuals with atypical histories** and who are difficult to examine should have ultrasonography.
   3. **A Papanicolaou** (Pap) **smear** and **gonococcal and chlamydial cultures** should be done routinely and if indicated.
   4. **Laparoscopy, with or without hysteroscopy, may be indicated** to determine the cause.
      a. **If pelvic disease is discovered,** then appropriate treatment is indicated.
      b. **Dilation and curettage (D & C) may be both diagnostic and therapeutic.**
E. **Management.** Treatment should be individualized according to the severity of pain, contraception desired, and the existence of concurrent medical disease.
   1. **Nonsteroidal antiinflammatory drugs** (NSAIDs). Since increased production of endometrial prostaglandins appears to be a significant factor in the development of primary dysmenorrhea, compounds that inhibit their synthesis may offer effective relief. In fact, for women who **do not use oral contraception, the drug of choice for primary dysmenorrhea is** one of the **NSAIDs.** Presently, a number of groups exist, including:
      - Indoleacetic acid derivatives (indomethacin).
      - Fenamates (mefenamic acid, flufenamic acid).
      - Arylpropionic acid derivatives (ibuprofen, naproxen sodium).
      - Benzoic acid derivatives (aspirin).
      - Butyrophenones (phenylbutazone).
      - Oxicams (piroxicam).
      - Pyrrolo-pyrrole group (ketorolac tromethamine).
      The first three have been 70% to 100% effective in relieving dysmenorrhea. However, **indomethacin is associated with more gastrointestinal side effects.** Clinical trials have indicated that **aspirin is no better than a placebo but is worth trying** because of its low cost.
      a. Only four drugs are **approved by the Food and Drug Administration** (FDA) for treatment of dysmenorrhea.

    (1) **Ibuprofen** (Motrin), 400 mg, 600 mg, or 800 mg, PO tid to qid PRN.

    (2) **Mefenamic acid** (Ponstel), 500-mg PO loading dose followed by 250 to 500 mg PO q6h PRN.

    (3) **Naproxen sodium** (Anaprox), 550-mg loading dose, followed by 275 mg PO q6–8h PRN **or** Anaprox DS, 500 mg PO bid PRN **or** Naprosyn, 500-mg loading dose followed by 250 mg q6–8h up to 1,250 mg/day.

    (4) **Rofecoxib** (Vioxx), 50 mg qd.

  b. The NSAIDs are **generally well tolerated;** however, they can cause hepatic, renal, hematologic, gastrointestinal, and central nervous system (CNS) **toxicity including** indigestion, nausea, abdominal pain, constipation, diarrhea, vomiting, headache, vertigo, visual disturbances, rashes, and bronchospasm. **Contraindications to their use** include ulcers, asthma, hypersensitivity to NSAIDs and hepatic or renal disease.

  c. Some practitioners have recommended using NSAIDs prophylactically approximately 1 to 3 days prior to menstruation. The **drawbacks of prophylactic treatment** can include:

    (1) **Irregular menses.**

    (2) **Prolonged periods of drug intake increasing the possibility of side effects.**

    (3) **Exposing an early pregnancy to drugs. The effects on the fetus are still unknown.**

  d. **Ketorolac tromethamine (Toradol), 30 to 60 mg IM once is an injectable NSAID that can be used to treat severe episodes of dysmenorrhea.**

  e. **A trial of up to 6 months with a NSAID** is sufficient to demonstrate whether relief will be obtained. Different types and dosages should be tried.

  f. **If the patient does not respond to NSAIDs or oral contraceptives,** the **diagnosis** of primary dysmenorrhea should be **reconsidered.**

  g. **Rofecoxib (Vioxx)** has been approved for the treatment of primary dysmenorrhea. It is a Cox-2 inhibitor. The recommended dose is 50 mg qd.

2. Inhibition of ovulation. Oral contraceptives should be considered for treatment of dysmenorrhea in women who **desire contraception in addition to pain control, obtain no relief from or cannot tolerate NSAIDs, and have no contraindications to pill use.**

  a. **Combination** (i.e., high-progesterone, low-estrogen) **oral contraceptive pills** have been used to treat primary dysmenorrhea with good results. Though not FDA approved continuous use can achieve amenorrhea.

  b. **Pills containing progesterone only** (the "minipill") appear to be less effective.

  c. **Medroxyprogesterone acetate** (Depo-Provera), 150 mg IM every 12 weeks, can inhibit ovulation and eventually cause **amenorrhea** with prolonged use.

  d. Gonadotropin-releasing hormone agonists can be tried for a short time (<6 months) (see Endometriosis, Chapter 16).

3. Progesterone-containing intrauterine device (IUD). A progesterone-containing IUD (Progestasert) may relieve primary dysmenorrheic pain. However, it can also cause pain and other undesirable side effects.

4. Betamimetic agents, such as terbutaline (up to 1.5 mg in an oral spray six times daily) give **significant relief** in some women. However, they have **many side effects** including tremors, palpitations, flushing, and increased menstrual blood loss.

5. Calcium antagonists, such as nifedipine, are being tested and look promising but are **not currently approved** for use.

6. **Psychiatric help may be appropriate for a small number of patients** with no evidence of secondary dysmenorrhea for whom medical treatment has failed.
7. **Acupressure or acupuncture** may provide relief from dysmenorrhea. The **sites** for acupressure include the web of the hand between the thumb and first finger, the lumbosacral area, and 3 cm superior to the medial malleolus.
8. **Presacral neurectomy** has been used as a **last-resort method in the past.** It is associated with a **high rate of complication,** and there is little assurance of good response of the dysmenorrhea.
9. **Laparoscopic ablation** of the uterosacral nerves has been studied in a small group of women (8).
10. Nutrition.
    a. **Vitamin B6,** 50 to 100 mg PO qid throughout the cycle, with an additional 100 mg PO q2h PRN for pain, can be given as a trial for two cycles.
       (1) Since there can be significant side effects for some people, the lower starting dose should initially be recommended.
       (2) Patients receiving 2 to 7 gm a day or 0.2 gm/day for 2 months have been reported to have developed neuropathy with ataxia and numbness of the hands and feet (7).
       (3) Symptoms may take up to 6 months to resolve after discontinuation (7).
    b. **An increased dietary intake of calcium, magnesium, and caffeine** may be beneficial.
11. The use of **sedatives and narcotics should be limited** in treating primary dysmenorrhea.
12. **Miscellaneous.** Aerobic exercise, heat or cold, vitamins, a change of environment, orgasms, herbs, chiropractic intervention, dietary changes (decrease alcohol, caffeine, salt, fats, sweets), massage, meditation, and other relaxation techniques such as transcutaneous electrical nerve stimulation (TENS) or biofeedback may be helpful.

II. **Secondary dysmenorrhea** (extrinsic, acquired) is defined as **menstrual pain due to pelvic pathologic processes.** For pain occurring with the first menses or after the age of 25 without the previously mentioned symptom complex, **anatomic abnormalities should be considered.**
   The causes are numerous, and the **differential diagnosis should include adenomyosis, endometriosis,** intramural or submucous **fibroids,** endometrial and endocervical **polyps, IUDs, pelvic inflammatory or infectious diseases** (PID), **congenital uterine abnormalities, ovarian cysts, psychogenic origins, pelvic congestion syndrome, endometrial casts or membranes, true cervical stenosis, endometrial carcinoma, tuberculosis, and pelvic adhesions.** Several of the more common causes are discussed in more detail.
   Symptomatology and patterns of pain will depend on the etiology of the secondary dysmenorrhea. It is important to **determine the age of onset of pain, duration in years, associated symptoms, character of the discomfort, and its relationship in time to the menstrual cycle.** Secondary dysmenorrhea should be suspected if menstrual pain begins after the age of 20. It is characterized by constant pelvic pain that often extends to the back and thighs. Sometimes it is associated with infertility and dyspareunia. For general history and physical examination, see sections I.B and C.
   A. **Adenomyosis** is a condition characterized by **ingrowth of endometrium into the uterine musculature.**
      1. **History**
         a. It is more common in **multiparous middle-aged women** and can produce a picture of **colicky, labor-like pain** that occurs only during the menses.
         b. **Menorrhagia** is also a common complaint.

    2. Physical examination. A woman with adenomyosis may have a **tender, slightly enlarged uterus.**

    3. Investigative procedures

      a. A **presumptive diagnosis** can be made based on the **history and physical findings.**

      b. An **endometrial biopsy or a fractional D & C** should be done to rule out cancer.

      c. Hysteroscopy can aid in making the diagnosis.

      d. Final diagnosis is usually not made until **pathologic examination of the uterus** has been done.

    4. Treatment. Adenomyosis can be treated with **oral contraceptives.** However, in women who do not desire to have any (more) children, a **hysterectomy or endometrial resection or ablation** may be a realistic alternative.

B. Endometriosis (see Chapter 16)

    1. History. Endometriosis is **more common in nulliparous women.** It may present as pain increasing in severity for 2 to 3 days premenstrually, peaking on the first and second days of bleeding or on the day of heaviest menstrual flow. Endometriosis may also be associated with **dyspareunia, rectal pain, tenesmus, backache,** and occasionally **urgency of urination.**

    2. Physical examination. Endometriosis is **suggested by enlarged, tender ovaries, fixation of the uterus, tender uterosacral nodules,** or a combination of these findings.

    3. Investigative procedures. Laparoscopy and biopsy are the definitive diagnostic procedures.

    4. Management. Depending on the extent of endometriosis and its association with infertility, treatment may be **surgical or medical.**

      a. Medical treatment includes **oral contraceptives; danazol,** 200 mg PO qid; **Provera, 10 to 30 mg PO qd; medroxyprogesterone acetate,** 100 mg IM q4wk; **or** gonadotropin-releasing hormone agonists such as intranasal **nafarelin acetate** bid, **or leuprolide acetate** (see Chapter 16, Endometriosis).

      b. Surgical treatment (see Chapter 16, Endometriosis).

C. Myomas are **benign growths derived from smooth muscle cells.**

    1. History

      a. Uterine myomas usually cause dysmenorrhea only when they are **submucosal or protrude into the uterine cavity.**

      b. They can cause excessive or **prolonged bleeding.**

      c. The larger myoma can produce **frequency of urination, constipation, or edema of the lower extremities.**

    2. Physical examination. Larger myomas can be **palpated through the abdominal wall.** On bimanual examination, one or more nodular growths may be palpable.

    3. Investigative procedures. In women who are difficult to examine, **anesthesia may be helpful.**

      a. Curettage can be used to diagnose submucous fibroids by revealing an irregular contour within the endometrial cavity.

      b. Hysteroscopy, ultrasound, or hysterography may also be helpful.

    4. Management

      a. In premenopausal women, mildly symptomatic myomas can be **watched with periodic examination.**

      b. If infertility is a problem, myomectomy can be performed.

      c. Very large, multiple, or very painful myomas can be handled with **hysterectomy when fertility is not an issue.**

      d. It is important to remember that most myomas involute postmenopausally.

      e. Uterine artery embolization is being done by radiologists at some hospitals.

    f. Gonadotropin-releasing hormone agonists can temporarily decrease the size and bleeding caused by fibroids. These medications are usually reserved for preoperative use or in the perimenopausal period.

D. Intrauterine devices
1. **History.** IUDs are **one of the most common causes** of dysmenorrhea. Thus, it is important to determine what the patient is using for contraception.
2. **Physical examination** may reveal a **slightly tender uterus.** The **string should be visible from the os.**
3. **Investigative procedures.** If the string is not visible, a **flat plate x-ray film or ultrasonogram** may be helpful in locating the IUD. However, if lost, **IUD hooks** should be used first.
4. **Management**
   a. IUD-induced dysmenorrhea may be alleviated by **NSAIDs.**
   b. **Progesterone-containing IUDs cause less pain than copper or plastic ones** but need to be changed yearly.
   c. A **combination copper/progesterone IUD** may decrease dysmenorrhea.
   d. **Removal** of the IUD **may be necessary.**

E. Pelvic inflammatory disease (see also Chapter 5)
1. **History.** PID produces dysmenorrhea that is often **maximal premenstrually and relieved with the onset of flow.** It may be accompanied by **fever and purulent discharge.**
2. **Physical examination.** PID is suggested if **fever, purulent cervical discharge, cervical motion tenderness, fixation and adnexal tenderness, masses,** or a combination of these are present.
3. **Investigative procedures**
   a. **A complete blood cell count** (CBC) may show an elevated white blood cell count with a left shift.
   b. The **erythrocyte sedimentation rate** (ESR) may be elevated.
   c. **Cervical cultures** should be done to rule out gonorrhea and chlamydial infection.
   d. **Management.** The treatment of PID includes **bedrest** and administration of the **appropriate antibiotics** (see Chapter 5).

References

1. *A.M. Journal Health Syst Phar* 1999;56:1294.
2. Coco AS. Primary dysmenorrhea. *Am Fam Physician* 1999;60:2.
3. Dawood MY. Current concepts in the etiology and treatment of primary dysmenorrhea. *Contemp Obstet Gynecol* 1987;70:785.
4. Dawood MY. Dysmenorrhea. *Compr Ther* 1982;8:9.
5. Dawood MY. Dysmenorrhea. *Clin Obstet Gynecol* 1990;33(1).
6. Dingfelden JR. Primary dysmenorrhea treatment with prostaglandin inhibitors: a review. *Am J Obstet Gynecol* 1981;140:874.
7. *Drug facts and comparisons, facts and comparison,* 55th ed. 2000.
8. Golub LJ. Exercise that alleviates primary dysmenorrhea. *Contemp Obstet Gynecol* 1987;29(5):51.
9. Helms JM. Acupuncture for the management of primary dysmenorrhea. *Obstet Gynecol* 1987;69:51.
10. Lennane JK. Social and medical attitudes toward dysmenorrhea. *J Reprod Med* 1980;25:202.
11. Lichten EM. Surgical treatment of primary dysmenorrhea with laparoscopic uterine nerve ablation. *J Reprod Med* 1987;32(1).
12. Smith RP. Cyclic pelvic pain and dysmenorrhea. *Obstet Gynecol Clin North Am* 1993;20:4.

15. DYSPAREUNIA AND CHRONIC PELVIC PAIN

Kenneth Griffis

Dyspareunia differs from chronic pelvic pain in that it is a **situation-specific event occurring with intercourse.** However, both of these conditions can be, and often are, concurrent. The cause and pathogenesis span a continuum from organic to psychogenic and most often are multifactorial.

I. **Dyspareunia** refers especially to **painful intercourse that frequently interferes with sexual satisfaction.** It can be primary (present throughout one's sexual history) or secondary (arising as a result of some specific event or condition). It can occur only during certain sexual situations, in particular positions, or with certain partners. Clinicians are often reluctant to discuss intimate details of a woman's sex life. However, this data may provide important information leading to diagnosis and appropriate treatment.

   A. **Types.** It is useful to differentiate between the different types of dyspareunia to arrive at the appropriate diagnosis, treatment, and eventual prognosis.

      1. **Superficial dyspareunia. Vaginismus** is a specific type of dyspareunia that refers to spasms of the levator ani and perineal muscles, making intercourse difficult, painful, undesirable, and often impossible. Many clinicians have defined vaginismus as an almost certain psychogenic illness. However, **organic disorders** of the **external genitalia** and **introital areas can cause** such **severe discomfort** that any attempt at **penetration** can **lead** to **spasm.** This particular cycle, primarily caused by situational and anticipatory anxiety, can become self-perpetuating after the original organic cause has resolved. Therefore, vaginismus is **often both organic and functional** and can be solely a result of recognized disease entities.

      2. **Deep dyspareunia** refers to a deeper pelvic pain that is experienced at any time during intercourse. Again, this may be secondary to pelvic abnormality, or it may be functional in origin. It also tends to overlap more with chronic pelvic pain syndrome.

   B. **Etiology.** The presence of **organic disease** is often the cause of dyspareunia. Virtually all gynecologic disease entities list dyspareunia as a possible symptom. The **differential diagnosis is long and the evaluation must be thorough.**

      1. **Prominent** in the list of diseases associated with dyspareunia are the following:

         a. **Chronic pelvic infection.**
         b. **Endometriosis.**
         c. **Pelvic carcinoma.**
         d. **Extensive prolapse or organ displacement.**
         e. **Episiotomy or surgical sequelae.**
         f. **Acute vulvovaginitis.**
         g. **Cystitis.**
         h. **Urethral syndrome or other urinary tract disorders.**
         i. **Introital, vaginal, and cervical scarring.**
         j. **All space-occupying lesions.**
         k. **Levator ani myalgia.**
         l. **Vulvar vestibulitis.**

      2. As with chronic pelvic pain syndromes, **gastrointestinal (GI) diseases** (e.g., bowel motility disorders) **must be excluded.**

      3. **Estrogen deprivation, irritating vaginal medications, sympathomimetic drugs, amphetamines, and cocaine** are also causes, **primarily in superficial dyspareunia** and vaginismus.

This chapter is a revision of the third edition chapter by Siobhane Parry and Anna Macias.

4. The most common causes of **superficial dyspareunia** include **vaginitis** (atrophic or infectious) or **lack of lubrication** (either caused by physiologic conditions or suboptimal sexual technique).
5. **Lesions in the cul-de-sac are said to correlate most often with deep-penetration dyspareunia.**
6. **Women who have deep-penetration dyspareunia and who do not have superficial pain on penetration or vaginismus** usually **do not have a causative external inflammatory syndrome.**
7. Some individuals with external dyspareunia or vaginismus have small, almost imperceptible **scar tissue** secondary to surgery or childbirth.
8. Two clinical syndromes not usually recognized involve **broad-ligament varicosities** and the **broad-ligament tear syndrome** (see section I.C.9.a.).
9. Frequently unrecognized etiology, particularly on first interview, is a **history of sexual assault or abuse.**
C. **History.** The key to diagnosis often rests with the clinician's willingness to raise the issue of sexual dysfunction. A protocol should be followed to identify causative organic and psychogenic factors using the psychosexual and medical history, a comprehensive physical examination, psychological assessment instruments, laboratory tests, and special procedures.
   1. It is necessary to ascertain first whether the dyspareunia is of the **superficial or deep type.**
   2. It is important to **delineate all of the usual pain parameters** such as onset, duration, location, radiation, timing, chronicity, recurrence, cyclic nature, and character.
   3. **Timing of the pain in relation to sexual intercourse** is particularly vital. It is important to inquire about **other times that pelvic pain may appear.**
   4. Existence of **concomitant GI or urinary complaints** should be sought.
   5. **Psychological factors and history of abuse or assault** should be investigated in a gentle, nonjudgmental manner.
   6. **Relationship to the menstrual cycle** can be very helpful in diagnosis.
   7. **A history of discharge or dry vaginal mucosa** would lead the clinician to suspect atrophic or inflammatory vaginitis or a lack of lubrication.
   8. **History of surgery or difficult episiotomy repair** could lead to the diagnosis of scar tissue that is the cause of the superficial dyspareunia.
   9. Some specific syndromes have **unusual historic presentations:**
      a. **Patients with broad-ligament varicosities and the broad-ligament tear syndrome** usually have deep pelvic aching developing progressively throughout the day after prolonged weight bearing, as well as deep-penetration dyspareunia.
      b. Historic presentation for **endometriosis and chronic pelvic inflammatory disease** (PID) are reviewed in section II.C.
D. **Physical examination** should be thorough and gentle and should include abdominal, external genital, vaginal, bimanual, and rectal examinations for every patient evaluated for dyspareunia.
   1. **Superficial dyspareunia of psychogenic etiology** will lead to an essentially **normal physical examination,** with the exception of the **typical spasms** previously described for vaginismus on speculum insertion or digital examination.
   2. **No mucosal abnormalities** should be present. If mucosal abnormalities are **discovered,** further tests may lead to the diagnosis of acute vaginitis, atrophic vaginitis, vulvar vestibulitis, or lack of physiologic lubrication.
   3. **Introital or vaginal scarring** causing pain with penetration can be apparent on careful physical examination.
   4. **Cystitis, urethral syndrome, or other urinary tract disorders** should be suspected if the urinary tract structures are **tender.**
   5. **Deep dyspareunia will depend more on the bimanual and rectal examination** for diagnosis.

6. Findings on physical examination for **pelvic infection and endometriosis,** two frequent causes of deep dyspareunia, are discussed in section II.D.
7. Physical examination should be able to suggest the **presence of extensive prolapse or organ displacement, pelvic carcinoma,** other **masses,** and **adhesions and other surgical sequelae** leading to deep dyspareunia.
8. **A thorough abdominal examination** must be included to assist in the diagnosis of **chronic bowel motility or other GI disorders** leading to dyspareunia or chronic pelvic pain.

E. **Investigative procedures**
1. **Gonorrhea and *chlamydia*** DNA probes should be taken to exclude inflammatory conditions of the vagina, uterus, and adnexa.
2. **Wet mounts and potassium hydroxide preps** can be useful.
3. A **urinalysis** should also be done. **If the urinary tract is especially suspect** because of certain historic or physical examination data, a **culture** should be done. **Cystoscopy, intravenous pyelogram, or renal ultrasound** may be indicated.
4. **GI symptoms may require contrast studies, sigmoidoscopic examination,** or both to rule out contributing GI symptomatology. However, this is usually **more applicable to chronic pelvic pain than to dyspareunia.**
5. **Measurements of estrogen status and a Papanicolaou** (Pap) **smear,** may be useful in **ruling out atrophic mucosal changes** not apparent on physical examination.
6. **Biopsy or colposcopy** may be indicated when **vaginal or vulvar lesions** are revealed on physical examination.
7. **Complex deep-penetration dyspareunia** may require **laparoscopy** for definitive diagnosis.
8. Investigative procedures for **endometriosis, chronic pelvic infection, and other organic abnormalities** are discussed in section II.E.

F. **Management** must be individualized for both the specific patient and the disease entity. Endometriosis, chronic pelvic inflammation, postsurgical syndromes, anatomic displacements, pelvic malignancies, and other space-occupying lesions deserve a well thought-out treatment plan that frequently **combines medical and surgical intervention.**
1. **Vulvovaginal inflammatory conditions** are usually **easily remedied by the office-based clinician.** Specific treatments are detailed in Chapters 1 and 2.
2. **Lack of lubrication** (due to either physiologic conditions or suboptimal sexual technique) is usually amenable to **additional lubrication** (water-based jellies or mucoadhesives) and **patient education** in sexual arousal techniques.
3. **Vulvar or introital scar tissue** may be treated by dilation or, infrequently, by **surgical intervention.** These conditions need to be quickly identified before a psychological pain-apprehension-avoidance cycle sets in. It should be emphasized that **repeat surgical procedures** (i.e., revisions) **are rarely indicated** for external scarring and should never be used as a last-chance approach in the absence of an identifiable pathologic process.
4. Since the fear of sex resulting from chronic dyspareunia is a conditioned response, **careful psychosocial intervention may be necessary** to unlearn the pain-apprehension-avoidance cycle, even if the problem is physiologic.
   a. Increasingly, **systematic desensitization techniques** dealing directly with pain and muscle spasm have been utilized.
      (1) Often, **direct contact is too threatening initially. Fantasy** can be utilized for gradual reduction of the dysfunctional response (i.e., instruct the patient to imagine a sexual situation without pain or other undesirable results).

(2) True **behavior modification** involves a slow, nonstressful approach to the desired behavior through physical acts until complete coitus can be achieved without discomfort. This typically evolves through fantasy to nonsexual physical touching with a partner, to vaginal self-dilation and self-stimulation, then to partner use of finger stimulation, to partial partner penile entry, and finally to complete sexual intercourse.

(3) **Vaginal muscle exercises** (i.e., Kegel exercises) **and traditional relationship counseling,** including nonsexual issues, are often useful therapeutic adjuncts.

(4) These relatively simple desensitization procedures and behavior modification techniques may permit symptom alleviation **without requiring formal referral to a more specialized therapist.** Even severe, disabling vaginismus is often very responsive to short-term behavioral treatment. Current psychological treatment includes one or more of the following components: **sensate focus exercises, cognitive-behavioral therapy, relaxation training, hypnosis** and **guided imagery,** and **group therapies.**

b. **If the etiologic factors are complex,** such as sexual assault or early sexual abuse, **more formal psychological evaluation and treatment** may be helpful.

c. **If the vaginismus is an active attempt by a woman to block intercourse** with an undesirable or inappropriate partner, all intervention may be unsuccessful until the **underlying problem is discovered and resolved.**

II. **Chronic pelvic pain** has been defined as nonmenstrual pain of at least 3 months duration or menstrual pain of at least 6 months duration. Diagnosis of the etiology of chronic pelvic pain is dependent on a thorough history and physical. The evaluation should be as noninvasive as possible to rule out the myriad of gynecologic and nongynecologic causes. The differential diagnosis of chronic pelvic pain is similar to the differential diagnosis of deep-penetration dyspareunia (see section I.B.).

A. **Types.** There are two broad categories of chronic pelvic pain: **functional and organic.**

1. **Functional pelvic pain** is real to the patient. It can be defined as a nonmenstrual pain of **3 or more months duration** that localizes to the anatomic pelvis, is severe enough to cause **functional disability,** and **requires medical or surgical treatment.** Lack of a specific diagnosis and treatment plan leads to "doctor-shopping" and unsatisfactory results for the patient.

2. **Organic. Pelvic pain** of organic etiology is **usually secondary to a well-defined physical entity.** This type of chronic pelvic pain is usually caused by **inflammation or a mass in the pelvis** resulting in displacement, torsion, obstruction, or congestion.

B. **Etiology**

1. **Functional chronic pelvic pain** is, by definition, **psychogenic,** and the **causes are multifactorial.** As with dyspareunia, sexual abuse or assault can lead to chronic pelvic discomfort. Pelvic pain is unlikely to be specifically and psychodynamically related to sexual abuse in childhood. However, the pernicious nature of abuse, whether physical or sexual, may promote the chronicity of painful conditions. In addition, problems that were originally organic can lead to residual psychogenic pain of a functional nature.

2. Disease entities causing **organic pelvic pain syndrome** include:

a. **Malignant or benign tumors.**

b. **Ovarian cysts** with adhesion or torsion.

c. **Severe uterine malpositions.**

d. **Chronic PID.**

       e. Chronic or recurrent urinary tract infection or inflammation (i.e., interstitial cystitis).

       f. Chronic bowel or GI inflammations.

       g. Endometriosis.

C. History. As with dyspareunia, history is the cornerstone of accurate diagnosis. The diagnosis is strongly influenced by **symptom variables of chronicity, timing, and associated features.**

An **organic etiology should be actively sought** in all patients **before a functional cause is presumed.** Pain that is appropriate and consistently localized, follows recognized patterns of radiation, displays a relatively acute or distinct onset, and shows a reasonable progression of signs and symptoms is more consistent with organic disease. The clinician should consider the **possibility of a psychogenic etiology** when there is vague discomfort of a continuous, unvarying quality unrelated to actual organ location or with bizarre patterns of radiation that are accentuated by stressful situations. Neither description, however, is exclusionary of functional or organic etiology.

   1. Endometriosis.

      a. Historical findings are controversial but are said to include **delayed pregnancy, pelvic surgery, and injury to the pelvic structures.**

      b. Acquired or secondary dysmenorrhea is classic. Pain begins 5 to 7 days prior to menstruation, increases during menstruation, persists throughout the period, and slowly resolves after cessation of menses. Variations of this classic pattern are innumerable.

      c. Specific symptom complexes are related to the actual site of endometrial implants.

         (1) Lesions in the cul-de-sac are said to correlate most frequently with deep-penetration dyspareunia.

         (2) Endometrial implants in either bladder or bowel areas can lead to hematuria, rectal bleeding, obstruction, or all of these.

         (3) Endometriosis **involving abdominal structures** can frequently lead to intermittent GI complaints of a cyclic nature.

   2. Chronic pelvic infection. Historical findings include **intrauterine device** (IUD), **uterine procedures,** increased incidence of **sexually transmitted diseases** (STDs), exposure to **multiple partners,** and previous significant psychosexual trauma.

      a. Predisposition to chronic PID resulting in pain is **directly related to a history of acute salpingitis, other pelvic infection, or postpartum or posttherapeutic abortion infection.**

      b. When questioning the patient about these illnesses, it is important to remember that the **original episode may have been subacute** (especially common in chlamydial PID) **or erroneously diagnosed.**

D. Physical examination. A thorough physical examination of the abdomen, external genitalia, vagina, uterus, adnexa, and rectum is necessary for evaluation.

   1. Findings in a patient with functional or **psychogenic chronic pelvic pain** are likely to be highly **diffuse, nonspecific, and nondiagnostic for any organic entity.**

   2. Pelvic masses, uterine malposition, and other physical findings specific for certain organic illnesses may be found on examination.

   3. Women with **endometriosis** will probably have increased pain and tenderness, which may be cyclic, during the pelvic examination.

      a. Endometrial implants may be **palpated or visualized.** Frequently, these are **firm, nodular type lesions** that increase in tenderness just prior to and during menstruation.

      b. Pelvic structures may be fixed.

   4. Women with **chronic PID** will usually have generalized tenderness on examination (less severe than with acute infection), equivocal and mild cervical motion tenderness, generalized adnexal tenderness, and cyclically or recurrently increased findings on examination.

5. Since many of these **entities will have overlapping physical examination findings, other investigative procedures will almost certainly be necessary** to diagnose the problem definitively.

E. **Investigative procedures.** Depending on the findings of the history and physical examination, many diverse laboratory, radiologic, ultrasound, direct visualization, or surgical techniques may be necessary for diagnosis.

1. When history and physical examination strongly point to **functional illness, extremely invasive procedures should be avoided.**
   a. **Laboratory studies,** such as an erythrocyte sedimentation rate (ESR), can usually help rule out chronic pelvic inflammation.
   b. **Pelvic ultrasound** can provide assurance that no important lesion has been missed on physical examination.
   c. **Screening urinalysis, wet-mount preparation,** and **Pap smear** should usually be performed.
   d. **Cultures** should be performed as appropriate for history.

2. Between 71% and 87% of **reproductive-**aged patients who present with chronic pelvic pain will have **endometriosis.** When the history and physical examination strongly point toward endometriosis, empiric treatment with nonsteroidal antiinflammatory drugs (NSAIDs), oral contraceptives, depot medroxyprogesterone acetate, or gonadotropin releasing agonist (GnRH-a) can be successful in approximately 50% of patients. For the remainder, laparoscopy to confirm the diagnosis would be appropriate (see Chapter 16).

3. When **chronic pelvic inflammation** is suspected, the following procedures are useful:
   a. **Laboratory analysis** should include:
      (1) **A complete blood cell count** (CBC).
      (2) **ESR** may be useful but is very **nonspecific.**
      (3) **Gonorrhea and *chlamydia* DNA probes.**
      (4) **Wet-mount preparations** as they can diagnose other chronic inflammatory conditions.
   b. **Ultrasound** can be helpful in suggesting chronic inflammatory changes in the pelvic structures.
   c. **Laparoscopy** may be necessary for definitive diagnosis.
   d. **Specific investigative and diagnostic procedures** appropriate for pelvic pain believed to be caused by chronic PID are covered in Chapter 5.

4. When **mass lesions or anatomic abnormalities** are suspected by history and physical examination, **pelvic ultrasound** is initially used, followed by **diagnostic laparoscopy or direct surgical visualization.**

F. **Management** of functional pelvic pain can be difficult and frustrating for both patient and clinician. The management plan must **emphasize to the patient that every care has been taken to exclude treatable organic disease.** However, repeated complex radiologic and surgical explorations or diagnostic procedures usually confirm the patient's self-definition of illness and frequently perpetuate the pain-apprehension-avoidance cycle.

1. The clinician must help the patient through **regular supportive visits.** When the patient realizes that the practitioner will not become angry or abandon her, even with a lack of strictly defined therapeutic success (complete cessation of symptoms), marked improvement in pain control or daily functional adaptation often occurs.

2. **Pain management is with nonaddictive medications,** such as NSAIDs or oral contraceptives. Empiric antibiotics are rarely beneficial. Other agents currently being used in chronic pain syndromes are tricyclic antidepressants, selective serotonin reuptake inhibitors, gabapentin, and lithium.

3. Current data suggest that availability of a **multidisciplinary pelvic pain clinic** can **reduce** the **frequency** of **surgical interventions.**

4. Some clinicians have success with **injecting local anesthetics** (i.e., bupivacaine hydrochloride [Marcaine]) **or normal saline** into various trigger points.
5. Other treatment modalities that may be helpful include acupuncture and massage therapy.
6. The management of organic pelvic pain is dictated by the specific disease entity. The management of PID and endometriosis is covered in Chapters 5 and 16, respectively. **Other specific conditions, mass lesions, or anatomic abnormalities** are usually referred for **surgical consultation and intervention.**

G. **Resources.** The following Web sites provide additional reading and resources:
  1. www.acog.org
  2. www.endometriosisl.com
  3. www.endozone.org
  4. www.obgyn.net
  5. www.pelvicpain.org

References

1. Committee on Practice Bulletins–Gynecology, American College of Obstetricians and Gynecologists. Medical Management of Endometriosis (ACOG Practice Bulletin No. 11, December 1999). *Compendium of selected publications* 2000:959–971.
2. Committee on Technical Bulletins, American College of Obstetricians and Gynecologists. Chronic Pelvic Pain (ACOG Tech Bull No. 223: December 1999). *Compendium of selected publications* 2000:337–345.
3. Delancey JO, et al. Dyspareunia. *Obstet Gynecol* 1993 [Suppl 4] 82:658.
4. Gambone JC, Reiter RC. Nonsurgical management of chronic pelvic pain: a multidisciplinary approach. *Clin Obstet Gynecol* 1990;33:205.
5. Halvorsen JG, Metz ME. Sexual dysfunction, part I: classification, etiology and pathogenesis. *J Fam Pract* 1992;5:51.
6. Halvorsen JG, Metz ME. Sexual dysfunction, part II: diagnosis, management, and prognosis. *J Fam Pract* 1992;5:177.
7. Halvorsen JG, Metz ME. Sexual dysfunction, part II: diagnosis, management, and prognosis. *J Fam Pract* 1992;5:177.
8. Howard FM. The role of laparoscopy in chronic pelvic pain. *Obstet Gynecol Surg* 1993;48:357.
9. Kames LD, et al. Effectiveness of an interdisciplinary pain management program for the treatment of chronic pelvic pain. *Pain* 1990;41:41.
10. Levy BS. How many operations are too many? *OBG Manage* 2000;12:8–10.
11. Ling FW. For the Pelvic Pain Study Group. Randomized controlled trial of depot leuprolide in patients with chronic pain and clinically suspected endometriosis. *Obstet Gynecol* 1999; 93:51–58.
12. Moody GA, Mayberry JF. Perceived sexual dysfunction amongst patients with inflammatory bowel disease. *Digestion* 1993;54:256.
13. Nolan TE, Elkins TE. Chronic pelvic pain. Differentiating anatomic from functional causes. *Postgrad Med* 1993;94(8):125, 131, 138.
14. Olive DL, Schattman GL, et al. Chronic pelvic pain an evidence-based approach to evaluation and initial management. In: Barbieri RL, ed. *OBG Manage* 2000 [Suppl] February.
15. Rapkin AJ, et al. History of physical and sexual abuse in women with chronic pelvic pain. *Obstet Gynecol* 1990;76:92.
16. Reiter RC, Gambone JC. Demographic and historic variables in women with idiopathic chronic pain. *Obstet Gynecol* 1990;75:428.
17. Scialli AR, Barbieri RI, et al., eds. Chronic pelvic pain: an integrated approach. In: APGO educational series on women's health issues. Washington, DC: Association of Professors of Gynecology and Obstetrics (APGO), 2000.

16. ENDOMETRIOSIS

Stephen E. Thorn

Endometriosis is defined as the presence of ectopic implants of tissue that look and act like endometrium and are found outside the uterine cavity. It is one of the most common gynecologic conditions requiring both medical and surgical treatment. It remains an incompletely understood condition that can result in infertility, chronic pelvic pain, a combination of both, or no associated symptoms or clinical consequences. Endometriosis should be suspected when any patient, regardless of age or social economic status, has progressive dysmenorrhea, dyspareunia, infertility or a combination of these symptoms.

I. **Incidence and prevalence**
   A. Endometriosis occurs in 7% to 10% of women in the general population and up to 50% of perimenopausal women. In infertile women, the prevalence is 38% (range 20%–50%) and in women with chronic pelvic pain, the prevalence is 71% to 87%. There are no data to support the view that the incidence of endometriosis is increasing, although improved recognition of endometriosis lesions may have led to an increase in the rate of detection.
   B. Some studies show that Japanese women have a prevalence that is double that among caucasian women, otherwise there is no apparent racial predisposition.
   C. There may be a hereditary factor since there is a 10% risk of developing endometriosis if a first-degree relative has been affected. Kindred studies have demonstrated a polygenic and multifactorial mode of inheritance.
   D. Malignancy in endometriosis is rare. Fewer than 50 cases of carcinoma arising in ovarian endometriosis have been reported and many of these have been adenoacanthomas.
   E. The median age of patients at the time of diagnosis is 25 to 29 years of age and is rarely found in postmenopausal women. Among pelvic conditions encountered at the time of surgery, endometriosis ranks a close second in frequency to uterine fibroids in those over the age of 30.

II. **Pathogenesis.** Archives are full of articles that have been written on the etiology of endometriosis. At least 12 theories have been proposed to explain how it develops. The following theories are the most accepted; however, none of them fully explains the complete etiology of this disease.
   A. **Implantation.** The first known reported case of endometriosis was reported by Von Rokitansky in the 1860s followed by scattered works until 1921, when Sampson recorded his theory of implantation as the causative factor. It is still the most widely embraced theory. The theory states that during menstruation, endometrial cells are passed through the tubes and implant on the posterior cul-de-sac, the uterosacral ligaments, the ovaries, and the peritoneal surfaces.
      The continued question with this theory is why don't all women develop endometriosis since most normally menstruating women experience some retrograde menstruation with each cycle. Some experts feel that an altered cellular immune response predisposes some women. This theory also does not explain why women who have had their tubes "tied" or who have had a hysterectomy get endometriosis.
   B. **Vascular and lymphatic dissemination.** Halban's theory of vascular and lymphatic dissemination of endometrial glands helps to explain the findings of endometriosis in such areas as the lungs, pleura, kidney, mediastinum, and brain.
   C. **Coelomic metaplasia** theory proposed by Myers and others at the turn of the 20th century states that the peritoneal mesothelial cells undergo

This is a revision of the third edition chapter by Alex Locke.

metaplastic transformation into endometrial cells as a result of some unspecified stimulus. At present, scientific evidence supporting this theory is lacking.

D. **Direct transplantation of endometrial cells** may occur iatrogenically following gynecologic surgery, such as cesarean section, myomectomy, or hysterectomy.

III. **Signs and symptoms.** The clinical manifestations of endometriosis are **variable** and **unpredictable** in both presentation and cause. **Dysmenorrhea, chronic pelvic pain, dyspareunia, uterosacral ligament nodularity, and adnexal mass (either symptomatic or asymptomatic) are among the most well recognized symptoms.** A significant number of women with endometriosis remain asymptomatic.

Endometriosis occurs most frequently in the pelvis with 50% of the cases involving the ovaries. Other common locations include the uterosacral ligaments, rectovaginal septum, sigmoid colon, serosal surface of the uterus, bladder, fallopian tubes, cervix, vulva, and vagina. It rarely occurs in the appendix, ileum, abdominal scars, umbilicus, ureter, or more distal sites such as the diaphragm, pleura, lungs, spleen, gallbladder, kidney, and brain.

A. **Dysmenorrhea** is a common symptom which may be cyclic and commence prior to the onset of menses. Endometriosis should be considered if symptoms of dysmenorrhea are refractory to antiprostaglandins or those who develop dysmenorrhea after years of pain-free menstruation (Fig. 16.1). The pain is usual bilateral in the lower abdomen and is associated with a sense of rectal pressure.

B. **Infertility** and its association to endometriosis remains a subject of considerable debate. Endometriosis is found in 25% of infertile women and an estimated 50% to 60% of those with endometriosis may be infertile. Infertility may be the first indication that the endometriosis is present. Invasive endometriosis may induce infertility as the result of anatomic distortion and related pelvic ovarian-tubal adhesions.

In patients who have minimal to mild endometriosis and no alteration of pelvic anatomy, the infertility is much more difficult to explain. It is hypothesized that the prostaglandins secreted by the endometrial implant or other chemicals secreted by white cells may interfere with the reproductive organs by causing contractions or spasms. The fallopian tube may or may not be able to pick up the egg, and the stimulated uterus may reject implantation.

In addition sperm motility may be adversely affected along with the ability of the sperm to penetrate the egg. Some researchers suggest that the woman's body may form antibodies against this transplanted endometrial tissue. These antibodies may attack the uterine lining and cause an increase in the spontaneous abortion rate, up to three times the normal rate. Fortunately removal of the endometriosis with medication or surgery will reduce this risk to normal.

C. **Adnexal masses.** A pelvic examination may exhibit ovarian masses which may be endometriomas in otherwise asymptomatic patients. Abdominal or vaginal ultrasounds show a unilateral or bilateral cystic mass in the ovary and homogeneous internal echoes. They may be unilateral or bilateral. An elevated CA-125 level will usually decrease with removal of the endometrioma. Malignancy is rare in association with endometriosis.

D. **Other symptoms include:**
   1. Dyspareunia.
   2. Bowel or bladder symptoms (i.e., painful defecation, dysuria).
   3. Premenstrual spotting.
   4. Menorrhagia.

E. Other signs include:
   1. Excessive pain on pelvic examination.
   2. Thick and retroverted uterus.
   3. Friable perineal implants.
   4. Uterosacral ligament nodularity.
   5. Laterally deviated cervix.

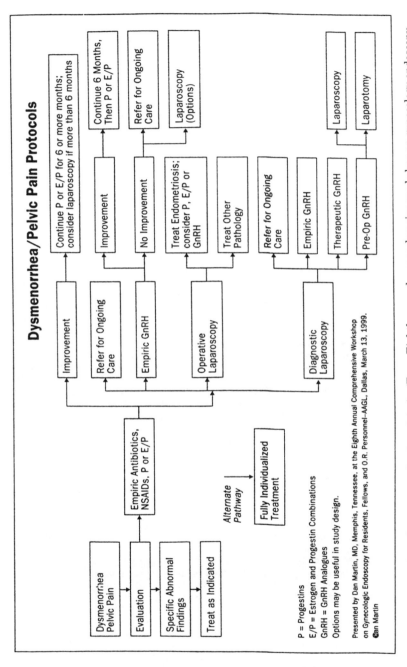

FIG. 16.1. Diagnosis and treatment of endometriosis. (From Eighth annual comprehensive workshop on gynecology endoscopy, *Ob Gyn News* 1999 [Suppl], with permission.)

IV. Diagnosis can be suggested after completing a thorough history and physical (including pelvic) examination. The only reliable method of diagnosing endometriosis with certainty is by inspecting the implants at the time of laparoscopic or laparotomy surgery or by obtaining biopsies of the pelvic peritoneum.

   A. Pelvic examination reveals nodularities in the uterosacral ligament or an induration in the cul-de-sac on rectovaginal examination and is generally accompanied by pain during the examination.

   B. Laparoscopy and biopsy. The appearance of the implants at the time of surgery varies. The most common are the reddish-blue nodules and the classic "powder burn" lesions. These areas may be accompanied by scarring or fibrosis and when biopsied, will show histologically the presence of endometrial glands and stroma.

   C. Ultrasound in many women may show the presence of an ovarian mass possibly representing endometrioma.

   D. Since the actual diagnosis of endometriosis requires a surgical procedure with accompanying biopsy, many investigators are searching for **noninvasive alternatives.** The blood test, CA-125, has been shown to be elevated in patients with severe endometriosis but its clinical utility as a diagnostic marker for endometriosis appears limited. It is of questionable value in detecting women with minimal and mild disease.

     Although no single laboratory test has shown reliable clinical utility, it is possible that eventually a combination of biochemical markers and clinical assessment will decrease the need for surgical confirmation.

V. Staging. The American Society of Reproductive Medicine (ASRM) (formerly the American Fertility Society) classification was revised for the third time in 1996, but still has its limitations (Fig. 16.2). This system is not a good predictor of pregnancy following treatment and does not correlate well with the symptoms of pain and dyspareunia. The true value is the uniform recording of operative findings and possibly the ability to compare results of various therapies.

VI. Treatment. In managing endometriosis, it is important to consider that the **disease** appears to be **progressive** and **recurrent.** Although a variety of treatment options exist, the **only** cure for endometriosis is a hysterectomy with bilateral oophorectomy. This is **not** a **viable option** for women who wish to **preserve** their fertility and hormonal status. For these patients, medical management entails inducing anovulation and surgery is conservative and generally performed laparoscopically.

   A. Medical treatment should be reserved for patients with pain or dyspareunia since no pharmacologic method appears to restore fertility.

      1. Oral contraceptive pills (OCPs) suppress luteinizing hormone (LH) and follicle-stimulating hormone (FSH), prevent ovulation, and render the endometrial tissue thin and compact. Combination OCPs (estrogen-progesterone) alleviate symptoms in 75% of women with endometriosis.

        a. They can be taken continually or cyclically and either discontinued after 6 to 12 cycles or continued indefinitely.

        b. Adverse effects may include headaches, nausea, and rarely hypertension.

      2. Danazol (Danocrine) has been highly effective in relieving the symptoms of endometriosis but adverse effects may preclude its use. It is a synthetic androgen that inhibits LH and FSH. This results in a hypoestrogenic state and endometrial atrophy which is a likely mechanism for the relief of pain.

        a. The preferred dosage is 200 to 400 mg bid for up to 6 months.

        b. Side effects are androgenic including acne, edema, hirsutism, deepening of the voice, and weight gain.

        c. The overall response rate is 84% to 92%, with beneficial effects lasting up to 6 months after treatment has stopped.

      3. Progestational agents.

        a. Medroxyprogesterone suspension (Depo-Provera) helps to suppress growth of endometriosis and is very inexpensive.

American Society for Reproductive Medicine
Revised Classification of Endometriosis

Patient's name _____ Date _____

Stage I (minimal)   —   1–5
Stage II (mild)   —   6–15
Stage III (moderate) —   16–40   Laparoscopy _____ Laparotomy _____ Photography _____
Stage IV (severe)   —   >40   Recommended treatment _____

Total _____   Prognosis _____

Peritoneum	Endometriosis		<1 cm	1–3 cm	>3 cm
		Superficial	1	2	4
		Deep	2	4	6
Ovary	R	Superficial	1	2	4
		Deep	4	16	20
	L	Superficial	1	2	4
		Deep	4	16	20

	Posterior cul-de-sac obliteration	Partial		Complete	
		4		40	

	Adhesions		<¹/₃ Enclosure	¹/₃–²/₃ Enclosure	>²/₃ Enclosure
Ovary	R	Filmy	1	2	4
		Dense	4	8	16
	L	Filmy	1	2	4
		Dense	4	8	16
Tube	R	Filmy	1	2	4
		Dense	4*	8*	16
	L	Filmy	1	2	4
		Dense	4*	8*	16

*If the fimbriated end of the fallopian tube is completely enclosed, change the point assignment to 16.
Denote appearance of superficial implant types as red [(R), red, red-pink, flamelike, vesicular blobs,
clear vesicles], white [(W), opacifications, peritoneal defects, yellow-brown], or black [(B), black,
hemosiderin deposits, blue]. Denote percent of total described as R__%, W__%, and B__%. Total
should equal 100%.

FIG. 16.2. Revised classification of endometriosis. American College of Obstetrics
and Gynecologists Compendium 2001. (Modified from the revised American Fertility
Society classification of endometriosis. Reprinted with permission from the American
Society for Reproductive Medicine. *Fertility and Sterility* 1996;67(5):819–820.)

  (1) The dosage is 100 mg IM is given every 2 weeks for 2 months
      then 200 mg IM every month for 4 months **or** 150 mg IM every
      3 months.
  (2) Side effects include weight gain, irregular periods, or amen-
      orrhea.
  b. **Medroxyprogesterone** (Provera) 5 to 20 mg orally per day has the
     same side effects as Depo-Provera and works in the same way.
  c. **Norethindrone acetate** (Aygestin), in numerous studies, has been
     shown to be most effective in alleviating symptomatic dysmenor-
     rhea and has fewer side effects.
    1. **At the start of the menstrual cycle,** 5 mg is given, and continued
       daily unless abnormal vaginal bleeding occurs.

2. If abnormal vaginal bleeding does occur, increase the dose by 2.5 mg until bleeding stops, then gradually tapers the dose by 2.5 mg every 2 weeks to a 5 mg maintenance dose.
4. **Gonadotropin-releasing hormone** (GnRH) **agonists.** These agents, nafarelin (Synarel), leuprolide (Lupron), and gosarelin (Zoladex), inhibit the secretion of gonadotropin and are comparable to danazol in relieving pain.
   a. **Symptoms** include hot flashes, mood changes, and other menopausal symptoms.
   b. Use is limited to 6 months because of the loss of bone density. Some studies have increased its length of treatment but careful consideration has to be given to bone loss.
   c. Because of severe hypoestrogenic symptoms, low-dose estrogen replacement therapy has been used to decrease the side effects.
   d. GnRH agonists are an expensive therapy but induce regression of implants, alleviate pain, and can allow pregnancy to occur.
B. **Surgical treatment** of endometriosis at the time of diagnostic laparoscopy has dramatically increased. With operative laparoscopy the endometriosis can be surgically resected with an experienced surgeon, thus sparing the patient a laparotomy. Adhesions can be lysed without any major complication and lysis has been shown to enhance fertility rates. If endometriomas are noted they can be resected and removed.
   1. Surgery should be done conservatively, especially on women who wish to retain fertility. The surgeon should try to remove adhesions and restore mobility of fallopian tubes.
   2. Women with severe pain who do **not** desire pregnancy can undergo surgical excision of the implants at the time of laparoscopy.
      a. Many educators believe in giving GnRH analogs 3 to 6 months following the surgery.
      b. Some feel uterosacral ligament nerve ablation (LUNA) will help relieve discomfort related to menstrual cramps in up to 85% of patients.
      c. For more severe pain a presacral neurectomy (TSN) can be performed.
   3. Women who remain symptomatic despite all modes of therapy and who do not wish to bear children, a total abdominal hysterectomy with bilateral salpingo-oophorectomy (BSO) or laparoscopic assisted vaginal hysterectomy with BSO may be their best treatment.
VII. There is an endometriosis association that has a **Web site** (www.endometriosisassociation.org) where women can obtain further information or support while going through treatment of their endometriosis.

References

Adamson GD. Diagnosis and clinical presentation of endometriosis. *Am J Obstet Gynecol* 1990;162:568–569.

American College of Obstetrics and Gynecologists (ACOG). *Compendium of selected publications* 2001.

American Family Physician. *Diagnosis and treatment of endometriosis.* Author, 1999.

Baker B. Cut treatment cost for unexplained infertility. *Ob Gyn News* 1998;33(12):24.

Hurst BS, Rock JA. Endometriosis: pathophysiology, diagnosis, and treatment. *Obstet Gynecol Surg* 1989;44:297–304.

Ly PY, Ory SJ. Endometriosis: current management. *Mayo Clin Proc* 1995;70:453–463.

Ending the cycle of pain, diagnosis and treatment of endometriosis. *Ob Gyn News* 1999.

Speroff L, et al. *Endometriosis: clinical gynecologic endocrinology and infertility,* 5th ed. Baltimore: Williams & Wilkins, 1994:853–871.

The female patient: understanding endometriosis. *Ob Gyn* 24(6).

Winkel C. Laparoscopy plus GnRH analogues: a practical approach to endometriosis. *Contemp Ob/Gyn* 1999;99–110.

17. DIETHYLSTILBESTROL

Carol S. Havens

I. **Past use of diethylstilbestrol (DES) to prevent spontaneous abortions.** DES is a **synthetic estrogen** that was first synthesized during the 1930s. By 1940, its clinical use was approved in the United States. It then gained acceptance as a way to prevent spontaneous abortion and was widely used for this purpose during the 1940s and early 1950s. A review of records at the Mayo Clinic shows that 7% of all pregnant women between 1943 and 1959 received DES (16). In the late 1950s, controlled studies failed to show any benefit from this use of DES, and its popularity declined. However, it continued to be used until 1971, when the first study linking DES exposure *in utero* with clear cell adenocarcinoma was published. At that time, the use of DES for threatened abortion was proscribed by the Food and Drug Administration (FDA).

   A. **Incidence and prevalence.** The exact prevalence of DES exposure is unknown. However, it has been estimated that as many as 6 million people, including mothers, sons, and daughters, were exposed to DES between 1940 and 1971. There may be as many as 2 million women who were exposed to DES *in utero*. Whenever possible, **medical records should be obtained to ascertain whether DES exposure actually occurred.**

   B. **Problems associated with DES exposure in mothers who took DES**
      1. The relative risk of **breast cancer in DES mothers is 1.35.** This is a small but statistically significant increase in risk (4). There is no increased risk of endometrial cancer (17).
      2. Psychiatric disorders are more common in DES-exposed mothers, daughters, and sons than in nonexposed individuals. Mothers are more disturbed than daughters, with guilt being the most common symptom (19).

   C. **Problems associated with DES exposure of men *in utero*.** The effects on DES sons are now being investigated.
      1. There are **reports of an increased incidence of certain genital tract abnormalities,** including an increased incidence of meatal stenosis, hypospadias, epididymal cysts, hypoplastic testes, cryptorchidism, and microphallus.
      2. **Pathologic changes** have also been described in sperm, including decreases in total sperm count, percentages of motile sperm, motility grade, percentage normal morphology, and overall quality score. However, there has been no documented evidence of impaired fertility or sexual function (11).
      3. The incidence of **testicular cancer** has been less well studied, but several studies have documented an increased risk (13). Other studies have not documented an increased risk of malignancy, and the National Cancer Institute is currently conducting a case-control follow-up study of the health of DES sons (11).

   D. **Problems associated with DES exposure of women *in utero***
      1. **Structural changes. Noncancerous changes** have been found in both the upper and lower reproductive tract, including transverse vaginal and cervical ridges that have been described as cockscombs, collars, and pseudopolyps, as well as vaginal adenosis, cervical eversion, endocervical stenosis, abnormally shaped uterine cavities, and uterine hypoplasia. As many as one third of women exposed may have vaginal changes, and most will have cervical changes. As many as two thirds of the women exposed to DES *in utero* will have uterine abnormalities. Fallopian tubes can be foreshortened, sacculated, or convoluted. The incidence of endometriosis may be increased.

159

  a. **Vaginal adenosis** refers to the presence of columnar epithelium on
     or beneath the vaginal mucosa. Generally, by age 30, this epithe-
     lium has been transformed by squamous metaplasia into mature
     squamous epithelium. Remodeling of the vaginal and cervical ridges
     to a more normal appearance often occurs with time.
  b. Adenosis and subsequent metaplasia and structural abnormalities
     are **more frequent when the DES exposure was started early
     in pregnancy or given at a higher dosage.** The **critical time
     for abnormalities** occurring from DES appears to be **prior to
     20 weeks gestation.**
  c. Clear cell adenocarcinoma developed in ten patients being followed
     for adenosis. **Atypical adenosis** (glands resembling the epithelium
     of the fallopian tube or endometrium) is **probably a precursor** of
     clear cell adenocarcinoma.
2. **Cancer**
  a. **Clear cell adenocarcinoma of the vagina** is the malignancy most
     commonly reported in the DES-exposed population. The risk for this
     malignancy has been estimated to be 1:1,000 in DES-exposed daugh-
     ters (13). The **peak incidence is in the late teens and early 20s,**
     followed by a rapid decline. The age at which the diagnosis has been
     made ranges from 7 to 48. If clear cell adenocarcinoma develops in
     non-DES-exposed women, it usually occurs postmenopausally. In ad-
     dition, recurrences have been reported as long as 20 years after pri-
     mary treatment, so prolonged follow-up is necessary (11). DES-
     associated clear cell adenocarcinomas behave less aggressively than
     those that develop without a history of exposure (10).
  b. The 1985 DES task force concluded that a relation between expo-
     sure to DES *in utero* and the subsequent development of squamous
     cell carcinoma of the cervix had not been proven, but needed further
     study (18). Additional studies have **not** documented an increased
     risk (13).
  c. **Vaginal intraepithelial neoplasia** also occurs in DES-exposed
     women at a younger age than in nonexposed women. This is probably
     due to the large transformation zone seen as a result of exposure to
     DES. It also may be triggered by human papillomavirus infection (3).
3. **Decreased fertility.** There appears to be a small decrease in fertility
   in DES-exposed daughters. Poor cervical mucus may be more common
   in DES-exposed daughters (7).
4. **Increased prematurity rate.** The rates of **premature delivery and
   perinatal death** are significantly increased in DES-exposed daughters. As many as 40% of these pregnancies terminate prior to 37 weeks
   gestation. The incidence is highest in those women whose exposure to
   DES occurred earlier *in utero,* was of longer duration, or was to a higher
   total dosage.
  a. It is **controversial whether gross structural abnormalities of
     the vagina and cervix** put a woman at higher risk. However, the
     incidence of uterine abnormalities is not enough to explain the in-
     creased incidence of prematurity. The increased rate of prematurity
     may be secondary to incompetent cervix.
  b. **Although still controversial,** several studies have shown that
     DES-exposed daughters have **higher incidences of spontaneous
     abortion, ectopic pregnancy, premature cervical dilation,
     and premature rupture of membranes** than age-matched con-
     trols. These studies also indicate that although the **incidence of
     premature labor was increased** in DES-exposed daughters, this
     did **not** lead to an increase in fetal demise.
5. **Menstrual abnormalities.** Several studies have shown a significant
   increase in complaints of menstrual irregularities in DES-exposed
   daughters, especially **oligomenorrhea, dysmenorrhea, and hypo-**

menorrhea. Others have shown a decreased duration and amount of menstrual bleeding but no effect on cycle length or variability and no increase in dysmenorrhea.

6. **Psychiatric abnormalities.** The incidence of psychiatric disease, especially depression and anxiety, was reported approximately twice as often in DES-exposed offspring as in controls. DES daughters also reported having more difficulties in relationships with spouses or mates (6).

E. There are **no known effects in children of DES-exposed daughters or sons.**

F. **Investigative procedures.** In addition to the routine pelvic examination, including inspection of the vulva, speculum examination of the vagina and cervix, Papanicolaou (Pap) smear of the cervix (see section I.F.3.), and bimanual and rectovaginal examination, there are several procedures that should be included.

1. **Palpation of the vagina may provide the only evidence of malignancy** since there are rare cases of carcinoma that are submucosal only.

2. **Speculum examination.** The entire vagina must be visualized.
   a. Areas of **adenosis** may appear red and granular and are often ulcerated.
   b. Areas undergoing **squamous metaplasia** are undetectable.

3. **Cytologic studies.** Smears should be taken **from** the **vaginal fornices,** the **endocervix,** and the **exocervix.** It is unclear whether these need to be placed on separate slides or if a single circumferential smear of the vagina is sufficient. Women with the eventual diagnosis of clear cell adenocarcinoma of the vagina who had negative Pap smears only had a cervical smear done (8). **Any areas of gross changes in the lower or middle part of the vagina** should also be sampled (14).

4. **Iodine stain.** The entire vagina and cervix should be stained with iodine (either Schiller's or Lugol's solution) if the Pap smear is abnormal, to determine the boundaries of epithelial changes. **Only normal, highly glycogenated surface epithelium will stain.** This stain does not delineate intramural lesions.

5. **Biopsy.** A biopsy should be taken of all areas of induration, thickening, or palpable nodules.
   a. Any discrete area that appears **different in color or texture** than surrounding areas or has an atypical appearance on colposcopy should also be sampled.
   b. **Clear cell adenocarcinoma** has consistently developed near the distal border of vaginal or cervical mucosa that fails to stain with iodine, and biopsies should be taken of this area.
   c. **Random sampling** of normal mucosa is not recommended.

6. **Colposcopy** permits a more accurate assessment of the extent of epithelial changes in the vagina and cervix and can aid in directing biopsies. Colposcopy is not necessary to diagnose adenocarcinoma and should be done only by someone specially trained and competent in the technique. In addition, it should be done only as indicated by Pap smears.

G. **Management**

1. The **initial examination** should include all of the investigative techniques discussed in F. (colposcopy is optional **but** recommended) **at the time of menarche or age 14,** whichever comes first. However, it must be performed at a younger age in any patient with vaginal bleeding, spotting, or abnormal vaginal discharge. This examination should be done by someone experienced in evaluating DES-exposed women.

2. **For women with minimal changes,** including structural changes or adenosis and a negative initial examination, **yearly follow-up is adequate** and need only include palpation, inspection, and cytologic workup. This examination can be done by anyone experienced in these examinations.

3. **Vaginal cytologic studies can be omitted in those patients who have no epithelial changes in the vagina in the initial examination.** Those patients with **more extensive changes should be followed more frequently** by someone experienced in following DES-exposed daughters.
4. **Any abnormal Pap smears or biopsies should be reviewed by a pathologist** experienced in DES changes and referred to a gynecologist for definitive treatment.
5. **Thorough examination** should also be done any time a woman complains of **abnormal bleeding or discharge.**
6. The patient should also be **educated about the possible consequences of DES exposure.** Counseling should be provided for any psychological effects of being exposed to DES.
7. **Contraceptive choices for DES daughters may differ from the general population. Intrauterine devices are not recommended because of the possible structural alteration in the uterus (21). Also, pregnancy and use of oral contraceptives appeared to be associated with an increased risk of clear cell adenocarcinoma in those whose cancer was diagnosed before age 20. However, this may have been due to increased surveillance (17).**

II. **Current use of DES.** DES is currently used in the United States for **some cases of advanced carcinoma** of the breast or prostate gland, the management of which is beyond the scope of this manual. DES may still be given to pregnant women in Eastern and Central Europe, Africa, Asia, and Latin America, where the risks are less well known.

References

1. Barnes AB, et al. Fertility and outcome of pregnancy in women exposed in utero to diethylstilbestrol. *N Engl J Med* 1980;302:609.
2. Bibbo M, et al. A twenty-five year follow-up study of women exposed to diethylstilbestrol during pregnancy. *N Engl J Med* 1978;298:763.
3. Bornstein J, et al. Human papillomavirus associated with vaginal intraepithelial neoplasia in women exposed to diethylstilbestrol in utero. *Obstet Gynecol* 1987; 70:75.
4. Colton T, et al. Breast cancer in mothers prescribed diethylstilbestrol in pregnancy. *JAMA* 1993;269:2096.
5. Cousins L, et al. Reproductive outcome of women exposed to diethylstilbestrol in utero. *Obstet Gynecol* 1980;56:70.
6. Ehrhardt AA, et al. Psychopathology in prenatally DES-exposed females: current and lifetime adjustment. *Psychosom Med* 1987;49:183.
7. Goldberg JM, Falcone T. Effect of diethylstilbestrol on reproductive function. *Fertility and Sterility* 1999;72:1.
8. Hanselaar AGJM, et al. Cytologic examination to detect clear cell adenocarcinoma of the vagina or cervix. *Gynecologic Oncology* 1999;75:338.
9. Herbst A. Current health status of DES-exposed mothers, daughters, and sons. *Consultant* 1980(Feb):219.
10. Herbst AL. Diethylstilbestrol and adenocarcinoma of the vagina. *Am J Obstet Gynecol* 1999;181:1576.
11. Herbst AL. Behavior of estrogen-associated female genital tract cancer and its relation to neoplasia following intrauterine exposure to diethylstilbestrol (DES). *Gynecologic Oncology* 2000;76:147.
12. Hornsby PP, et al. Effects on the menstrual cycle of in utero exposure to diethylstilbestrol. *Am J Obstet Gynecol* 1994;170:709.
13. Marselos M, Tomatis L. Diethylstilbestrol. I: pharmacology, toxicology, and carcinogenicity in humans. *Eur J Cancer* 1992;28A:1182.
14. Mittendorf R, Herbst A. Managing the DES-exposed woman: an update. *Contemp Obstet Gynecol* 1994;39:62.
15. Ng A, et al. Natural history of vaginal adenosis in women exposed to diethylstilbestrol in utero. *J Reprod Med* 1977;18:1.

16. Noller K, Dish C. Diethylstilbestrol usage: its interesting past, important present, and questionable future. *Med Clin North Am* 1974;58:793.
17. Palmer JR, et al. Risk factors for diethylstilbestrol-associated clear cell adenocarcinoma. *Obstetrics and Gynecology* 2000;95:814.
18. Report of the recommendations of the 1985 DES task force of the U.S. Department of Health and Human Services. *MMWR* 1986;35:155.
19. Robboy S, et al. *Prenatal diethylstilbestrol (DES) exposure: recommendations of the diethylstilbestrol-adenosis (DESAD) project for the identification and management of exposed individuals.* Mar 1981; NIH pub. no. 81-2049.
20. Saunders EJ. Physical and psychological problems associated with exposure to diethylstilbestrol (DES). *Hosp Community Psychiatry* 1988;39:73.
21. Tedeschi C. Ties that bind: mothers, daughters and sons continue to feel effects of DES. *ADVANCE Nurse Pract* 1999(Nov):28–34.

18. ABNORMAL PAPANICOLAOU SMEAR

Richard H. Oi

I. **Purpose of the Papanicolaou (Pap) smear.** The death rate from cervical cancer has decreased significantly over the last 40 years as a result of widespread cervical cancer screening. Cervical squamous cell cancer is preceded by a precursor lesion, the identification and eradication of which will prevent progression to cancer. The precursor can be readily detected by a painless, reproducible, and reasonably accurate screening test, the **Pap smear,** which has been the basis for the significant decrease in cervical cancer mortality.

   A. **Physiologic features.** The cervical epithelium consists of stratified squamous cells on the ectocervix that transitions into mucinous columnar epithelium in the endocervix with the interface between the two tissues designated as the **squamocolumnar junction (SCJ).** The natural history of the endocervical columnar epithelium is to undergo metaplastic transformation to squamous epithelium, i.e., **squamous metaplasia,** this change being especially active during adolescence and during pregnancy. **The area involved with this metaplastic change is designated the <u>transformation zone</u> (TZ) and is the tissue at risk of being influenced by oncogenic factors, principally human papillomavirus (HPV), to initiate neoplastic change.** It is this area, which includes the SCJ, that **must be sampled when obtaining a Pap smear.**

   B. **HPV.** Investigations have established a very significant association between **HPV infections and cervical cancer precursors and invasive squamous cell carcinoma** (1). Some 70 genotypes have been identified and approximately 27 are associated with anogenital lesions. HPV genotypes may be broadly classified into two groups: (a) those associated with lesions that are at low risk for cancer progression (types 6 and 11), are more often associated with condylomatous lesions alone or with minimal degrees of dysplasia, and often regress spontaneously and (b) those that demonstrate a greater propensity for malignant progression (types 16 and 18) and are more often associated with higher grades of dysplasia and invasive carcinoma. However, presence of high-risk HPV types does not imply inexorable progression to cancer. Risk of neoplasia with types 31, 33, and 35 appears to be greater than with types 6 and 11, but less than with types 16 and 18 (see also Chapter 4).

II. **Guidelines for screening.** The following recommendations are a consensus of the American Cancer Society, American College of Obstetricians and Gynecologists, National Cancer Institute, American Medical Association, American Nurses' Association, American Academy of Family Physicians, and the American Medical Women's Association (2). **All women who are or who have been sexually active or who have reached age 18 should have an annual cervical smear and pelvic examination.**

   A. **Pap smear recommendations for women not considered to be at high risk for cervical cancer**

      1. A Pap test may be performed less frequently after three or more consecutive, satisfactory, normal annual examinations at provider discretion.

      2. There is no upper limit at which screening is discontinued.

   B. **High-risk women should be screened annually.** High-risk factors include:

      1. **Early age at first intercourse** (<17 years). In the adolescent, the TZ is especially active and may be more susceptible to oncogenic factors.

      2. **Multiple sexual consorts.** Multiple sexual partners increases the risk of exposure to HPV and perhaps other oncogenic cofactors that are sexually transmitted. Promiscuity of a male partner is also a risk factor.

      3. HPV infection. There is a strong association of genital HPV infections with squamous cancer precursors and squamous carcinomas.

      4. HIV infection. Decreased immunity increases the incidence of HPV-related lesions.

      5. Women who are smokers.

III. **Classification of Pap smears**

  A. **Descriptive.** The terms "mild, moderate, and severe dysplasia and carcinoma in situ" are used to designate precursor epithelial changes that untreated may progress to invasive squamous cell carcinoma. More recently, the term **cervical intraepithelial neoplasia** (CIN) has been suggested to designate these changes such that mild dysplasias are designated as CIN I, moderate dysplasias as CIN II, and severe dysplasias and carcinoma in situ as CIN III (3).

  B. **Cytologic reports**

    1. A National Cancer Institute workshop was convened and produced a consensus report, *The 1988 Bethesda System for Reporting Cervical Vaginal Cytologic Diagnoses,* (4) recommending the Bethesda System (TBS) as a guideline for reporting cytologic findings. Most cytopathology laboratories have adopted this terminology to ensure that communication of cytopathologic findings to the clinician will be in "unambiguous diagnostic terms that have clinical relevance."

    2. A second conference was convened in 1991 to evaluate initial TBS use and to consider appropriate modifications (5). Minor revisions were proposed but the general format was retained (Table 18.1).

IV. **Screening methodology**

  A. **Conventional Pap smear**

    1. Technique.

      a. The vaginal speculum should be moistened with water only. Lubricants should not be used since they will interfere with cytologic interpretation.

      b. The area sampled must include the TZ, which will also include the SCJ.

      c. If the patient has recently douched or if there is blood or lubricant present, the cytologic interpretation is compromised.

      d. When possible, avoid obtaining smears within 7 to 10 days of menses because the endometrial "exodus" may interfere with cytologic interpretation.

    2. Method.

      a. A sample from the endocervical canal and a spatula scraping of the ectocervix should include material from the TZ, the area at risk of neoplastic change.

      b. The **endocervical sample** is best obtained first, using an endocervical brush that is rotated a quarter-turn within the endocervical canal; and the material is smeared across the top half of a glass slide. Cervical cytology is exfoliative cytology and does not require vigorous scraping to obtain an adequate sample. As an alternative, a **saline-moistened noncotton swab** may be used to gather the endocervical material.

        (1) The presence of endocervical cells in the Pap smear ensures that the TZ and SCJ have been sampled.

        (2) The endocervical brush may be used in pregnant women, recalling that the normal endocervical canal is 2 to 3 cm in length and that vigorous manipulation is not necessary to obtain an adequate sample.

        (3) There appears to be an increasing incidence of adenocarcinomas of the cervix, especially relative to squamous cell carcinomas. The specific use of techniques to obtain material from the endocervical canal may improve detection of early glandular dysplasias and neoplasias.

Table 18.1. The Bethesda System for reporting cervical/vaginal cytologic diagnoses

FORMAT OF THE REPORT:
a. A statement on Adequacy of the Specimen for Evaluation
b. A General Categorization which may be used to assist with clerical triage (optional)
c. The Descriptive Diagnosis

ADEQUACY OF THE SPECIMEN
Satisfactory for evaluation
Satisfactory for evaluation but limited by ... (specify reason)
Unsatisfactory for evaluation ... (specify reason)

GENERAL CATEGORIZATION (OPTIONAL)
Within normal limits
Benign cellular changes: See descriptive diagnoses
Epithelial cell abnormality: See descriptive diagnoses

DESCRIPTIVE DIAGNOSES
Benign cellular changes
Infection
    Trichomonas vaginalis
    Fungal organisms morphologically consistent with *Candida* spp
    Predominance of coccobacilli consistent with shift in vaginal flora
    Bacteria morphologically consistent with *Actinomyces* spp
    Cellular changes associated with herpes simplex virus
    Other
Reactive changes
    Reactive cellular changes associated with:
    Inflammation (includes typical repair)
    Atrophy with inflammation ("atrophic vaginitis")
    Radiation
    Intrauterine contraceptive device (IUD)
    Other

Epithelial Cell Abnormalities
Squamous Cell
    Atypical squamous cells of undetermined significance: Qualify[a]
    Low-grade squamous intraepithelial lesion encompassing:
    HPV[b]
    Mild dysplasia/CIN 1
    High-grade squamous intraepithelial lesion encompassing:
    Moderate and severe dysplasia
    CIS/CIN 2 and CIN 3
    Squamous cell carcinoma
Glandular Cell
    Endometrial cells, cytologically benign, in a postmenopausal woman
    Atypical glandular cells of undetermined significance: Qualify[a]
    Endocervical adenocarcinoma
    Endometrial adenocarcinoma
    Extrauterine adenocarcinoma
    Adenocarcinoma, not otherwise specified (NOS)
Other malignant neoplasms: Specify
Hormonal evaluation (applied to vaginal smears only)
    Hormonal pattern compatible with age and history
    Hormonal pattern incompatible with age and history: Specify
    Hormonal evaluation not possible due to: Specify

---

[a] A typical squamous or glandular cells of undetermined significance should be further qualified as to whether a reactive or a premalignant/malignant process is favored.
[b] Cellular changes of human papillomavirus (HPV)—previously termed kollocytosis atypia, or condylomatous atypia—are included in the category of low-grade squamous intraepithelial lesion.
From: National Cancer Institute Workshop. The revised Bethesda system for reporting cervical and/or vaginal cytologic diagnoses report of the 1991 Bethesda workshop. *Acta Cytol* 1992;36: 273–275, with permission.

c. **The ectocervical sample** is then obtained with a plastic or wooden spatula that is shaped to include and to pass over the SCJ and TZ. This material may be smeared over the bottom half of the same slide and may overlap the endocervical material.

d. Immediate fixation in 95% alcohol or with fixative spray is important and necessary to prevent any spurious changes caused by drying.

e. Pap smear should be obtained prior to samples taken for sexually transmitted disease testing.

B. **Thin Prep Pap test** (6,7)

1. Thin Prep is a liquid-based, thin-layer preparation approved by the Food and Drug Administration in 1996.

2. A broom-like spatula and fixative solution is used.

3. The specimen is collected by rinsing cervical-vaginal material obtained with the broom-like spatula into a fixative fluid, and the vial is delivered to the laboratory.

4. Slides are prepared by manual pipetting or by an automated system resulting in a thin-layer preparation that is then manually screened.

5. Advantages.

   a. Produces slides that are superior to a conventional Pap smear in finding cases of abnormalities.

   b. Optimizes fixation and staining and eliminates poorly fixed material or drying artifact.

   c. Randomization ensures a more representative sampling of the cells obtained versus direct Pap smear sample.

   d. Clear cellular visualization makes evaluation easier and perhaps quicker.

   e. Residual material in the vial can be used for other tests, e.g., HPV DNA testing.

6. Disadvantages.

   a. Logistics of a card with a slide versus a vial with fluid to be delivered to the laboratory.

   b. More sample preparation time.

   c. Increased laboratory costs.

7. Many more laboratories are beginning to convert to Thin Prep Pap testing.

C. **Screening automation (AutoPap, PapNet)** (8)

1. Liquid-based material as in thin-layer preps are introduced into the automated Pap scanning instrument system that produces a computerized review of given numbers of images for each slide, which demonstrate areas with the highest likelihood of abnormalities. A cytotechnician then triages the material into a review or no review category.

2. This is likened to automated blood smear analyzers in that a machine is used to review a cytopathology specimen and changes conventional Pap smear screening methodology.

3. Early studies have demonstrated significant improvements in the detection of abnormal slides and improvement in the false-positive rate.

D. **HPV DNA testing** (9)

1. A hybridization technique assay (Hybrid Capture).

   a. Detects the presence or absence of HPV DNA.

   b. Determines whether low risk (HPV 6, 11) or intermediate risk (HPV 31, 33, 35) or high risk (HPV 16, 18) oncogenic viruses are present.

   c. Provides a quantitative assessment of viral load.

2. Potential role.

   a. Screening women, such as HIV patients, who are at high risk of having a cancer precursor.

   b. Identifying high-risk oncogenic HPV in women with persistent minor grades of Pap smear abnormality [atypical squamous cells of undetermined significance (ASCUS) and low-grade squamous intraepithelial lesion (LSIL)].

   c. Quality control of cytologic and histologic diagnosis.

3. Studies are ongoing to address sensitivity and specificity of HPV DNA testing as influenced by factors such as age of the patient, oral contraceptive use, pregnancy, immunosuppressed **states, and so on.**

VI. Clinical responses. With TBS (Table 18.1), appropriate actions are as follows.

A. A statement of specimen adequacy is required, addresses the problem of false-negative smears, and ensures that the TZ has been sampled. This section has three elements.

   1. Satisfactory for evaluation. Smear can be properly interpreted and the cytologic findings can be acted on as reported.

   2. Unsatisfactory for evaluation. The specimen is unreliable for the detection of any cervical abnormality. Repeat smear.

   3. Satisfactory for evaluation, but limited by is in most cases resulting from absence of an endocervical or metaplastic cell presence (i.e., the TZ may not have been sampled). Repeat smears, however, may not demonstrate endocervical elements because of physiologic reasons.

   a. Repeat smear in a high-risk patient.

   b. A low-risk patient (e.g., a monogamous woman without a previous abnormal smear and no history of sexually transmitted diseases including HPV) would not require a repeat sample, especially if it is unequivocally known that the TZ was sampled.

B. General categorization and descriptive diagnosis. "Benign cellular changes" and "epithelial cell abnormality" categories are followed by a descriptive diagnosis.

   1. Within normal limits. There are no abnormalities and the patient should return at an appropriate interval for routine screening.

   2. Benign cellular changes.

   a. Inflammatory or infectious process: Treat the specific agent if symptomatic (i.e., **candidiasis, trichomoniasis**). Cellular changes associated with **herpes simplex** should have culture confirmation, especially if childbearing is still a consideration.

   b. Reactive changes or atrophic changes. Nonspecific changes are probably not significant except if the patient is symptomatic.

C. Epithelial cell abnormality-squamous cells

   1. ASCUS cases are those in which cytologic findings are of uncertain significance. Cytologic changes are more than reactive changes but are without features of dysplasia.

   a. Repeat smears should be obtained every 4 to 6 months, until two negative smears have been reported; then the clinician should return to routine screening. A second ASCUS smear requires colposcopic evaluation.

   b. A high-risk patient or one with a history of previous abnormal smears or dysplasia on biopsy should be referred.

   c. In postmenopausal women who are not receiving estrogen replacement, the smear should be repeated after 3 weeks of daily intravaginal estrogen therapy. With a normal second smear the patient returns to routine screening. A continued equivocal smear is referred for colposcopy.

   2. LSIL

   a. Generally referred for colposcopy.

   b. Evaluation most often identifies a reversible viral lesion that may undergo spontaneous regression. A reliable, low-risk patient may therefore be followed with repeat smears every 4 to 6 months until she experiences two negative smears, after which she may return to annual screening. **If repeat smear shows LSIL, the patient should be referred for colposcopy.**

   c. Colposcopy in the pregnant patient.

   (1) If normal, the patient should be followed with repeat evaluation at least once more, usually in the late second trimester.

   (2) Changes consistent with HPV or CIN I and entire lesion seen. The patient may be followed with repeat smears **without** biop-

sies and thus not jeopardize the pregnancy. Repeat smears and colposcopy should be done in the late second trimester and if there is not any evidence of progression, the patient may deliver as obstetrically indicated with **definitive evaluation and management postpartum.** Low-grade lesions often undergo spontaneous regression after the pregnancy.

   4. **High-grade squamous intraepithelial lesion** (HSIL). These patients are all colposcopically evaluated and managed appropriately.
   5. **Squamous cell carcinoma.** An obvious lesion should have been biopsied even prior to obtaining the Pap smear; patients with covert lesions are referred for colposcopy.
   D. **Epithelial cell abnormality-glandular cell**
      1. **Atypical glandular cells of undetermined significance** (AGUS). These are cytologic changes in endocervical or endometrial cells showing more than reactive changes but lacking features of adenocarcinoma. AGUS should be subcategorized as of endocervical or endometrial origin.
         a. Endocervical glandular atypia.
            (1) A repeat smear may be considered in a low-risk patient.
            (2) The patient should be referred for colposcopy, directed cervical biopsies, and specifically a vigorous endocervical curettage.
            (3) If normal findings, smear should be reviewed before deciding on cone biopsy or follow-up repeat smear.
         b. Endometrial glandular atypia.
            (1) Requires endometrial biopsy and/or dilation and curettage and hysteroscopy in patients at risk for endometrial hyperplasia or neoplasia.
            (2) In low-risk patients such as a young patient, consider that the atypical glandular cells may be part of the menstrual exodus.
         c. Rarely, the source of atypical glandular cells is the fallopian tube or an epithelial tumor of the ovary.
      3. **Adenocarcinomas,** whether the suspected site is cervical, endometrial, ovarian, or no organ specified, should be referred for full evaluation.
VI. **Diagnostic methodology**
   A. **Colposcopy.** The technique involves examining the cervix with a well-illuminated binocular microscope while bathing the cervix with a dilute solution of vinegar.
      1. Examination should be considered satisfactory, i.e., the entire TZ can be visualized.
      2. CIN lesions are identified by acetowhite changes within the TZ bordering the SCJ. Directed biopsies are taken from the worst area identified in a lesion that is seen in its entirety, as determined by the degree of acetowhite changes with or without abnormal vascular patterns.
      3. Endocervical curettage is performed to complement the directed biopsy.
      4. A patient with a lesion that was seen in its entirety and that had a directed biopsy from its worst area showing CIN and a negative endocervical curettage can be managed by outpatient cryotherapy or LEEP excision.
   B. **Cone biopsy**
      1. Colposcopy has largely replaced cone biopsy as the first step in the investigation of an abnormal Pap smear. However, cone biopsy is still necessary to rule out cervical cancer in the following circumstances.
         a. The colposcopic examination is unsatisfactory because the entire TZ and SO cannot be visualized.
         b. An acetowhite lesion is identified, but the entire lesion cannot be seen, often because it extends into the endocervical canal.
         c. The endocervical curettage is positive for CIN (dysplasia) and therefore, an invasive lesion within the endocervical canal cannot be ruled out.
         d. There is a discrepancy among the cytologic, colposcopic, and histologic findings.

    e. Microinvasive carcinoma is identified in either the cervical or endo-cervical biopsy and conization is required to rule out a frankly invasive carcinoma.

    2. Cone biopsy is often **therapeutic,** as well as diagnostic because it will ascertain the presence of an invasive lesion and, if absent, will surgically remove any residual CIN.

C. LEEP is an office procedure often used as an alternative to cone biopsy. If endocervical evaluation is important as indicated in the need for cone biopsy (see section VI.B.), consider that the excised material may show thermal artifact at the endocervical margin that may make endocervical histology and involvement of endocervical margins difficult to ascertain. It is preferable to use LEEP as a treatment rather than a diagnostic procedure.

VII. Treatment

  A. Condyloma or condylomatous atypia

    1. These lesions rarely proceed to cancer, often undergo spontaneous regression, and thus may be observed over a variable period even up to 12 months.

    2. Eradication is by cryotherapy or LEEP excision if the lesions persist.

  B. CIN

    1. This precursor lesion is usually eradicated by outpatient therapy using cryosurgery or LEEP excision.

    2. If cone biopsy is necessary, it would be therapeutic in the absence of invasive disease.

    3. Hysterectomy may be offered only if there are other indications to remove the uterus.

    4. Whichever modality is used, extended follow-up with repeat Pap smears or colposcopy is indicated, anticipating recurrence or development of a new genital tract lesion.

  C. Invasive carcinoma is promptly referred for gynecologic oncology consultation and appropriate treatment.

References

1. Duggan MA. Human papillomaviruses in gynecologic cancer. *Curr Opin Obstet Gynecol* 1996;8:56.
2. Fink DJ. Change in American Cancer Society Checkup Guidelines for detection of cervical cancer. *CA* 1988;38:127.
3. Richart RM. Natural history of cervical intra epithelial neoplasia. *Clin Obstet Gynecol* 1968;10:748.
4. The 1988 Bethesda system for reporting cervical vaginal cytologic diagnoses. *JAMA* 1989;262:931.
5. The Bethesda system for reporting cervical vaginal cytologic diagnoses. Report of the 1991 Bethesda workshop. *Am J Surg Pathol* 1992;16:914.
6. Wilbur DC, Bonfigho TA, Rukowski MA, et al. Sensitivity of the AutPap 300 QC system for cervical cytologic abnormalities: biopsy data confirmation. *Acta Cytol* 1996;40:127.
7. Lee DR, Ashfag R, Birdsong GG, et al. Comparison of conventional Papanicolaou smears and fluid-based thin layer systems for cervical cancer screening. *Obstet Gynecol* 1997;90:278.
8. Team PPM. Assessment of automated primary screening on PAPNET of cervical smears in the prismatic trial. *Lancet* 1999;353:381.
9. Coy JT, Schiffman MH, Winzelberg DJ, et al. An evaluation of humanpapillomavirus testing as part of referral to colposcopy clinics. *Obstet Gynecol* 1992;80:389.

19. SPECIMEN COLLECTION AND INTERPRETATION

Gerald W. Upcraft

There are several laboratory procedures that are important in establishing or confirming specific gynecologic disorders. Knowledge of these procedures will enable the examiner to obtain adequate specimens and to choose the proper culture medium or fixative for transporting them to the laboratory. **Even in the absence of an obvious discharge, specimens for smears and cultures can be obtained from prospective sites.**

I. Microscopic examination
   A. Gram stain
      1. **Indication** is **any purulent discharge** from the vagina, urethra, Skene's or Bartholin's glands, rectum, or cervix.
      2. **Procedure.** A small amount of the discharge is **smeared on a glass slide, heat-fixed, and then flooded with crystal violet** washed off with distilled water and followed by **Gram iodine.** After 1 minute, the iodine is washed off, and the slide is **decolorized with acetone and counterstained with safranine.**
      3. Interpretation
         a. **Identification of intracellular gram-negative diplococci supports the diagnosis of gonorrhea** in women and is diagnostic in penile discharge specimens.
         b. **Small pleomorphic gram-negative variable bacilli or coccobacilli are characteristic of bacterial vaginosis.** Clue cells, which are vaginal cells with adherent coccobacilli on their surfaces, may be demonstrated in bacterial vaginosis (see Fig. 1.2).
         c. *Trichomonas vaginalis* is identified as **a pale-staining, pear-shaped parasite** with long flagella at the narrow end (see Fig. 1.3).
         d. **Polymorphonuclear leukocytes and bacteria are commonly found in routine vaginal smears** and may be part of the normal flora. Consequently, these findings are not helpful in the diagnosis of specific infections.
         e. **Occasionally, sperm** may be identified in the vaginal smears.
         f. **Yeast can be visualized as gram-positive budding organisms.**
   B. Dark-field examination
      1. **Indications. Ulcerated lesions of the vulva,** especially those found in the labia minora, may represent a chancre that occurs during the primary stage of syphilis. The identification of *Treponema pallidum* under dark-field examination is absolutely diagnostic.
      2. **Procedure.** The examiner should **wear gloves** when performing this test.
         a. **The lesion is compressed from the sides while cleansed** with a piece of sterile gauze moistened with saline.
         b. **The base of the lesion is gently scraped** with a sterile blade **until serum exudes** on the surface.
         c. The serum from the base of the lesion is then placed on a **glass slide under a coverslip and examined under oil immersion with dark-field illumination.**
         d. **Several samples** should be obtained and examined.
      3. **Interpretation.** *T. pallidum* will appear as **motile, corkscrew organisms with purposeful motion** across the microscopic field. Treponemes will be absent from lesions within a few hours after starting antibiotic treatment.

C. **Potassium hydroxide preparation** (KOH prep) for fungi
   1. **Indications are suspected yeast or fungal infections.**
   2. **Procedure. Skin scrapings or vaginal discharge** is placed on a **microscopic slide. One drop of 10% KOH** is added, **and a coverslip** is placed before examining under a microscope.
   3. **Interpretation.** Microscopic examination revealing **budding yeast, germinal tubes,** or **fungal hyphae** is diagnostic.
D. **Saline wet-mount preparation**
   1. **Indications include suspected trichomonal or bacterial vaginosis.**
   2. **Procedure.** A small amount of **vaginal discharge** is placed on a **microscopic slide,** a drop of **physiologic saline** is added, **and a coverslip** is placed. The slide is **examined immediately using a microscope.**
   3. **Interpretation.** Microscopic examination revealing characteristic **motile pear-shaped flagellate protozoans** is diagnostic for *T. vaginalis* infection. **Epithelial cells coated with bacteria,** giving a ground-glass appearance, are called **clue cells.** Clue cells are suggestive of bacterial vaginosis. **Spermatozoa** can also be identified in this manner. Fungal elements are occasionally seen but are better viewed using the KOH preparation described in section I.C.

II. **DNA/PCR test and cultures.** Cultures have largely been replaced by very sensitive and rapid DNA/PCR tests. In January of 2001, the Food and Drug Administration granted clearance to market a system for the direct qualitative detection of *Chlamydia trachomatis* and *Neisseria gonorrhoeae.* The test has been approved for use with endocervical swabs, male urethral swabs, and with male and female urine. The system employs strand displacement amplification technology.

Many culture techniques are organism specific. Some cultures can be cultivated in the office by persons experienced in microbiologic technique. Most require specialized handling and equipment. **Transport media are designed to keep organisms in a proper environment until they can be set up in specific culture media.** Transport media are commercially available as plated agar media or tube media in agar or broth form. Examples of these include Stuart's transport medium, which is brain-heart infusion broth for cultivation of bacteria, yeasts, and molds and Mycosel or Sabouraud's dextrose agar for isolation of fungi. Transgrow agar with vancomycin, colistin, and nystatin and carbon dioxide is recommended for the transportation and cultivation of *N. gonorrhoeae.* Gen-bec plates are a self-contained selective media for gonorrhea with a carbon dioxide source. They can be used for transport or culture in the office. Transport media do not contain carbohydrate or nitrogen sources necessary for replication, thereby preventing overgrowth of fastidious organisms by contaminating flora. **Gonorrhea, herpesvirus,** and **_Chlamydia_ require special handling**.

A. **Gonorrhea.** The **endocervical canal is the best site** to obtain specimens for DNA/PCR testing or cultures. Urinary tests for both gonorrhea and *Chlamydia* are available for women and men. These tests simplify testing of male partners of infected women and decrease the discomforts of testing for both men and women. Thirty percent of women who are culture-positive for *N. gonorrhoeae* from the endocervix, vagina, or rectum are asymptomatic and constitute a reservoir for the disease as do untreated male partners. Positive testing after treatment with recommended schedules is uncommon and is usually due to reinfection. Sensitive tests, such as DNA/PCR, may remain positive for 2 weeks despite successful treatment because of the presence of DNA in dead organisms. Interval culture in several months **is preferred** over reculture immediately post treatment.
   1. **Indications** include the presence of **purulent vaginal discharge, history of exposure** to gonorrhea, or **symptoms of pelvic inflammatory disease.**

a. **Urethral or vaginal swabs or urine testing** is indicated when cervical testing is unsatisfactory (i.e., in children or in posthysterectomy patients).

b. **Rectal or pharyngeal specimens** can also be cultured when indicated by history. At present, cultures should be prepared since test kits for DNA/PCR testing are not approved for these sources.

2. **Procedure.**

  a. **Sources of specimen.**

    (1) **Endocervical canal.** Through the speculum, **remove cervical mucus** preferably with a cotton swab.

      (a) Insert the small-tipped specimen swab into the endocervix and rotate for 15 to 30 seconds.

      (b) Insert the swab into the transport tube and break the swab at the score line.

      (c) Replace the cap and screw into place.

      (d) The endocervical swab should be kept between 3 to 30°C (38 to 86°F).

      (e) Transport to the laboratory within 24 hours.

    (2) **Urethral specimen. Strip the urethra toward the orifice to express exudate.** Use a sterile loop or **rayon** swab to obtain the specimen for culture or use the swab provided for DNA/PCR testing.

    (3) **Urine specimen.** The patient should **not** have urinated within 1 hour prior to collection.

      (a) The patient should collect the first 15 to 20 mL of voided urine (use the first part of the stream) in a plastic, preservative-free, sterile urine specimen cup.

      (b) Refrigerate the urine immediately at 2 to 8°C (36–46°F).

      (c) Transport to the laboratory on wet ice within 24 hours.

    (4) **Rectal culture.** Insert sterile **rayon** swab **approximately 1 in. into the anal canal.**

      (a) If the swab is **contaminated by feces, use another** swab to obtain the specimen.

      (b) Move swab from side to side in the anal canal to sample crypts.

      (c) Allow 10 to 30 seconds for absorption of organisms to the swab.

  b. **Culture media.**

    (1) **Thayer-Martin plates.** This is a culture medium for selective isolation of *N. gonorrhoeae*. It is composed of chocolate agar containing vitamins, cofactors, and antibiotics. Storage life of this medium at room temperature is 2 weeks. To get maximum recovery, the medium **must be at room temperature prior to inoculation.**

      (a) The swab is **rolled directly on the medium** in a large Z pattern and **cross-streaked immediately** with a sterile wire loop.

      (b) It is then **placed in a candle jar or carbon dioxide incubator** within 15 minutes.

      (c) **Begin incubation of plates the same day at 35 to 36°C.**

    (2) **Transgrow bottles.** This is a **selective medium for transport and cultivation of** *N. gonorrhoeae*. **It is recommended when specimens cannot be delivered to the laboratory (or incubator) on the day they are obtained.** This medium maintains viability of pathogenic *Neisseria* for more than 48 hours at room temperature. Storage life at room temperature is approximately 3 months. It may be stored in the refrigerator at 4°C until used, but it is important that it be warmed either to room temperature or preferably to 35 to 36°C before inoculation.

(a) To inoculate, remove the cap of the bottle, **soak up all excess moisture in bottle with specimen swab, then roll the swab from side to side** across the medium starting from the bottom, and tightly cap the bottle immediately.

(b) The Transgrow bottle is **stored in an upright position at 35 to 36°C for no more than 16 to 18 hours** and sent to the laboratory with the incubation time noted.

3. **Interpretation.** Ideally, all cultures should be sent to the laboratory for interpretation. In most states, this service is provided free of charge by the public health department. However, if one has to interpret the cultures in the office, after 24 to 48 hours of incubation at 35 to 36°C **growth on the medium will show convex, glistening, elevated, creamy, mucoid colonies 1 to 5 mm in diameter that are oxidase-positive. Gram stain** of smears from these colonies will show **gram-negative diplococci** approximately 0.8 µm in diameter.

B. *Candida.* The patient complains of **pruritus** and a **thick white or curdy discharge.** A drop of 10% KOH on a small amount of the discharge may show **thread-like (hyphae) or yeast-like structures microscopically.** In the event of a treatment failure or a negative microscopic examination, culture for yeast can be taken from the vaginal secretion. **Yeasts are part of the normal vaginal flora** and **need not be treated in asymptomatic** culture-positive patients.

   1. **Transport media.** Swabs taken from the discharge are placed in **Sabouraud's dextrose broth** or **Stuart's medium** and sent to the laboratory.

   2. If the cultures are done in the office, swabs from the discharge are **streaked on Sabouraud's glucose agar and incubated at room temperature.** After 48 to 72 hours, presence of **soft, cream-colored colonies with a yeastlike odor** is noted. Microscopically, these appear as long, budding cells adherent to one another.

C. *T. vaginalis.* The vaginal discharge is characteristically **thin, bubbly, yellowish, and has a foul odor.** A drop of saline mixed with a small amount of the secretion confirms the clinical impression by demonstrating the **pear-shaped, motile parasites with long flagella.** They are commonly two to three times the size of a white blood cell.

   Cultures for *T. vaginalis* are generally unnecessary and **not** easily done in the office. Rarely, cultures will demonstrate the organism when wet preparations are unrevealing.

D. **Bacterial vaginosis** is a common condition. The vaginal discharge is **thin, gray-white,** and **malodorous.** A saline preparation microscopically reveals clue cells, and a KOH preparation emits a fishy amine odor. This constellation of findings **is diagnostic.** Cultures for *Gardnerella vaginalis* are of limited value but can be helpful in difficult or recurrent cases.

E. *C. trachomatis.* Men and women are frequently infected with gonorrhea and *Chlamydia* at the same time. In men, *C. trachomatis* is the most common cause of nongonococcal urethritis. Both sexes may harbor the organism without exhibiting any clinical symptoms. In women, the **cervix, fallopian tubes, and urethra are common sites of infection** (see Chapter 5).

   1. Swabs obtained from the urethra or cervix provide specimens used to inoculate tissue cultures. These are sent to the laboratory in a transport medium specific for *Chlamydia.* Since *C. trachomatis* is an intracellular organism **some abrasion of the mucosal surfaces may be necessary to procure the specimen.**

   2. Cervical swabs or urine specimens may be used with newer more sensitive strand amplification tests. These tests provide results much faster and the tests are more specific and sensitive than culture methods.

F. **Genital herpes simplex virus (HSV).** In women, the most frequent sites of infection are the **mucosal surfaces of the labia, fourchette, and**

cervix. The early lesions consist of vesicles on the mucosal surfaces. The older lesions are ulcerated.

1. **Indication is any lesion consistent with the preceding description.**
2. **Procedure.** A specimen swab of a skin or genital lesion is collected during the acute stage of symptomatic infection and placed in a special transport media. The specimen may be placed in cell cultures to replicate for identification or it may be identified by monoclonal antibodies that detect early antigens of HSV. Serotyping of the virus (type 1 or 2) may also be done. Results are available within 16 hours to 7 days of receipt of the specimen, depending upon the culture method used. **The specimen must be collected during the acute phase of the infection.**
   a. Swabs from fresh lesions (vesicle content or ulcerated areas) are **placed in a viral culturette transport medium** (e.g., buffered Hank's balanced salt solution) **and must be delivered as rapidly as possible to the laboratory.**
   b. **If immediate delivery is not possible, specimens may be kept in the refrigerator no more than 24 hours.**
3. **Serologic tests** may be used to aid in the diagnosis of primary infections or to type viral strains. Two samples of patient's serum (1 mL each), placed in plastic vials and collected 2 weeks apart, represent **acute and convalescent serum.**
   a. **In primary infections,** the neutralizing antibody appears at 5 to 7 days and rises to a peak level at 10 to 21 days. This rise is maintained for many weeks and then falls to a level that is maintained for years.
   b. **Complement-fixing antibodies** follow a pattern similar to neutralizing antibodies. A **fourfold increase in titer is diagnostic of primary infection.** Recurrent infection shows only a slight increase in antibody levels.
4. **Papanicolaou** (Pap) **smears** from the cervix or lesion may demonstrate large multinucleate cells with intranuclear eosinophilic inclusions.

III. **Pap smears.** Important information can be derived from Pap smears from the genital tract. In addition to the differentiation between a benign and malignant lesion, they may be used as **screening procedures for cytohormonal evaluation by utilizing smears obtained from the vaginal pool.**

A. **Vaginal**
1. **Evaluation of endocrine status of women** can be assessed by examination of the squamous cells from the vaginal smears. The **maturation index** refers to maturation of the squamous epithelium comparing parabasal, intermediate, and superficial cells based on a 100-cell count. Several factors may influence the status of the squamous epithelium and **may yield inaccurate results.** These are the **presence of inflammatory processes** caused by bacterial or trichomonal infection, **cytolysis** caused by certain microorganisms, **or drugs other than hormones.**
2. **Procedure.** Vaginal smears for hormonal evaluation should be obtained from the **proximal portion of the lateral wall of the vagina.**
3. **Interpretation.** A normal menstruating woman at the time of ovulation will show a maturation index of 5 : 35 : 60 (5% parabasal cells, 35% intermediate cells, and 60% superficial cells). In postmenopausal women, the maturation index is approximately 90 : 10 : 0. **Predominance of superficial cells indicates high estrogen effect, and predominance of parabasal cells indicates low estrogen effect.**

B. **Cervical**
1. **Indications.**
   a. **Routine Pap smears.** Routine Pap smears should be performed (see Chapter 32 for guidelines). In patients with cervicitis, a repeat smear is recommended 6 weeks to 2 months **after** treatment of the infection.

      b. Suspicion of malignancy based on a visible lesion or previous diagnosis of dysplasia should prompt colposcopically directed cervical biopsy and endocervical curettage.

  2. Procedure. Scrapings should include **both exocervical and endocervical areas.**

      a. An endocervical swab can be obtained with a cotton-tipped applicator moistened with physiologic saline. **Better results** have been obtained using a specialized **endocervical brush** to collect the specimen.

      b. The exocervical scrapings may be obtained by the use of a **wooden or plastic spatula.** A special spatula designed to obtain both endocervical and exocervical material is available commercially.

      c. Fixation of the smears on glass slides is obtained by either placing them immediately in 95% alcohol or using special fixative sprays.

      d. Thin Prep Pap smears. Rather than smearing the cervical sample onto a slide as is done with the conventional Pap smear, the collection device provided in the kit is rinsed in a vial of preserving solution.

        (1) The specimen is then sent to a laboratory where a processor is used to disperse and filter the contents to reduce blood, mucus, and inflammation.

        (2) A thin, even layer of the cervical cells is then automatically deposited onto a slide.

        (3) The result is a uniform preparation of well-preserved cells ready for microscopic examination.

        (4) The Thin Prep **improves** the **detection** of low-grade and more severe lesions and **reduces** the number of less-than-adequate specimens submitted.

      e. Human papillomavirus (HPV) DNA testing with Hybrid Capture. The **combination** of **Pap smear and HPV DNA testing** is **more effective in detecting invasive cancers and high-grade lesions than either test alone.** It is know that women whose Pap smears have been read as negative **and** who have negative HPV DNA testing are at **virtually no risk** of developing cervical cancer or a high-grade precursor in the next 5 to 10 years.

        (1) Specimens may be collected with specially provided kits or the test can be performed on the cellular residues of liquid-based cytology collection kits for Thin Prep Pap smears.

        (2) Patients whose cervical Pap smears have been read as atypical and who also have positive HPV DNA testing can be triaged for colposcopy.

        (3) Specific HPV genotypes have been shown to be associated with certain anogenital diseases.

          (a) Types 6, 11, 42, 43, and 44 (low-risk group) are associated with benign condylomas (warts).

          (b) Types 16, 18, 31, 33, 35, 45, 51, 52, and 56 (high-risk group) are associated with cervical carcinoma and its predisposing lesions: cervical atypia, severe dysplasia, cervical intraepithelial neoplasia, and carcinoma in situ.

  3. Interpretation.

      a. See Chapter 4 (HPV) and Chapter 18 (Abnormal Pap Smear) for test interpretation.

C. Breast

  1. Indications.

      a. Any nipple discharge or crusted lesions of the nipple should be investigated to **rule out malignancy.**

      b. Prior to biopsy, cystic or solid masses in the breast can be investigated in the office.

  2. Procedure.

      a. When there is **obvious nipple discharge,** express a small amount and smear it on a glass slide. **Prepare the slide as for a Pap smear.**

    b. In cystic or solid breast masses, fine-needle aspiration may be used.

      (1) A syringe holder is available commercially but is not necessary. A disposable 20-mL syringe fits in this holder. Using a 21-gauge needle, **an aspirate is easily obtained from a cystic mass.**

      (2) The liquid aspirate is transported to the laboratory for **immediate cytologic processing or fixed in 50% alcohol** and processed later.

      (3) With a solid mass, the same instrument is used for obtaining specimens for cytologic examination. The syringe holder allows the examiner to hold the syringe with one hand and use the other hand to localize and fix the mass as the aspiration is being performed.

        (a) The **needle is directed to the mass** and the syringe plunger is withdrawn, creating a negative pressure in the barrel of the syringe. As one maintains a negative pressure, **multiple punctures** are done in the mass. Release the plunger and withdraw the needle and syringe. All the aspirated cellular material is concentrated in the barrel of the needle.

        (b) Squirt the aspirated material onto a **glass slide and make smears** for cytologic examination. The smears may be **air-dried and stained with Wright's stain for immediate interpretation or fixed in 95% alcohol solution or sprays** for Pap staining.

   3. Interpretation. The smears stained with Wright's stain are examined immediately.

    a. Benign lesions will show mainly inflammatory cells and occasional normal columnar epithelial cells.

    b. If the lesion is malignant, abnormal epithelial cells with increased nuclear-cytoplasmic ratio and prominent nucleoli are identified. Sometimes a necrotic background with nuclear fragments gives a clue to the diagnosis of malignancy.

IV. Endometrial specimens: biopsy

  A. Indications

    1. Abnormal uterine bleeding.

    2. Infertility investigations.

    3. Surveillance of hormonal replacement.

    4. To collect specimens for culture.

  B. Procedure

    1. For infertility studies and dating of the endometrium, only a small sample is necessary. It may be obtained using a commercially available, small, plastic cannula aspiration device.

    2. For other purposes, a Novak biopsy curette or other plastic curette can be used. First, the cervix is stabilized with a single-tooth tenaculum. The curette is passed gently through the undilated cervical os to the uterine fundus. **The cavity is curetted systematically,** obtaining samples from anterior, posterior, and both lateral walls. Vacuum is maintained using a syringe. Endocervical curettage should also be done, if indicated.

    3. The specimen is fixed in 10% buffered formalin or other suitable fixative for histologic examination. **The clinical history, including date of last menstrual period, hormonal therapy, and purpose for the biopsy, should accompany the specimen to the laboratory.**

  C. Interpretation

    1. The pathologist should report the apparent menstrual dating of the endometrium. The patient must report the date of onset of her next menses. The pathologic and clinical dating are compared retrospectively.

2. **Simple, cystic, or adenomatous hyperplasia** is a reversible change of the glandular lining of the uterus. It is considered to be the result of excessive or unopposed estrogen stimulation. Left untreated, a small percentage of patients with these lesions will eventually develop endometrial adenocarcinoma. Most lesions of this type will regress spontaneously or with progestogen therapy. **Follow-up biopsy is required 3 months after progestin therapy has been started.**

3. **Metaplasia** of the endometrium is indicative of excessive estrogenic stimulation.

4. **Atypical adenomatous hyperplasia** is a precancerous change. Hyperplasias with atypia carry a substantial risk for development of endometrial adenocarcinoma but may also regress spontaneously. This result should prompt consideration of hysterectomy.

5. **Endometrial carcinoma** (true malignancy).
   a. **Adenocarcinoma** is an invasive malignancy characterized by abnormal glandular proliferation. It is graded from well-differentiated to poorly differentiated.
   b. **Adenoacanthoma** is an adenocarcinoma with **benign** squamous metaplasia.
   c. **Adenosquamous carcinoma** is an invasive malignancy of endometrial glands with **malignant squamous components.** It carries a **poor prognosis.**
   d. **Papillary serous adenocarcinoma is a highly malignant** lesion that behaves similarly to epithelial ovarian carcinoma. It too carries a **poor prognosis.**

6. **Stromal sarcoma** is an invasive malignancy of poor prognosis that spreads by contiguous extension and lymphatic metastasis.

V. Biopsy

A. Vulvar

1. **Indications. Biopsies should be taken of any visible subcutaneous mass or epidermal lesions of the vulva** if malignancy is suspected.

2. **Procedures.**
   a. **Movable subcutaneous nodules are easily excised** with or without an ellipse of overlying skin.
   b. **An elliptic skin biopsy** with adequate margins is used for **epidermal lesions.**
   c. **Punch biopsies can be used on larger lesions.**
   d. **Biopsy specimens** are fixed in **10% buffered formalin** for histologic processing.

3. **Interpretation.**
   a. **Benign epidermal lesions** include chronic dermatitis, nevi, actinic keratoses, and vulvar dystrophies.
   b. **Benign subcutaneous lesions** include epidermal inclusion cysts, Bartholin's cysts, fibromas, and granular cell myoblastomas.
   c. **Malignant lesions** include noninvasive or invasive squamous cell carcinoma, Paget's disease, basal cell carcinoma, malignant melanoma, and Bartholin's gland carcinoma.

B. Vaginal

1. **Indications. Any palpable mass or ulcerated lesions** of the vagina should be biopsied.

2. **Procedure. Excisional biopsy** of the mass or mucosal lesion is done for histologic diagnosis.

3. **Interpretation.**
   a. **Mucosal lesions** include inflammatory, dysplastic, and neoplastic processes.
   b. **Malignant lesions** consist primarily of squamous cell carcinoma, either noninvasive or invasive.

c. **Vaginal adenosis or well-differentiated clear-cell adenocarcinoma** of the vaginal wall can be seen in young women of mothers who had diethylstilbestrol during pregnancy. It is believed to be of müllerian duct origin (see Chapter 17).

d. **Sarcoma botryoides** is a vaginal tumor seen in infants and children. It is **invasive and highly malignant**.

C. **Cervical**

1. **Indications.**

   a. **Following a routine Pap smear with cytologic diagnosis of malignancy or dysplasia.**

   b. **Nonspecific cervicitis unresponsive to medical treatment or any other ulcerative or papillary cervical lesions.**

2. **Procedure.**

   a. **Three percent acetic acid (fresh common household vinegar)** is used to **identify areas suggestive of dysplasia, metaplasia, or malignancy.** These areas undergo a color change described as the acetowhite reaction.

   b. **Small biopsies** are taken from areas showing dyskaryotic areas by colpomicroscopy. **Schiller's test** aids in localizing these areas. The principle involved in the Schiller's test is that the glycogen-containing cells of normal squamous epithelium stain dark brown with Lugol's iodine solution. Nonglycogenic epithelium becomes yellow-white. Glycogen is absent or minimal in malignant cells. The **squamocolumnar region of the cervix is a frequent site of early squamous carcinoma formation.**

   c. **Conization is a surgical procedure that includes total ablation of the squamocolumnar junction of the cervix and its epidermal surface** by means of a cone-shaped excision. A black silk suture may be placed at the 12 o'clock position on the cone biopsy specimen, to use as a reference point for the pathologist to use in localizing the site and margins of the neoplastic process. Conization is performed in the hospital operating room.

3. **Interpretation.**

   a. **Nonspecific chronic cervicitis is a benign lesion.**

   b. **Mild, moderate, and severe dysplasia.**

      (1) **All degrees of dysplasia** are premalignant lesions and are usually treated with cytodestructive procedures such as cryotherapy, excision, or laser vaporization.

      (2) **Dysplasias, carcinoma in situ** (CIS), **and microinvasive squamous cell carcinoma** are frequently **asymptomatic** and **may not exhibit any gross abnormalities of the cervix.** They are diagnosed by routine Pap smears, colposcopy, and biopsies.

   c. **CIS and microinvasive squamous cell carcinoma** are early stages of cervical carcinoma (see section V.C.3.d). They are localized in the cervical epithelium. In microinvasive squamous cell carcinoma, the abnormal epithelial proliferation has broken through the basement membrane in a few areas and has invaded the superficial stroma.

   d. **Invasive squamous cell carcinoma.** The neoplastic process has **invaded the deeper portion of the underlying stroma.** These tumors usually show **gross erosions or ulcerated areas.**

VI. **Colposcopy and colpomicroscopy.** The colposcope was originally designed by Hinselmann in 1926. It consists of a binocular magnifier incorporating a powerful light source. The colposcope enables the examiner to view the structure of the superficial cervical epithelium at magnification of up to × 200.

   Since colposcopy should be done only by clinicians specially trained in this technique, interpretation is beyond the scope of this book.

The **procedure** for colposcopy is as follows:

A. **Pap smears need to be done first.**

B. **The cervix is cleansed** with a cotton sponge and the **entire area is then scanned** with the colposcope.

C. **The vascular pattern** is visualized by the use of a green filter.

D. A 3% acetic acid solution causes a color change reaction and helps differentiate normal epithelium from metaplastic or abnormal epithelium.

VII. **Pregnancy tests.** Tests for pregnancy are based on detection of **human chorionic gonadotropin** (hCG). This hormone is produced by the placenta and is **detectable about 10 days after fertilization.** The use of monoclonal antibody technology has rendered biologic and agglutination tests for pregnancy obsolete. False-positive tests and confusing results attributable to interfering substances have been virtually eliminated as a source of error. Since the sensitivity of the urine and serum pregnancy tests are essentially the same, the serum tests are used only when the level of hCG must be quantified or the urine sample is not satisfactory.

A. **Urine**

  1. **Indications.** This specimen is used for the **detection of early uterine or ectopic pregnancy.**

  2. **Procedure and interpretation.**

    a. **A freshly voided early-morning urine specimen** is recommended.

    b. **Restrict intake of fluids** from midnight until morning collection, if possible.

    c. A specific gravity of 1.015 is desirable for this pregnancy test.

    d. A positive test is **positive even with low specific gravity.** A dilute urine could produce a false-negative result.

B. **Serum tests**

  1. **Quantitative hCG analysis.**

    a. **Radioimmunoassay (RIA) or microparticle enzyme immunoassay** are used to detect very low levels of hCG in serum. These assays can be easily and accurately quantitated. The methodology is complex and performed only in clinical laboratories.

    b. **Indications** are to determine the viability of an intrauterine pregnancy, to determine timing of early sonographic examination, or to manage trophoblastic diseases.

  2. **Interpretation.**

    a. hCG values during normal pregnancy can reach 100,000 mIU/mL or more during the first trimester. Values decrease in the second and third trimesters.

    b. hCG levels higher than 2 mIU/mL can be detected.

    c. hCG levels higher than 100,000 mIU/mL can be found in trophoblastic diseases.

    d. **Intrauterine pregnancy can be demonstrated by direct pelvic ultrasound when hCG levels exceed 6,500 mIU/mL.** Failure to detect intrauterine pregnancy at this level is suggestive of ectopic pregnancy or trophoblastic disease.

    e. **In early normal pregnancy, hCG levels double every 2 to 3 days.** Failure to do so suggests ectopic pregnancy, missed abortion, or "blighted ovum."

    f. Serial determinations of hCG are useful to assess response to treatment by surgery or chemotherapy and to detect recurrences of trophoblastic diseases. It is important that the same methodology and laboratory be used for comparison of consecutive specimens.

  3. **Qualitative hCG analysis.** Serum pregnancy tests are occasionally useful when urine specimens are inadequate or unsuitable for evaluation.

VIII. **Immunofluorescent techniques**

A. **Indications**

  1. **Identification of chlamydial and viral organisms.**

  2. **Identification of *Treponema pallidum.***

B. Procedure and interpretation. The fluorescent antibody method is an **in vitro measurement of antibody response.** In general, infected cells are exposed to the patient's serum, washed, and then exposed to fluorescent antibody directed against human immunoglobulins. If the patient's serum has antibodies against the virus (e.g., herpesvirus) that infects the cells, the tissue will be stained by the fluorescent antihuman gamma globulin. In the absence of antibody, specific staining will not occur.

IX. Serologic tests

    A. Venereal Disease Research Laboratory (VDRL) test is a slide microflocculation test used in screening for syphilis. It is an antigen-antibody reaction using cardiolipin combined with lecithin and cholesterol (commercially available) as the antigen and the patient's serum as the antibody. The serum of the patient must be incubated at 58°C for 30 minutes to inactivate complement and other inhibitors. Presence or absence of flocculation is observed.

        1. Results are nonreactive if there is no flocculation, weakly reactive if there is slight flocculation, and reactive if definite flocculation occurs.

        2. A positive result suggests syphilis infection; therefore, specific tests for syphilis should be carried out.

        3. False-positive results may occur in patients with infectious **mononucleosis, hepatitis, or leprosy** and for several months following a **smallpox vaccination.**

    B. Rapid plasma reagin (RPR) card test is a modified Wasserman or VDRL test. Ethylenediaminetetraacetic acid (EDTA) and choline chloride have been added to the cardiolipin-lecithin-cholesterol complex to inactivate the substances in unheated sera. Therefore this is used as another **screening test for syphilis and has been replacing the standard VDRL test.**

        The **procedure** consists of **mixing** the plasma of the patient and the reagent in a rotating motion with an applicator stick on a hard-faced piece of white cardboard and **observing** for flocculation. The interpretation of the results is similar to the VDRL. The test has also been automated for processing large numbers of specimens efficiently.

    C. Fluorescent treponemal antibody absorption test (FTA-ABS) is a test for antitreponemal antibody based on the principle of the indirect fluorescence procedure. If a virulent *T. pallidum* from an infected rabbit testis is placed on a glass slide and overlaid with serum from a patient with antibody to treponemes, an antigen-antibody reaction will occur with the antibody binding firmly to the surface of the treponeme. If the treponeme-antibody mixture is then exposed to an antibody against human gamma globulin tagged with fluorescein isothiocyanate and viewed under a fluorescent microscope, all human antitreponemal-antibody binding to the spirochete will be tagged with fluorescein dye and will outline the treponeme (antigen).

        The original FTA used a 1:5 serum dilution, and it was very sensitive but not very specific. It gave a positive result in 30% of patients with no known history of syphilis. Currently used is the FTA-ABS, which is a modification of the FTA by absorbing **the nonspecific treponemal antibodies which then gives a higher sensitivity.** The FTA-ABS can be **performed in most clinical laboratories, and the results are available within a day.** It is a specific test for syphilis and is used for confirmation.

        Indication is a **positive VDRL or RPR or the presence of a hard, nontender ulcer in the vulva, posterior vaginal fornix, or exocervix** after history of syphilis contact, which may represent a lesion in the primary stage of syphilis.

    D. Microhemagglutination assay for antibodies to *T. pallidum* (MHA-TP)

        1. Indication. This test is used both to **screen for and confirm syphilis.**

        2. Procedure. The MHA-TP is **automated.**

        3. Interpretation. The reactivity of this test has 90% to 95% agreement with the FTA-ABS test. Results are similar to FTA-ABS.

E. FTA-cerebrospinal fluid (CSF) test is the FTA test without the absorption step, using CSF instead of serum. It is considered **highly sensitive for neurosyphilis.** It is **lacking somewhat in specificity** since as many as 5% of those with a negative serum FTA-ABS have a positive FTA-CSF test. **False-positive results** are believed to result from blood contaminating the CSF at the time of collection or by alteration in the blood-brain barrier, which permits serum proteins to enter the CSF.

References

1. Cox JT. Clinical role of HPV DNA testing. In: Lorincz AT, Reid R, eds. Human papillomavirus 1, 2nd ed. *Obstet Gynecol Clin North Am* 1996;23(3):811–851.
2. Frenczy A. The Bethesda system (TBS): advantages and pitfalls. In: Franco E, Monsonego J, eds. *New developments in cervical cancer screening and prevention.* 1997:151–158.
3. Henry JB. *Clinical diagnosis and management,* 16th ed. Philadelphia: WB Saunders, 1991.
4. Jolly JLS. Minimal criteria for the identification of *Gardnerella vaginalis* isolated from the vagina. *J Clin Pathol* 1983;36:476.
5. Koss L. *Diagnostic cytology and its histopathologic bases,* 4th ed. Philadelphia: Lippincott, 1992.
6. Oates JK. Genital herpes. *Br J Hosp Med* 1983;29:13.
7. Peter JB, Lovett MA. Genital infection from *Chlamydia trachomatis. Diagn Med* Nov–Dec; 1982.
8. Tietz NW. *Clinical guide to lab tests,* 3rd ed. Philadelphia: WB Saunders, 1995.

20. ADNEXAL MASSES

Kathleen E. Taylor

An adnexal mass is an **abnormality of the tubes or ovaries.** The differential diagnosis must include other abdominopelvic structures, such as bowel, bladder, uterus, and lymph nodes and their pathologies, and will vary somewhat with the age of the patient. Ovarian cysts and neoplasms can occur at any age.

I. **History.** This is the most important part of any workup. A careful history of **symptoms, time course, relationship of problems to menstrual cycles, and bowel and bladder function** will direct diagnostic tests.
   A. **Sexual history.** Adolescent women should be **interviewed alone** for at least part of the time without parent, guardian, or friend present. It is important to obtain an accurate sexual history that includes the following:
      1. Number of partners.
      2. Coital frequency.
      3. Method of contraception.
      4. Dyspareunia.
      5. Partner's symptoms.
   B. **Gynecologic history** should include questions on the following:
      1. Menarche.
      2. Cycle length.
      3. Length and heaviness of flow.
      4. Any change in the menstrual pattern.
      5. Intermenstrual and premenstrual symptoms.
      6. Irregular bleeding or spotting.
      7. History of vaginitis, vaginal discharge, or irritation.
      8. History of sexually transmitted diseases.
      9. Pregnancy history including any complications.
      10. Genitourinary procedures including any complications.
      11. Any abdominal surgery including any complications.
   C. **General history**
      1. A general history should be obtained with an **emphasis on the endocrine system** including the following:
         a. Temperature intolerance.
         b. Hair and skin changes.
         c. Nervousness or tremor.
         d. Tiredness or weakness.
         e. **Breast changes, discharge, or both.**
         f. Weight change.
         g. Urinary frequency or dysuria.
         h. Bowel patterns: diarrhea, constipation, flatulence, mucus, or blood in stools.
      2. A **history of any mental or emotional stress,** recent and past, should be elicited.
      3. A **complete drug use history,** specifically asking about nonprescription items such as laxatives, antacids, vitamins, and analgesics as well as recreational drugs, smoking, and alcohol, is important.
      4. A **history of illnesses, medications, hospitalizations, and surgeries** should be obtained.
      5. A careful family history on **both** paternal and maternal sides should be taken, **especially** for **breast, endometrial,** and **ovarian cancers. Two or more first- or second-degree relatives with these cancers may indicate a familial syndrome** with a genetic risk of up to 50% for development of ovarian cancer. So far, all families registered in the Familial Ovarian Cancer Registry are caucasian.

II. **Physical examination.** The following should be particularly emphasized in the general physical examination since some ovarian neoplasms are hormonally active.
   A. **Skin and hair**
      1. Skin and hair should be examined for signs of **virilization** including acne, temporal balding, and male-pattern hair distribution.
      2. **In the preadolescent patient,** Tanner stage of pubic hair development should be determined.
      3. The skin should be examined for **dryness, eruptions, or other lesions.**
   B. **Breasts.** The following should be noted:
      1. Tanner stage in girls (Table 20.1).
      2. Tenderness.
      3. Gland enlargement.
      4. Areolar pigmentation.
      5. Breast masses.
      6. Discharge.
   C. **Lymphatics. Careful palpation** of supraclavicular, axillary, and inguinal nodes and examination for **hepatosplenomegaly** should be done.
   D. **Abdomen.** Abdominal examination should include listening to **bowel sounds** and **checking for organomegaly, tenderness, guarding, and rebound.**
   E. **Genital and pelvic examinations** should be done with the following emphasized.
      1. **Clitoromegaly.** The normal size is 2 to 4 mm wide and **larger than 10 mm is significant virilization.**
      2. **Vagina.**
         a. **Evaluate moistness and rugosity,** which indicate an estrogen effect.
         b. The presence of unusual odor, color, and consistency of **discharge** should be noted.
      3. **Cervix.** Discharge should be cultured for gonorrhea and *Chlamydia.* A mucopurulent discharge can be present with either infection.

Table 20.1. Tanner staging in girls*

Stage	Breast	Pubic hair
Stage 1 (prepubertal)	Elevation of papilla only	No pubic hair
Stage 2	Elevation of breast and papilla as small mound, areola diameter enlarged Median age: 9.8 years	Sparse, long, pigmented hair chiefly along labia majora Median age 10.5 years
Stage 3	Further enlargement without separation of breast and areola Median age: 11.2 years	Dark, coarse, curled hair sparsely spread over mons Median age: 11.4 years
Stage 4	Secondary mound of areola and papilla above the breast Median age: 12.1 years	Adult type hair, abundant but limited to the mons Median age: 12.0 years
Stage 5	Recession of areola to contour of breast Median age: 14.6 years	Adult type spread in quantity and distribution Median age: 13.7 years

* From: Speroff L, Glass RH, Kase NG. *Clinical gynecologic endocrinology and infertility*, 4th ed. Baltimore: Williams & Wilkins, 1989, with permission.

F. Bimanual and rectal examinations are most important.
  1. The **anterior and posterior vaginal walls** should be palpated and evaluated for pain or a mass.
    a. A **rectovaginal wall dissection** may occur with abscess. This is a soft, tender widening of the septum and is best felt on rectovaginal examination.
    b. Also, the patient should be evaluated for **bladder tenderness, distention, and fecal impaction.**
  2. **Cervical motion tenderness.** Referred pain in one or both adnexa indicates inflammation whether from pus, cyst fluid, or blood.
  3. **Uterine position.**
    a. A **mass anterior to the uterus** displacing it backward may be a full bladder with a urethral obstruction. **Dermoid cysts** may present in this position, floating anteriorly because of the relatively higher fat content.
    b. **Parovarian and ovarian masses** may deviate the uterus to one side.
    c. If the **uterus is fixed posteriorly** and cannot be easily manipulated, **adhesions, endometriosis, or cancer** is suspected.
    d. **Tender nodularity felt on the uterosacral ligaments** by rectal examination is also seen commonly in **endometriosis.**
    e. An **irregular uterine outline** that is firm, nontender, and fairly mobile is usually indicative of **fibroids.** They may vary in size from a few millimeters to a mass that reaches above the umbilicus.
    f. If the irregularities extend into the adnexa, they may make ovarian evaluation impossible. It is **difficult to distinguish between a lateral fibroid and an ovarian mass by palpation.**
    g. A **smooth uterine enlargement** that may be slightly tender indicates **the most common pelvic mass—pregnancy.** Even if the pregnancy is in the fallopian tube, the hormonal changes will cause some uterine enlargement (approximately 6 weeks size).
  4. **The adnexa need to be gently evaluated,** particularly if there is pelvic pain. Too vigorous an examination may rupture a cyst or ectopic pregnancy. Size, shape, mobility, consistency, fluctuance, and tenderness should be noted.
    a. **An ectopic pregnancy** may be felt as a 2- to 3-cm, soft swelling just lateral to the uterine fundus.
    b. A **diffuse, thickened, tender area** is often found with **salpingitis.**
    c. An **ovarian neoplasm** usually will not be tender unless it has undergone torsion, has hemorrhaged within itself, or has leaked fluid.
    d. A **follicle or corpus luteum cyst** is mildly tender and is usually smaller than 5 to 6 cm in diameter.
    e. A **fixed adnexal mass** can indicate scarring or adhesions secondary to infection, endometriosis, or metastasis.
  5. **Pelvic side walls.** Masses that are fixed to the side wall have **significance in staging and management of cancers.** Nodularity may indicate nodal enlargement, tumor implantation, or endometriosis.

III. Investigative procedures
  A. Laboratory tests
    1. **Pregnancy test. Any woman with an adnexal mass who is of reproductive age and any woman experiencing her first year of menopause** should have a urine pregnancy test done. If this test is negative, a serum pregnancy test may be indicated.
      a. Quantitative levels of the beta-subunit of human chorionic gonadotropin (hCG) are useful in determining ectopic pregnancy.
      b. Vaginal ultrasound visualization is expected at a hCG level of 3,000 mIU/mL or higher.

  c. If the level is higher than 6,000 mIU/mL, an intrauterine gestational sac should be visible on abdominal ultrasound.
2. **A complete blood cell count** is necessary for any patient with pain or bleeding.
  a. **A differential white blood cell count and erythrocyte sedimentation rate** may be helpful, although they are frequently within normal limits in salpingitis.
  b. **A low hemoglobin and hematocrit level** with normal indices may indicate fairly acute bleeding. Microcytic indices indicate chronic anemia.
  c. **A low platelet count** may be the result of bone marrow suppression secondary to malignancy or disseminated intravascular coagulation (DIC), which may accompany malignancy, sepsis, or severe bleeding.
3. **If DIC is suspected,** prothrombin and partial thromboplastin times, fibrinogen, fibrin split products, and a platelet count should be obtained.
4. **A type and cross-matching for whole blood or packed red cells** should be obtained in any patient with heavy bleeding or abdominal pain with rebound.
5. **Blood type and antibody screen should be obtained in a pregnant patient** since $RH_o(D)$ immune globulin (RhoGAM) should be administered to an Rh-negative woman with an ectopic pregnancy or miscarriage.
6. **Serum follicle-stimulating hormone (FSH) and luteinizing hormone (LH) levels should be obtained if signs of a virilizing tumor are present.** Polycystic ovarian syndrome may have a higher LH and a normal FSH as contrasted to the normal FSH/LH ratio of about 2 : 1.
7. **Serum testosterone, dehydroepiandrosterone sulfate (DHEA-S), and urinary 17-ketosteroid levels** will help differentiate between ovarian and adrenal abnormality.
  a. **Ovarian tumors** produce relatively more testosterone than DHEA-S and have normal or only mildly elevated urinary 17-ketosteroid levels.
  b. **Adrenal tumors** produce high levels of DHEA-S and urinary 17-ketosteroids.
8. **In an adolescent or young woman with a solid tumor,** check serum **alphafetoprotein** (AFP). Virtually all endodermal sinus tumors excrete AFP, which is used as a tumor marker for follow-up.
9. **CA-125 levels** should be drawn prior to surgery on any adnexal mass. This test is elevated in more than 70% of ovarian malignancies. However, it can be elevated in many other conditions such as endometriosis or pelvic inflammatory disease (PID). The levels are useful in following treatment progress if ovarian cancer is indeed found.
B. **Ultrasound** is useful in characterizing the **size, consistency, and relative position of any adnexal and pelvic masses.**
  1. **If ectopic pregnancy** is a concern, ultrasound can identify the presence or absence of an intrauterine gestational sac as early as 5 to 6 weeks.
    a. **Visualization of a uterine sac** essentially rules out ectopic pregnancy since the incidence of both uterine and ectopic pregnancy is about 1 : 40,000.
    b. **Demonstration of a gestational sac** in the tube or other pelvic location is frequently possible with vaginal ultrasound.
  2. **Fluid collections can be identified** and may indicate cysts, abscesses, or hemorrhage.
  3. **Free fluid in the pelvis and abdomen** can also be identified and quantified to some degree. The presence of the fluid may represent a ruptured cyst, blood, or ascites.
  4. **Both cystic and solid masses** can be measured and characterized. **Septae, excrescences, and components** such as calcifications and fat can be identified.
  5. **Uterine fibroids** produce a typical sonographic echo. Thus, they can frequently be differentiated from masses arising from the ovaries.

6. **A solid adnexal mass** that is clearly not part of the uterus requires surgical evaluation.
7. Ultrasound may also be helpful in **identifying salpingitis and endometritis** as well as **hydrosalpinx, pyosalpinx, and pelvic abscess.**

C. **Culdocentesis.** For women with acute pelvic pain **and** in whom fluid is demonstrated in the cul-de-sac on ultrasound, culdocentesis is a valuable tool that can be used to differentiate among infection, hemorrhage, and cyst rupture. This procedure can be painful; therefore, **many physicians prefer to perform it while the patient is under general anesthesia.**
   1. With the woman in a semisitting position on the edge of the examining table with feet in stirrups, any **intraabdominal fluid** should collect in the cul-de-sac.
   2. A **speculum** is placed in the vagina, exposing as much of the posterior fornix as possible.
   3. The cervix and vaginal vault is prepared with povidone-iodine (**Betadine**).
   4. The **posterior lip of the cervix** should be grasped with a toothed tenaculum and traction applied.
   5. **Raising** a superficial skin wheal in the posterior fornix with 1-mL 2% lidocaine through a 25-gauge needle **and waiting** several minutes before proceeding **render this procedure minimally uncomfortable** since the anesthetic diffuses to the very sensitive peritoneum. Without local anesthesia, this is a painful procedure, particularly if peritoneal irritation is present.
   6. **The posterior cul-de-sac** is then entered with an 18- or 20-gauge spinal needle on a syringe.
   7. **Free flow of 2 to 3 cc of air** injected after entry indicates presence in a cavity.
   8. **The syringe is withdrawn slowly.** If no fluid appears, the needle is advanced and retracted a bit.
      a. The recovery of **nonclotting blood indicates intraabdominal hemorrhage.** This could be due to an ectopic pregnancy or a ruptured bleeding cyst.
      b. **Clear serous or serosanguineous fluid** usually indicates a **ruptured cyst.**
      c. **Cloudy or frankly pyogenic fluid** indicates either **salpingitis or ruptured appendix.**
   9. **Cultures of this fluid are not particularly helpful** since vaginal organisms often contaminate it. However, the cultures should **still** be obtained.
   10. A **negative result on culdocentesis does not necessarily rule out a ruptured ectopic pregnancy** since the cul-de-sac may be filled with clots that cannot be aspirated.
   11. **Blood that clots within 1 to 2 minutes** may indicate aspiration of a pelvic vessel, invalidating the test.

D. Abdominal x-ray films
   1. **Any woman with a solid adnexal mass, large cystic complex mass, or major uterine anomaly should undergo intravenous pyelogram** as part of the evaluation.
      a. **Renal and urinary tract anomalies,** such as a pelvic kidney, frequently accompany major reproductive anomalies. Involvement of ureters, their location in relation to the mass, and any possible hydroureter or hydronephrosis are important to evaluate prior to surgery.
      b. **Large or very low and lateral fibroids** can also cause ureteral deviation or compression.
   2. **Identification of calcifications** may be made in 40% of dermoid cysts on an abdominal x-ray film. Speckled calcifications can be seen in gonadoblastomas.

3. **When perforation of a viscus,** such as a ruptured appendix, perforated diverticulum, or even perforated ulcer is considered in the differential diagnosis, **flat and upright abdominal x-ray films** may demonstrate free air under the diaphragm. These films must be obtained **prior to performing culdocentesis,** which introduces air into the abdomen.
IV. **Differential diagnosis: prepubertal years.** Prior to puberty, one must have a **high index of suspicion of malignancy** if an enlarging pelvic or abdominal mass is felt (Table 20.2). Since the pelvis is small, abdominal complaints are common and abdominal tumors must be considered in the differential diagnosis. Tumors of the fallopian tubes and uterus are very rare in childhood. Dermoid cysts constitute 50% of ovarian tumors in childhood.
  A. **Congenital anomalies** are most likely to be noted at the time of the woman's first examination. **Uterine abnormalities** may not be noticed until pregnancy, when the uterus enlarges and the outline is more easily felt. The overall incidence of uterine anomalies is 1:1500.
    1. **Bicornuate uterus** is an incomplete fusion of the two uterine halves.
      a. It may be **arcuate** (indented fundus), **septate** in varying degree, or with **two separately palpable uterine cornua.**
      b. There may be **one or two cervical openings** (uniforate or biforate).
      c. **No treatment is necessary unless** the anomaly causes difficulty with pregnancy.
    2. **Uterus didelphys** is a complete uterine duplication.
      a. One side may be rudimentary and, in rare instances, **may lack communication with the cervix.** When menses begins, this will cause a cyclically painful, enlarging adnexal mass.

Table 20.2. Age-related incidence of adnexal masses

Preadolescent	Puberty	Reproductive	Menopause	Postmenopause
Uterine anomaly →	→	→	→	→
Pelvic kidney →	→	→	→	→
Paratubal cysts →	→	→	→	→
	Hematometrium →	→	→	→
	Tuboovarian abcess →	→	→	→
	Ovarian torsion →	→	→	→
		Pregnancy →	→	→
		Luteoma of pregnancy →	→	→
		Functional cysts →	→	→
		Endometriosis →	→	→
		Polycystic ovaries →	→	→
		Leiomyomas (fibroids) →	→	→
		Diverticular abcess →	→	→

Ovarian tumors

Preadolescent	Puberty	Reproductive	Menopause	Postmenopause
Dermoid cyst				
Solid teratoma →	→	→	→	→
Endodermal sinus tumor →	→	→	→	→
Dysgerminomas →	→	→	→	→
Gonadoblastomas →	→	→	→	→
Gonadal stromal tumors →	→	→	→	→
	Epithelial tumors (endometrioid, serous, mucinous) →	→	→	→
	Thecoma/fibroma →	→	→	→
	Sertoli-Leydig cell tumors →	→	→	→
	Granulosa cell tumor →	→	→	→
	metastatic GI tumors →	→	→	→

   b. This congenital anomaly **requires surgical intervention.** Further surgical alteration may become necessary to allow successful pregnancy.
   3. **A pelvic kidney** is sometimes felt as a solid, solitary mass in the posterior pelvis. The incidence is 1:600.
   a. This anomaly **should not be removed** since it may be the only functional kidney.
   b. **Intravenous pyelogram** is the diagnostic test that will both identify the kidney and reveal any other renal anomalies. Uterine and renal anomalies often occur simultaneously.
B. **Physiologic and functional disorders**
   1. **A distended bladder** is usually due to an obstruction of the urethra secondary to infection or stone.
   2. **Distended bowel or rectum** occurs from impacted feces.
   a. **On bimanual examination,** the mass is mobile, irregular, and located laterally or posteriorly.
   b. Both gaseous distention and feces give typical findings on **abdominal x-ray films. An abdominal x-ray film may also show free air under the diaphragm if bowel perforation has occurred.**
C. **Functional ovarian cysts** may occur at any age, but are rare after menopause. Benign simple cysts make up 15% of all adnexal masses in children.
   1. **Follicular cysts** are found even in the ovaries of young children (see section V.D.1.).
   2. **Germinal inclusion cysts** are small surface cysts of ovarian epithelial origin that are **benign,** usually simple cysts, and **generally asymptomatic.** They seldom become large enough to cause concern.
   3. **Parovarian cysts** can occur at any age, but are most common in the reproductive years (see section V.D.7.).
D. **Neoplasms**
   1. **Germ cell tumors.**
   a. **Dermoid cysts (benign cystic teratoma), solid teratomas, and dysgerminomas** may occur in this age group, but are more common in the reproductive years (see section V.G.1.).
   b. **Gonadoblastomas** are a rare mixed germ cell and sex-cord tumor occurring in intersex individuals, arising from immature abnormal gonads or streak gonads. Most of these patients are karyotypically 46XY or mosaic 45XO-46XY.
      (1) The patient may have **slight breast enlargement, clitoromegaly, hirsutism, and sometimes vaginal bleeding.**
      (2) An **x-ray examination of the abdomen** may demonstrate speckled calcifications.
      (3) They are **usually small,** sometimes not even palpable, but may grow to be as large as 10 to 15 cm.
      (4) These are of **low malignant potential. Prognosis after removal is good.**
   c. **Endodermal sinus tumors** arise from the yolk sac endoderm. They are seen mostly in children and adolescents and are solid, smooth, rubbery, and without adhesions. They are **highly malignant, metastasizing** early through the lymphatics. They secrete AFP, which can be measured in the blood both for diagnosis and follow-up. Surgery and chemotherapy are used for treatment with little success. These tumors are insensitive to radiation. The prognosis is poor.
   2. **Epithelial ovarian tumors** are primarily serous and mucinous cystadenomas and are very uncommon in childhood and early adolescence. They account for approximately 18% of ovarian neoplasms in late adolescence.
   a. Epithelial tumors arise from the **ovarian germinal epithelium,** which has the potential to develop into any of the germinal tract epithelium types.

       b. All have the potential to develop into **cystadenocarcinoma** and **require surgical exploration and removal.**

       c. **Serous cystadenoma** is the most common epithelial ovarian tumor and occurs in all age groups (see section V.G.2.a.).

    3. **Gonadal stromal tumors. Granulosa cell tumors** are infrequent in children and when present are **rarely malignant.** They occasionally produce precocious puberty (see section V.G.3.a.).

V. **Differential diagnosis: reproductive years. Physiologic or functional disorders are the most common etiology** of adnexal masses in this age group (Table 20.2). **Infectious causes** should be high on the differential diagnosis list in adolescents because both salpingitis and appendicitis are common during the reproductive years.

    Adnexal masses that occur in adolescence include those of lymphatic origin. Mononucleosis, lymphoma, and leukemia may cause enlarged pelvic lymph nodes that are palpated as adnexal masses. Uterine fibroids (leiomyomas), ovarian neoplasms, and tubal abnormalities become more common with increasing age. One in five women older than 30 years will have palpable leiomyomas.

    In adolescence, an adnexal mass is **most often benign. Benign dermoid cysts** are by far the most common neoplasms in adolescents. These and other germ cell tumors account for 80% of ovarian tumors requiring surgery. About one in ten ovarian neoplasms are malignant in adolescents. Borderline or low malignancy types are more common than anaplastic or virulent tumors. Epithelial ovarian tumors are more common in the reproductive years. Malignant changes are more likely to occur with increasing age.

A. **Pregnancy must be a primary consideration** in the differential diagnosis.

    1. **Menses are frequently irregular** during adolescence. Spotting or bleeding may occur in the first month or so of a pregnancy whether it is intrauterine or ectopic.

    2. **Sexual history may be unreliable** because of naiveté or fear of exposure.

    3. Therefore, a **pregnancy test should be performed on any post-menarchal young woman with a pelvic mass.**

    4. **Pregnancy-related masses** include the following:

       a. **Ectopic pregnancy** (see section V.E.).

       b. **Hydatidiform mole** (see section V.D.6.).

       c. **Choriocarcinoma** (with or without theca lutein cysts) (see section V.G.1.d.).

       d. **Luteoma of pregnancy** (see section V.D.3.).

       e. **Rapidly enlarging fibroids** during pregnancy.

B. **Congenital anomalies** are frequently found in this age group at the time of first pelvic examination. The **incidence is small** (about 1:1,500 for uterine anomalies and 1:600 for pelvic kidney).

C. **Physiologic disorders** are essentially the same as those found in the prepubertal age group (see section IV.B.).

    1. **A distended bladder** may occur in a woman with a 12-week pregnant uterus secondary to pelvic entrapment of the enlarging uterus in the sacral curve, which tilts the cervix anteriorly and compresses the urethra.

       a. The bladder is **felt as a tense, tender, smooth midline mass.**

       b. Since the bladder may be very distended, there may not be an urge to void on palpation.

       c. **Urinary catheterization** provides the diagnosis.

       d. The entrapped uterus can usually be **gently maneuvered out of the pelvis by bimanual pressure** while the patient is under anesthesia. Once the uterus is lifted from the sacral curve, **this problem generally does not recur.**

    2. **Diverticular abscess** must be considered when a tender, fluid-filled mass is found in the pelvis in older women.

D. Functional ovarian cysts are the most common cause of the adnexal mass in the reproductive years.
   1. **Follicular cysts** constitute 20% to 50% of ovarian masses in post-menarchal women during the reproductive years.
      a. Ruptured cysts present as **acute, severe pelvic pain that increases with movement.** Rupture also produces peritoneal inflammation, causing rebound tenderness.
         (1) The pain tends to **decrease over 1 or 2 days.**
         (2) **Torsion** will continue to cause symptoms unless it spontaneously untwists.
      b. Follicular cysts **smaller than 6 to 8 cm** will usually disappear after one or two menstrual cycles. If still present after two cycles, a trial of any oral contraceptive to suppress ovarian function should cause them to shrink or disappear over the next 1 to 2 months.
      c. If the cysts are **larger than 6 to 8 cm,** suspicion of neoplasm is increased, and the woman should be **evaluated by sonogram and either laparoscopy or laparotomy.** These cysts can cause pain either by rupture or by torsion, which can lead to bleeding and necrosis of the ovary.
      d. **Clear or serosanguinous fluid on culdocentesis is diagnostic** of a ruptured cyst. If torsion is suspected, surgery may save the involved ovary and tube.
   2. **Corpus luteum cysts** occur after ovulation, may contain serous or serosanguinous fluid, and can attain a size of 6 to 8 cm. Like follicular cysts, they **may disappear over one or two menstrual cycles or with ovarian suppression.** They occur in early pregnancy, almost always shrinking or disappearing by the end of the first trimester. In nonpregnant women, the management is the same as follicular cysts.
   3. **Luteoma of pregnancy** is reported to occur in 10% to 40% of pregnancies. It is usually discovered during ultrasound, cesarean section, or other abdominal exploration.
      a. It is a **benign, solid tumor** usually ranging from 5 to 10 cm.
      b. Occasionally, it **produces testosterone** causing mild maternal masculinization during pregnancy, and it has also been reported to cause masculinization in the female fetus.
      c. Luteomas **regress after pregnancy** leaving no residua.
   4. **A solid ovarian tumor discovered during pregnancy should be surgically evaluated because of the possibility of ovarian cancer.**
   5. **Germinal inclusion cysts** also occur in this age group (see section IV.C.2.).
   6. **Theca lutein cysts** are sometimes present in normal pregnancy, but more often accompany trophoblastic disease. However, only 30% of women with hydatidiform moles have enlarged ovaries.
      a. **Widespread luteinization of the ovaries** occurs with multiple cysts ranging from 1 to 15 cm.
      b. The ovaries **enlarge rapidly** and may continue growing for a short time after delivery of the molar pregnancy.
      c. Within 3 to 4 months, the ovaries will **return to their normal size** with no adverse effect.
      d. **Unless torsion occurs, they require no treatment** despite the size and may even have some protective effect against development of choriocarcinoma (probably because of the large amounts of estrogen they produce).
   7. **Parovarian cysts** are remnants of the wolffian ducts and account for approximately 10% of adnexal masses. These **benign** cysts may be found in any age group but are most commonly discovered in the 30- to 40-year-old group. They tend to expand within the mesosalpinx, displacing the uterus both out of the pelvis and away from the involved side. Since these cysts have no pedicle, they are **not subject to torsion.**

      a. They **require surgical removal only to differentiate them** from other ovarian neoplasms.

      b. The **hydatid of Morgagni** is a pedunculated cyst of müllerian origin found at the lateral end of the fallopian tube. It is usually smaller than 1 to 2 cm in diameter and **is of no concern.** However, it can expand to 10 to 15 cm and may cause torsion of the adnexa.

    8. **Endometriomas,** also called **chocolate cysts,** are a major consideration in this age group and are found by cyclic menstrual bleeding into endometrial tissue that has implanted on the ovaries or, less commonly, elsewhere in the pelvis.

      a. They are **typically immobile** since they form **extensive scarring.**

      b. They gradually enlarge over many months and may be associated with a **history of severe cyclic pain** and **severe dysmenorrhea** frequently starting 1 to 2 days prior to menses (see Chapter 14). However, they are **often asymptomatic.**

      c. Whereas lesser degrees of endometriosis are amenable to medical management, endometriomas **larger than 2 cm usually require surgical excision** (see Chapter 2).

    9. **Polycystic ovaries,** also known as the **Stein-Leventhal syndrome,** result from an abnormality in the hypothalamic-pituitary-ovarian axis. Elevated levels of **LH** cause hyperstimulation of the ovaries resulting in multicystic development and luteinization. The high levels of estrogen produced by the increased ovarian stromal tissue are unopposed by postovulatory progesterone and **may result in endometrial hyperplasia or even carcinoma.** Polycystic ovaries become **more apparent with each postmenarchal year.**

      a. Polycystic ovaries are typically felt as smooth, **enlarged unilateral or bilateral ovaries.**

      b. **Sonogram** may demonstrate numerous 2 to 3 cm subcapsular cysts.

      c. The FSH/LH ratio usually shows **LH increased several times above normal, instead of the usual ratio of 1:1 or 2:1.**

      d. **The typical patient** is somewhat obese and hirsute with irregular menses and infertility secondary to anovulation. However, some or all of these signs may be absent in less severe forms of the syndrome.

E. **Ectopic pregnancy** must be high on the differential diagnosis list of the adnexal mass in any woman of reproductive age. The incidence is about 1:200. However, in recent years that incidence has been rising probably secondary to an increase in PID and intrauterine device use. The rate of ectopic pregnancies is 1:40 in populations with a high incidence of PID. The death rate from ruptured ectopic pregnancies has declined primarily owing to increased suspicion and early intervention.

    1. The **most common site of occurrence is the fallopian tube,** but the ovary, abdomen, interstitial or cornual portion of the uterus, or the cervix may be involved.

    2. Classically, the patient presents with **irregular bleeding, late menses, abdominal pain, and symptoms of pregnancy.**

    3. **Physical examination** may reveal a normal or slightly enlarged uterus and a small, tender adnexal mass. If there is intraabdominal bleeding, the rectum, cul-de-sac, and pelvic organs will be very tender, and peritoneal signs may be elucidated. However, **any of the components of this picture may be missing.**

    4. **Symptoms usually occur during the second to third months of pregnancy** when distention of the tube causes bleeding and rupture.

    5. **With cornual pregnancy** there may be no symptoms until the third or fourth month of gestation. Rupture is usually sudden and disastrous.

    6. **Clinical diagnosis** of ectopic pregnancy is about 75% accurate. It is usually made by a **serum beta-hCG level that does not double in 48 hours and** with **an ultrasound,** preferably **vaginal,** demonstrating an **empty uterine cavity.**

With a **beta-hCG level greater than 3,000 mIU/mL** an intra-uterine pregnancy should be visualized on vaginal ultrasound. At a beta-hCG level greater than 6,000 mIU/mL the intrauterine gestational sac should be visualized on abdominal ultrasound.

    a. The addition of a **serum progesterone level lower than 8 mg/mL** identifies a nonviable or ectopic pregnancy with more than 80% accuracy. A **progesterone level greater than 15 mg/mL** indicates a normal pregnancy in more than 90% of patients.

    b. **Ultrasound** may also identify free fluid in the abdomen or cul-de-sac, which may indicate intraabdominal bleeding. **Culdocentesis** may be done to determine blood versus serous fluid, as from a ruptured cyst. A **negative culdocentesis result does not** rule out bleeding, since a clot may have formed that is too thick to aspirate. If there is evidence of intraabdominal hemorrhage, surgical intervention is indicated.

    c. If no gestational sac is seen and the foregoing criteria are met, a **suction curettage** can be done to ascertain if villi are present. This would indicate a spontaneous abortion. Concomitant ectopic and intrauterine gestations occur in only about 1:10,000 cases.

    d. **Methotrexate IM** is an alternative method for treating ectopic pregnancies of less than 9 weeks' gestation that meet the foregoing criteria. A single injection results in resolution of the pregnancy without surgical intervention in 96% of cases, if no fetal cardiac activity was identified in the tube. Methotrexate should be used only by practitioners familiar with its actions, potential toxicity, and complications. Recurrence and fertility rates are comparable with laparoscopic surgery (3,15).

    e. **Laparoscopy** should be performed if there is any doubt about the diagnosis.

F. Pelvic infections are seen primarily in women of reproductive age.

    1. **Acute salpingitis** can result in a thickening of the adnexa, progressing to a distinct mass if there is resultant scarring and adhesions of the tube and ovary. Pyosalpinx or hydrosalpinx is a frequent sequela of salpingitis. The latter may occur up to years later and may be asymptomatic.

    2. **Tuboovarian abscess** can also follow salpingitis.

        a. It may be **large** (10 cm or more in diameter) and sometimes be felt **pointing in the cul-de-sac or dissecting the rectovaginal septum.**

        b. **Appendiceal rupture and subsequent sequestration can mimic a tuboovarian abscess** (see Chapter 5, section VIII.D.).

G. Neoplasms. In adolescents about one in ten ovarian neoplasms are malignant. Borderline or low malignancy types are more common than anaplastic or virulent tumors.

    1. **Germ cell tumors** account for 80% of ovarian neoplasms requiring surgery in adolescents.

        a. **Benign cystic teratoma (dermoid cyst)** is the most common germ cell tumor. It is **benign** in greater than 99% of cases. In **less than 1%,** some type of **malignant** change occurs. Because of the totipotential nature, any type of malignancy may occur. However, squamous cell carcinoma is the most common.

            (1) All dermoid cysts contain **hair, sebaceous material,** and sometimes completely developed **teeth or other calcifications.**

            (2) Teratomas may **grow quite large before becoming symptomatic,** which is usually secondary to pressure on the bladder or bowel, unless torsion or leakage occurs.

            (3) **In rare instances, functional thyroid or carcinoid tissue is present.** If greater than 50% of the tumor is occupied by one of these tissues, the term **struma ovarii (thyroid)** or **ovarian carcinoid** would be applied. The hormone production may be enough to cause either **thyrotoxicosis or carcinoid syndrome** (diarrhea, flushes, bronchospasm, telangiectasia, or cardiac valvular disease).

(4) The overall incidence of **bilateral cysts** is 10% to 20%, although they may not occur simultaneously.

(5) Because of the **sebaceous material,** cysts frequently float outside the pelvis or anterior to the uterus.

(6) Identification may be tentatively made by **ultrasonic demonstration** of a cyst with sonolucent fatty material or areas of calcification. Calcifications and sebaceous material can also be seen on **abdominal x-ray films.**

(7) Since the cysts continue to grow and may cause torsion, rupture, bleeding, or fistula, they **should be removed.**

b. **Solid teratomas** are usually **malignant.** More than 50% of these tumors occur before the age of 20. They are **unilateral** in 98% of the cases, **usually free of adhesions, and mobile. Neural tissue** is a predominant component of solid teratomas.

(1) They are **rarely hormonally active.** Occasionally, one does produce hCG from embryonal or trophoblastic tissue, which may cause sexual pseudoprecosity, with breast or hair development, or both, in young patients.

(2) **Surgery plus chemotherapy** is the usual treatment.

(a) In young women, **preservation of the uterus and opposite ovary** may be considered if there is no evidence of metastasis.

(b) About one-third have already **metastasized intraabdominally at surgery**. Distant metastases are unusual. Overall 5- and 10-year survival is 60%. Age at the time of diagnosis is not correlated with survival.

c. **Dysgerminomas** arise from undifferentiated germ cells, usually occurring before 20 years of age. They may be **unilateral or bilateral** and are **hormonally inactive** in most cases. However, some may secrete hCG from choriocarcinomatous elements.

(1) **Most are asymptomatic.** Histories of elevated temperatures, night sweats, and leukocytosis have been reported in some patients.

(2) Dysgerminomas are frequently associated with **pseudohermaphroditism and sexual underdevelopment.**

(3) They tend to **appear at the time of menarche** and are found on routine physical examination. **Amenorrhea** is often the presenting complaint. However, they **may appear after menses are established** without interruption of normal cycles.

(4) Dysgerminomas are **freely mobile, smooth, solid, rubbery** adnexal masses varying in size from a few centimeters to filling the pelvic cavity.

(5) **They are always malignant. Surgical removal and chemotherapy** are the mainstays of therapy. Prognosis has improved markedly in the past few years. **With chemotherapy,** 95% disease-free survival is expected. Reproductive potential is maintained in most young patients.

d. **Choriocarcinoma arising without a pregnancy** is very rare and is **highly malignant.** It secretes hCG, which is followed as a tumor marker during chemotherapy. It does not respond as well to therapy as choriocarcinomas arising during pregnancy. The **prognosis is poor.**

e. **Gonadoblastomas and endodermal sinus tumors** are also found in this age group (see section IV.D.1.b. and IV.D.1.c.).

2. **Epithelial ovarian tumors. Serous cystadenomas** are most frequent during the third and fourth decades of life. **Mucinous and endometrioid types** peak between the ages of 30 and 50.

   a. **Serous cystadenomas** occur in all age groups, are frequently bilateral, and have a **greater potential for malignancy than mucinous cystadenomas.** They are similar to the fallopian tube epithelium, containing papillomatous, solid, and clear, thin, fluid components.

     (1) These tumors **vary in size,** but do not tend to grow as large as the mucinous cysts.

     (2) They are **irregular** and **may be smooth or rough,** depending on whether papillary growth has occurred on the outer capsule surface.

   b. **Mucinous cystadenomas** are composed of epithelium resembling endocervical cells, which produces a thick, sticky fluid. They are as common as serous tumors. They are rarely found before puberty, and 40% are found postmenopausally. Bilateral cysts occur in about 15% of cases. Their **malignant potential** is only 6%, with an additional 14% of borderline malignancy.

     (1) They can grow to **astonishing size** and have been recorded as weighing more than 100 lb (45 kg). On the average, they **exceed 15 cm at diagnosis.**

     (2) These tumors are **prone to torsion** and **adhesions.**

     (3) They are usually **smooth and irregular in outline** because of loculations or daughter cysts.

   c. **Endometrioid tumors** are much less common than the two preceding types. They may be cystic and up to 25 cm. They may arise in chocolate cysts. **The rare endometrioid cancer arising in endometriosis is a different diagnosis.** They are **usually malignant but have a good prognosis,** with a 70% overall survival.

3. **Gonadal stromal tumors** are also known as **sex-cord mesenchymal tumors.** They are **often hormonally active.**

   a. **Granulosa cell tumors** are most often found in adults, equally distributed between premenopausal and postmenopausal women.

     (1) They average 5 to 10 cm, but **may grow to fill the pelvis.**

     (2) They are usually **unilateral, smooth, round, occasionally lobulated, and generally solid.**

     (3) The larger tumors may undergo cystic **degeneration.**

     (4) **If hormonally active,** they may produce **dysfunctional bleeding** in women of reproductive age or postmenopausal cyclic or irregular bleeding.

     (5) Since they can produce excess estrogen (about 25% do), they are **associated with endometrial hyperplasia or carcinoma,** particularly in women older than 40 years with 80% showing endometrial changes.

     (6) **If malignant,** as 25% are, late recurrence beyond 5 years often occurs. **Both radiation and chemotherapy are effective.** Prognosis varies with differentiation and cell type.

   b. **Thecoma fibromas** are almost **never malignant.** They rarely appear before the age of 30 and are less common after menopause than granulosa cell tumors to which they are closely related. Thecomas are almost always **hormonally active,** whereas a pure fibroma may be inert.

     (1) Their presentation is identical to granulosa cell tumors and can be distinguished only by **histologic examination.**

     (2) They are **solid, bulky, rubbery masses.**

     (3) Another **variant of thecoma fibroma,** also closely related to granulosa cell tumors, is the **luteoma.** These may produce estrogen, androgen, or be inert. They are **more likely to become malignant.**

c. **Sertoli-Leydig cell tumors** were formerly called **arrhenoblastomas or androblastomas.** They are **very rare.** About 25% are hormonally active. Sertoli-Leydig cell tumors occur primarily in the reproductive years. They are bilateral in only 5%. Malignancy occurs in 3% to 20%.

(1) **If Sertoli cells are predominant,** there may be a feminizing effect.

(2) **With predominantly functional Leydig cells,** changes result from the testosterone produced by the Leydig cells.

   (a) The patient first becomes **defeminized,** with shrinkage of breasts and female fatty deposits and amenorrhea.

   (b) **Masculinization** then follows with clitoromegaly, hirsutism, and deepening voice.

   (c) In the rare instances of these tumors occurring in **childhood,** masculinizing may result. Adrenal tumors are much more common as the source of this syndrome.

(3) Variants of this group are **hilar cell tumors and mixed types** such as lipoid cell tumors and gynandroblastomas. The latter are rare tumors also containing granulosa cell elements. **Treatment is the same as for granulosa cell tumors.**

VI. **Differential diagnosis: menopause.** There are many nongynecologic causes of masses felt in the pelvis in this age group (Table 20.2). Abnormalities of both bladder and bowel, metastatic tumors, and lymphatic disorder must be considered in the differential diagnosis. **Thorough workup is important.**

A. **Physiologic disorders** are essentially the same as those found in the prepubertal-aged group (see section IV.B.). **Diverticular abscess** must be considered when a tender, fluid-filled mass is found in the pelvis.

B. **Functional cysts should not occur after menopause.** However, a simple cyst smaller than 5 cm may be observed with repeat ultrasound in 2 to 3 months. If unchanged, it may be observed with interval examinations as more than 90% of these are benign.

C. **Neoplasms.** Ovarian tumors are common in older women. Although benign dermoid and epithelial cysts do occur, **any ovarian mass in a postmenopausal woman should be considered potentially malignant and managed surgically.**

1. **Carcinoma of the fallopian tubes** is rare and difficult to diagnose. In a series of 898 cases, only 10 were correctly diagnosed preoperatively. They <u>occur most often</u> in <u>postmenopausal</u> women and are <u>more common</u> in <u>nulliparous</u> women.

2. **Epithelial ovarian tumors.**

   a. **Clear-cell mesonephroid tumors** are rare, epithelial, cystic, multiloculated tumors that may be **benign, borderline, or malignant.** Most of these are found after menopause. They are treated the same as the other epithelial tumors. If malignant, the 5-year survival is 40%. They are occasionally associated with hypercalcemia.

   b. **Serous and mucinous cystadenomas and endometrioid tumors** also appear in this age group (see section V.G.2.).

3. **Gonadal stromal tumors. Granulosa cell tumors and thecoma fibromas** are also found in this age group (see sections V.G.3.a. and V.G.3.b.).

VII. **Management.** When all the data have been gathered in the workup of an adnexal mass, the course to be followed is fairly simple. It is important to gather as much information as possible to ascertain the need for surgery or to avoid unnecessary surgery.

A mass that is solid, complex, or larger than 10 cm in any age group should be treated as possibly malignant.

Presurgical tests may include an intravenous pyelogram and possibly a **barium enema** if symptoms suggest bowel involvement. A CT scan or MRI may be helpful in diagnosing and staging and in the planning of surgery. Follow-up of any borderline or malignant neoplasm should be done by a specialist as therapy is always changing and advancing.

A. Prepubertal

1. A small mass, **less than 5 cm**, that is cystic on ultrasound can be watched safely **if the patient is asymptomatic.**
2. **A repeat ultrasound** in 1 to 2 months will indicate whether the mass is growing or shrinking.
   a. **An enlarging mass should be removed.**
   b. Any complex, solid, or large mass (≥8 cm) should be **surgically evaluated.**

B. Reproductive. After menarche and before menopause, the same basic rules apply to **asymptomatic masses** of 5 cm or less.

1. **Functional cysts** are the most commonly found masses.
   a. **They can be watched over one or two cycles** with repeated examination before any other workup is initiated.
   b. **If they persist unchanged,** try ovarian suppression with oral contraceptives for a cycle or two.
2. **An enlarging or persistent mass** should be evaluated (see section III).
3. **Any solid mass or mass larger than 8 cm should be evaluated surgically.** A cystic, simple mass in this age group is most likely benign. However, large ovarian masses are subject to torsion, rupture, hemorrhage, or infection as well as possible malignant change and **should be removed.**
4. **If a woman with a mass presents with acute symptoms of pain or fever, immediate diagnostic procedures must be done to determine the cause.**
   a. **Infections may result in permanent impairment of fertility** as well as long-term sequelae of pain, adhesions, abscess, and repeated infection. These can often be prevented by early diagnosis and effective therapy (see Chapter 5 for information on PID).
   b. **An ectopic pregnancy** may be diagnosed early enough to save the involved fallopian tube in some cases and **certainly presents one of the true emergencies in gynecology if ruptured or bleeding** (see section V.E.6.).
   c. **Any acute pelvic mass with hemoperitoneum,** as found on culdocentesis, requires at least laparoscopic evaluation.
   d. **Torsion of an adnexal mass** may result in necrosis of the involved adnexa with loss of one ovary if diagnosis and surgical intervention are delayed.
   e. **If clear fluid is found on culdocentesis** and the patient's history and laboratory workup are consistent with a **ruptured cyst,** an acutely painful episode with a cystic mass can be observed closely. The pain from spillage of functional cyst contents will resolve over several days of bedrest. **Mild analgesia is the only necessary treatment.**

C. Menopausal. In the group older than 40, particularly postmenopausally, **an adnexal mass should be considered malignant until proven otherwise.** Any adnexal mass, cystic or solid, in a postmenopausal woman requires immediate preparation and surgical removal by a specialist. Ovarian cancer has a much better prognosis if detected and removed in the early stages.

References

1. Cacciatore B, et al. Comparison of abdominal and vaginal ultrasonography in suspected ectopic pregnancy. *Obstet Gynecol* 1989;73:770.
2. Cancer of the ovary: a review article. *N Engl J Med* 1993;329:1550.
3. Chemotherapy for ectopic pregnancy. *Obstet Gynecol Clin North Am* 1991;18:123.
4. Clemens EM, et al. HCG, progesterone, AFP and estradiol in the identification of ectopic pregnancy. *Obstet Gynecol* 1993;81:5.
5. Ectopic pregnancy. *Obstet Gynecol Clin North Am* 1991;18:1.

6. Emans S, Goldstein DP. *Pediatric and adolescent gynecology,* 3rd ed. Boston: Little, Brown, 1990.
7. Gershenson D. Update on malignant ovarian germ cell tumors. *Cancer* 1993;71:4.
8. Lindblom B, et al. Serial hCG determination for differentiation between intrauterine and ectopic gestation. *Am J Obstet Gynecol* 1989;161:397.
9. Novak ER. *Textbook of gynecology,* 10th ed. Baltimore: Williams & Wilkins, 1981.
10. Abu-Rum N, Barakat RR, Curtin JP. Ovarian and uterine disease in women with colorectal cancer. *Obstet Gynecol* 1997;89(1):85–87.
11. Auslender R, Atlas I, Lissak A, et al. Follow-up of small, postmenopausal ovarian cysts using vaginal ultrasound and antigen. *J Clin Ultrasound* 1996;24(4):175–178.
12. Cancer. Progress report on ovarian cancer. *Harv Womens Health Watch* 2000; 7(9):2–4.
13. Eltabbakh GH, Yadev PR, Morgan A. Clinical picture of women with early stage ovarian cancer. *Gynecol Oncol* 1999;75:476–479.
14. Igoe BA. Symptoms attributed to ovarian cancer by women with the disease. *Nurse Pract* 1997;22(7):122, 127–128, 130.
15. Kozlowski KJ. Ovarian masses. *Adolesc Med* 1999;10:337–350, vii.
16. Menon IJ, Taalat A, Jeyarajah AR, et al. Ultrasound assessment of ovarian cancer risk in postmenopausal women with elevation. *Br J Cancer* 1999;80:1644–1647.
17. Mettler L, Semm K, Shive K. Endoscopic management of adnexal masses. *JSLS* 1997;1(2):103–112.
18. Moore RD, Smith WG. Laparoscopic management of adnexal masses in pregnant women. *J Reprod Med* 1999;44(2);97–100.
19. Panoskaltsis TA, Moore DA, Haidopoulos DA, et al. Tuberculous peritonitis: part of the differential diagnosis in ovarian cancer. *Am J Obstet Gynecol* 2000;182:740–742.
20. Partridge EE, Phillips JL, Mench HR. The National Cancer Data Base report on ovarian cancer treatment in United States. *Cancer* 1996;78:2236–2246.
21. Plaxe SC, Braly PS, Freddo JL, et al. Profiles of women age 30–39 and age less than 30 with epithelial ovarian cancer. *Obstet Gynecol* 1993;81[5 (Pt 1)]:651–654.
22. Rao GJ, Ravi BS, Cheriparambil KM, et al. Abdominal tuberculosis or ovarian carcinoma: management dilemma assoc. elevated CA-125 level. *Medscape Womens Health* 1996;1(4):2.
23. Rock JA, et al. Endometriosis. *Obstet Gynecol Clin North Am* 1989;16:1.
24. Ryan K, et al. *Kistner's gynecology.* 5th ed. Chicago: Year Book, 1990.
25. Scully RE. *Tumors of the ovary and maldeveloped gonad.* Bethesda, MD: Air Force Institute of Pathology, 1979.
26. Steven Piver M, et al. Epidemiology and etiology of ovarian cancer. *Semin Oncol* 1991;18:177.
27. Steven Piver M, et al. Familial ovarian cancer registry. *Obstet Gynecol* 1984;64:195.
28. Stovall TG. Single dose methotrexate therapy for treatment of ectopic pregnancy. *Obstet Gynecol* 1991.
29. Tanaka YO, Nishida M, Yamaguchi M, et al. MRI of gynaecological solid masses. *Clin Radiol* 2000;55:899–911.
30. Thompson SD. Ovarian cancer screening: a primary care guide. *Lippincott's Prim Care Pract* 1998;2:244–250.
31. Timor-Tritsch IE, et al. Use of transvaginal ultrasonography in diagnosis of ectopic pregnancy. *Am J Obstet Gynecol* 1989;161:157.
32. Tortolero-Luna G, et al. Epidemiology and screening of ovarian cancer: update on epithelial ovarian cancer. *Obstet Gynecol Clin North Am* 1994;21:1.
33. Underwood P. Adnexal masses in teenagers. *Contemp Obstet Gynecol* 1983.
34. Verheijen RH, von Mensdorff-Pouilly S, van Kamp GJ, et al. CA 125: fundamental and clinical aspects. *Semin Cancer Biol* 1999;9(2):117–124.
35. Zuranoski VR. Elevated serum CA125 levels in diagnosis of ovarian cancer. *Int J Cancer* 1988;42:677.

21. HIRSUTISM

Kenneth Griffis

Hirsutism is defined as **excessive androgen-dependent (male-pattern) terminal hair growth occurring in women.** Terminal hairs may be present over the upper lip, chin, cheeks, central chest, back, upper arms, lower abdomen, and thighs. Hairs in the axillae and lower pubic triangle respond to the normally low levels of androgen present in pubescent girls and are not indicative of hirsutism. An **increase in only vellus (fine and fair) hair is termed *hypertrichosis* and is not related to androgens.** Follicles producing vellus hair are normally present over most of the body. Under the influence of androgens, they **may be converted to terminal hair follicles** producing coarse, pigmented hair. Hypertrichosis may be seen in several disease states including anorexia nervosa, porphyria, and assorted nervous system disorders. Phenytoin, cyclosporine, minoxidil, penicillamine, and diazoxide use may also be associated with hypertrichosis.

The **amount of sexual hair normally seen does vary somewhat among different ethnic groups,** with increased amounts noted in women of Mediterranean extraction and decreased amounts seen in American Indians and oriental Asians. There is also **great individual variation** in the amount of sexual hair that is personally acceptable or normal. This is particularly pronounced in the United States where the feminine idea of beauty often includes removal of even nonsexual (i.e., axillary, leg) hair. The clinician may indeed be called on to assess and comfort a patient whose complaints of hirsutism are accompanied by a normal physical examination.

Hirsutism may occur by itself or may be accompanied by other signs of male hormone effect (virilization). These may include acne, deepening of the voice, temporal balding, increased muscle strength, and clitoromegaly as well as increased libido. When virilization accompanies hirsutism, a **significant excess in circulating androgens** will invariably be present, and a prompt and thorough evaluation is indicated.

I. **Andrology.** Androgens are **steroid hormones that stimulate male secondary sex characteristics.** In the nonpregnant woman, androgens are **secreted by the ovaries and the adrenal glands.** Serum androgens are not firmly regulated since adrenocorticotropic hormone (ACTH) and gonadotropin secretion, which control adrenal and ovarian hormone synthesis, respectively, are controlled by factors other than androgen levels. The 17-ketosteroids, which include dehydroepiandrosterone (DHEA), dehydroepiandrosterone sulfate (DHEA-S), androstenedione, androstanedione, and androsterone, are relatively weak prohormones. These exhibit biologic activity only by conversion to the 17-hydroxysteroids, which include androstenediol, testosterone, dihydrotestosterone (the most potent androgen), and androstanediol. Whether testosterone or dihydrotestosterone (which is primarily formed from testosterone by 5α-reductase in target cells) is the more important androgen in hair follicles has not been established and may differ among individuals.

   A. **Androgen secretion.** Although DHEA, DHEA-S, and androstenedione circulate in the highest concentrations in women, **testosterone is the most important androgen because of its potency and relatively high concentration.**

   1. In normal premenopausal women, approximately 50% of **serum testosterone** is derived from the **peripheral conversion of androstenedione.** The remaining 50% is secreted in roughly equal amounts from **the ovaries and the adrenal glands.**

This chapter is a revision of the third edition chapter by Robert M. Walter, Jr., Mahmoud M. Benbarka, and Pamela T. Prescott.

2. Approximately half of circulating **androstenedione** is secreted by the **adrenal glands** and the other half by the **ovaries**.

3. The **adrenal glands** are the source of 80% of **DHEA** and 95% of **DHEA-S**.

B. **Androgen levels.** Until recently, it was believed that most women with hirsutism, but without virilization, had normal circulating levels of androgens. With more precise, complete, and repetitive endocrine measurements, it is now apparent that **nearly nine in ten women with hirsutism will have hyperandrogenemia.** The 17-hydroxysteroids circulate bound primarily (nearly 80%) to sex hormone binding globulins (SHBGs); 20% are loosely bound to albumin, and 1% to 2% remain free or biologically active. The **SHBG levels are increased by estrogens and decreased by androgens.** As a result, although only 40% of hirsute patients have increased serum testosterone levels, more than 70% have **increased free testosterone levels.** When determinations of all the free 17-hydroxysteroids are performed, nearly 90% of patients will exhibit an abnormality. The **normal levels of total testosterone often seen in patients with increased free testosterone result from testosterone-induced lowering of the SHBG concentration and, therefore, the bound testosterone component.** Some patients with normal serum levels of the foregoing hormones will have increased serum 3α-androstanediol and its glucuronide conjugate, reflecting increased local metabolism of dihydrotestosterone.

II. **Ovarian etiology**

A. **Polycystic ovary syndrome** (functional ovarian hyperandrogenemia)

1. **Presentation.**

a. This is a **heterogeneous syndrome** with a clinical presentation **varying from mild hirsutism and regular menses to severe hirsutism, amenorrhea, and virilization.** This syndrome is the most common cause of hirsutism.

b. The onset of symptoms is often in the **teenage years** and **obesity** is often present.

c. **Ovarian pathologic findings vary** from the classic description by Stein and Leventhal of enlarged pearly white organs with many small follicular cysts and a markedly thickened tunica albuginea to hyperthecosis with luteinized cells within the ovarian stroma. **Ovarian stromal hyperplasia or nodular cell hyperplasia may occur in postmenopausal patients** with presentation of hirsutism late in life.

d. The **pathogenesis** of the polycystic ovary syndrome is **not yet clear,** but both the ovaries and the adrenal glands are typically involved. Hyperinsulinemia with insulin resistance is typically seen.

2. **Diagnosis** is suggested by **evidence of hirsutism occurring without evidence of cortisol or adrenal androgen excess.**

a. **Serum free testosterone and androstenedione** are often modestly elevated.

b. A **strong family history** may be present with dominant inheritance suggested.

c. **Serum luteinizing hormone** (LH) **levels** are typically elevated, whereas **follicle-stimulating hormone** (FSH) levels are below normal.

d. **Palpably enlarged ovaries** will further support the diagnosis in some cases. The presence of ovarian cysts on ultrasound may or may not be associated with the syndrome. Ovarian biopsy is not routinely indicated.

e. **Dexamethasone suppression** results in variable degrees of androgen suppression and is of limited diagnostic use.

3. **Management**

a. If infertility is an issue for the patient, **induction of ovulation** may be achieved with **clomiphene** (see Chapter 23).

   b. Other therapeutic modalities may include **glucocorticoids, gonadotropins, or gonadotropin-releasing hormone** (GnRH). Wedge resection of the ovary is ineffective and contraindicated in young women (9).

   c. Hirsutism may be treated by **suppressing ovarian steroidogenesis with combination oral contraceptives.**

     (1) The least androgenic have been those containing the progestins norethynodrel or ethynodiol diacetate. Newer progestins (norgestimate, desogestrel, gestodene) are even less androgenic. The **very low estrogen preparations may be inadequate.** Adequacy of estrogen dosage may be determined by measuring serum free testosterone and androstenedione (if previously elevated) to document suppression.

     (2) Patients with uteri should not receive long-term unopposed estrogen treatment but should be cycled with progesterone.

     (3) A **clinical response will not be seen for at least 6 months,** and additional nonspecific therapeutic measures that are discussed in section V may be required either in addition to or instead of the oral contraceptives.

B. Ovarian tumors

  1. Presentation. Androgens are secreted by several ovarian tumors including **Sertoli-Leydig cell (arrhenoblastomas), granulosa-theca cell, lipoid cell, hilus cell and adrenal rest tumors, dysgerminomas, and gonadoblastomas.**

   a. There is typically a **rapid development of hirsutism** with accompanying evidence of **virilization and a palpable ovarian mass** in at least half of cases.

   b. The greatest incidence occurs between the ages of 20 and 40, although the possible range is much wider.

   c. Hilus cell tumors typically occur in later life.

   d. Gonadoblastomas may occur before the teenage years, are often bilateral, rarely are palpable, and have a high malignant potential.

  2. Diagnosis.

   a. In women with ovarian tumors, **serum total testosterone levels** usually surpass 250 ng/dL (normal level for women is <90ng/dL) and are commonly in or above the normal male range (350–1,200 ng/dL).

   b. Androstenedione levels are usually markedly elevated.

   c. Suppression of hyperandrogenemia with estrogens does not rule out a tumor.

   d. Some ovarian tumors may show apparent dexamethasone suppressibility.

   e. Since nearly half of ovarian tumors may be nonpalpable, **ultrasound, CT scan, MRI, ovarian vein catheterization,** or **laparoscopy** may be needed for localization of the suspected tumor.

  3. Management. The treatment is **surgical removal.** Patients with nearly threefold increases in testosterone or androstenedione levels should be **evaluated rigorously for the presence of a tumor.**

III. Adrenal etiology

 A. Congenital adrenal hyperplasia

  1. Presentation. Hyperplasia of the adrenal glands may result from **enzymatic defects in the synthesis of cortisol.** A compensatory increase in ACTH release causes increased synthesis of precursors of the defect. **Inheritance is autosomal recessive.**

   a. Classically, the clinical presentation begins at birth when the diagnosis is suggested by the presence of **ambiguous genitalia.**

   b. Multiple **childhood symptoms** support the diagnosis:

     (1) Primary amenorrhea.

     (2) Absence of breast development.

(3) **Precocious pseudopuberty.**
(4) **Virilization.**
(5) **Hypoglycemia accompanied by cortisol insufficiency.**
(6) **Salt wasting and hypotension** in some patients.
(7) **Hypertension.**
c. It has recently been recognized that some patients have **mild enzymatic defects** and **present only with hirsutism and only after puberty.** Some studies report that up to 30% of patients with simple hirsutism have this late-onset, acquired adrenogenital syndrome.
2. **Pathophysiology.** There are **three enzymatic defects** that may cause hirsutism or virilization (Fig. 21.1):
   a. A **3β-hydroxysteroid dehydrogenase deficiency** may present in infancy with androgenic components as well as with **Addisonian crisis** (cortisol deficiency) and **salt wasting** (mineralocorticoid deficiency). **Simple postpubertal hirsutism** has also been reported.
   b. By far the **most common enzymatic defect is the 21-hydroxylase deficiency.** Androgenic presentation may have the range noted in foregoing section a. Patients with a marked defect will experience **salt wasting, hypotension,** and **hyperkalemia.**
   c. The **11-hydroxylase deficiency** will result in a spectrum of androgenicity but may be accompanied by **hypertension** and **hypokalemia** (mineralocorticoid excess).
3. **Diagnosis. DHEA, DHEA-S, and 17-ketosteroids are elevated** in all of the following defects:
   a. The **3β-hydroxysteroid dehydrogenase defect produces increased 17-hydroxypregnenolone levels.**

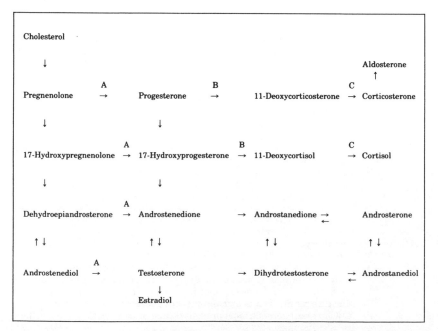

FIG. 21.1. Outline of steroid hormone synthesis including mineralocorticoids, glucocorticoids, and sex steroids. **A:** 3β-hydroxysteroid dehydrogenase. **B:** 21-hydroxylase. **C:** 11-hydroxylase.

      b. The **21-hydroxylase defect yields increased 17-hydroxyprog-esterone levels** with accompanying increased urinary levels of its metabolite, pregnanetriol.

      c. The **11-hydroxylase defect** is characterized by **increased levels of 11-deoxycortisol and 11-deoxycorticosterone.**

      d. If all studies are normal, a subtle defect may be identified by a marked increase in one of the metabolites discussed in III.A.3.a., III.A.3.b., or III.A.3.c. after ACTH stimulation (Cortrosyn stimulation test).

      e. **Serum testosterone and androstenedione may be mildly elevated with the 21-hydroxylase and 11-hydroxylase defi-ciencies.**

      f. With **all three enzymatic defects, cortisol levels will be sub-normal to normal and ACTH levels supernormal,** and the **hyperandrogenemia will be suppressible with physiologic amounts of glucocorticoid.**

    4. Management of patients with these enzymatic defects requires **ad-ministration of glucocorticoids and possibly mineralocorticoids** and should be managed by a specialist.

B. Adrenal tumors.

    1. Presentation. Functional tumors (adenomas and carcinomas) of the adrenal cortex **may present with hirsutism.** These tumors may present at any time from infancy to senescence. Clinical manifesta-tions develop rapidly with **virilization occurring in the majority of cases.** Indeed, hirsutism may be less significant than acne, tempo-ral balding, deepening of the voice, increased musculature, and clitoral hypertrophy.

      a. Many, but not all, patients will have evidence of **Cushing's syn-drome** reflecting concurrent overproduction of glucocorticoids.

      b. A **palpable adrenal mass** may be present in a few patients.

    2. Diagnosis.

      a. In patients with hirsutism caused by **adrenal adenomas and car-cinomas,** serum levels of **DHEA, DHEA-S, and androstenedione will typically be extraordinarily elevated as will urinary 17-ketosteroids.** DHEA-S levels greater than 900 µg/dL (normal ≤250 µg/dL) and total testosterone levels greater than 200 ng/dL (normal <90 ng/dL) may be seen.

      b. Patients with **adrenal adenomas and clinical presentation primarily of Cushing's syndrome** will have **elevated cortisol levels and suppressed ACTH levels and may not show sig-nificant androgen abnormalities.**

      c. Rarely, **adrenal tumors produce just testosterone in large amounts,** and DHEA, DHEA-S, and urinary 17-ketosteroids may be normal in those cases.

      d. Stimulation and suppression studies give conflicting results.

          (1) Adrenal carcinomas are not dexamethasone-suppress-ible even with high dosages (8 mg/day). Some adrenal adeno-mas may show suppression or at least erratic secretion, which can be confounding.

          (2) Human chorionic gonadotropin-responsive (hCG-respon-sive) adrenal tumors have been described.

      e. **CT scan, ultrasound, MRI, arteriography,** or **adrenal vein catheterization** may be required for localization of the suspected tumor.

    3. Management. The treatment is **surgical removal.** Discussion of further management is beyond the scope of this book.

C. Cushing's disease

    1. Presentation. Patients with **pituitary adenomas producing ACTH** will present primarily with symptoms of **glucocorticoid excess, or Cushing's syndrome,** such as **centripetal obesity, easy bruisabil-**

ity, diabetes mellitus, and hypertension but also may have hirsutism and even mild virilization. The development of symptoms and signs may be gradual and may occur at any age, although most commonly it occurs between the ages of 20 and 40.

   2. **Diagnosis.**
      a. Patients with Cushing's disease will **fail to suppress serum cortisol levels to less than 5 μg/mL the morning after taking dexamethasone,** 1 mg at bedtime.
      b. They will also **not suppress serum cortisol levels or urinary free cortisol excretion to low levels after dexamethasone,** 0.5 mg q6h for 2 days **(low dose).**
      c. They will, however, **suppress serum cortisol after dexamethasone,** 2 mg q6h for 2 days **(high dose), whereas most adrenal adenomas and all adrenal carcinomas will not.**
      d. **ACTH levels** are modestly elevated or normal but are always **inappropriately elevated for the simultaneously elevated cortisol levels.**
      e. A **CT scan or MRI** may confirm the presence of a pituitary adenoma.
   3. **Treatment.**
      a. **Transsphenoidal hypophysectomy** has been a highly effective mode of therapy in experienced hands.
      b. **Radiation therapy and pharmacologic therapy** (e.g., cyproheptadine, bromocriptine, o,p'-DDD [mitotane], ketoconazole, and metyrapone) may be of additional help.
D. **Ectopic ACTH**
   1. **Presentation.**
      a. The most common ACTH-producing carcinoma is **oat cell carcinoma of the lung.** However, **thymomas, islet cell tumors, carcinoid tumors, medullary lung carcinoma, and pheochromocytoma** also occur.
      b. The presentation is usually **rapid** with **mineralocorticoid effects,** such as hypertension and particularly hypokalemia, being dominant.
         (1) Signs of **glucocorticoid and adrenal androgen excess** may be seen.
         (2) **Hyperpigmentation** may be present.
   2. **Diagnosis.**
      a. **Serum levels of ACTH, cortisol, and adrenal androgens are extraordinarily elevated** and not suppressible with even high-dose dexamethasone except for bronchial carcinoid tumors, which typically do suppress.
      b. **A search for the primary tumor is critical.**
   3. **Treatment.**
      a. **Benign tumors should be resected** but, more commonly, this is not possible.
      b. Treatment is **chemotherapy of the primary tumor and control of adrenal steroidogenesis** with mitotane, metyrapone, aminoglutethimide, or ketoconazole.
IV. **Idiopathic hirsutism.** At least 50% of women with chronic hirsutism alone **do not carry a specific etiologic diagnosis;** although, as noted previously, hyperandrogenemia can usually be found with a careful evaluation. Overproduction of androgens by the ovaries, adrenal glands, or both, may be demonstrated with involvement of the adrenal glands alone being the least common. Probably **most patients with idiopathic hirsutism have mild polycystic ovary syndrome or mild congenital adrenal hyperplasia.** In the latter diagnosis, stimulation with ACTH will show hyperresponsiveness of the immediate steroid precursors of the particular enzyme deficiency in some patients who have normal levels in the nonstimulated state. Indeed, **stress has been associated with hirsutism** in some studies. Furthermore, there is evidence that adrenal hyperandrogenemia may lead to ovarian hyperandrogenemia and vice versa. An **association of hir-**

sutism with hyperprolactinemia has been noted but not confirmed. A reversible association of hyperandrogenemia and hirsutism with obesity is clear.

A. **Diagnosis.** If the patient has **no evidence of virilization and does not have a rapid progression of symptoms indicative of a tumor, the laboratory evaluation need not be exhaustive.** A **free testosterone level** (or preferably either a pooled specimen or several separate levels, in view of daily fluctuations) and a **DHEA-S level are useful screening tests.**

1. An **elevation of DHEA-S** suggests adrenal origin.
2. **An elevation of testosterone** is nonspecific but suggests ovarian origin if the DHEA-S is normal.
3. **Stimulation tests with hCG or ACTH need not be done routinely.**
4. **If free or total testosterone levels are higher than three times normal** and particularly if virilization is present, a search for an ovarian (rarely adrenal) tumor must be made.
5. **If DHEA-S levels are three to five times increased,** adrenal suppression with dexamethasone should be performed (see section III.C.2.). Failure of suppression should be followed by localization studies for an adrenal tumor.
6. **Modest elevations of testosterone, DHEA-S, or both** do not require further evaluation of possible polycystic ovary syndrome or congenital adrenal hyperplasia. Suppression tests with dexamethasone or oral contraceptives will not give reliable information about the site of origin of the hyperandrogenemia but may assist with selection of therapy.

B. **Management**

1. **If no diagnosis is made,** the response of hirsutism to **oral contraceptives** may be superior to the response to dexamethasone but **suppression tests** may help with this choice. Oral contraceptives should contain progestins with low androgen activity [see section II.A.3.c.(1)].

   If **dexamethasone** is chosen, a dose of 0.25 mg hs should be given, with incremental increases to 0.75 mg hs only if warranted by failure to suppress DHEA-S to normal. A **response to therapy will take 6 to 12 months.** Some patients with idiopathic hirsutism treated successfully with dexamethasone for at least 1 year will have a **prolonged remission of their hirsutism** following subsequent discontinuation of the drug.
2. A successful **weight reduction program** may ameliorate hirsutism in patients with significant obesity, although this relationship is poorly understood.

V. **Hirsutism: other therapies**

A. **Medroxyprogesterone acetate**

1. In patients who tolerate oral contraceptives poorly, 30 to 40 mg/day PO or 400 mg IM every 3 months may **significantly decrease ovarian androgen production and reduce hirsutism** in a majority of patients.
2. Patients can expect **amenorrhea** while receiving this treatment.

B. **Cyproterone acetate competes with androgens for the androgen receptor** and has been widely used in Europe for treatment of acne and hirsutism. It has yet to receive Food and Drug Administration approval in the United States because of **concerns over its side effects including possible adrenal insufficiency.**

C. **Spironolactone,** which **competes with aldosterone for renal mineralocorticoid receptors,** also **blocks the androgen receptor** as well as **increases the metabolic clearance rate of testosterone.**

1. A **reduction** in hirsutism is commonly seen within 6 months in women taking 50 to 200 mg/day.
2. **Patients at risk for hyperkalemia** (renal insufficiency, adrenal insufficiency, diabetes mellitus) must be monitored very closely and are best not given the drug at all.

D. **Cimetidine. Limited data** indicate that cimetidine, a histamine H_2-receptor antagonist, **weakly blocks the binding of androgen to its receptor.** It is not very effective in treating hirsutism.

E. **Flutamide,** a new agent that competes with androgens for the androgen receptor, has been shown to be well tolerated and more effective than spironolactone in recent trials. A marked reduction in hirsutism is seen within **3 months** in women taking 250 mg bid or tid.

F. **Finasteride,** a 5α-reductase inhibitor, inhibits conversion of testosterone to dihydrotestosterone, the active intracellular androgen and GnRH agonists.

G. **Gonadotropin-releasing hormone analogs** inhibit LH secretion and may be extremely effective. Long-term treatment can cause bone demineralization and negatively affect lipid profiles. However, "add-back" therapy with estrogen and progesterone may be able to overcome these adverse effects.

H. **Topical treatment**
   1. **Shaving** is transiently effective and does not stimulate hair growth, although regrown hair has a bristly appearance.
   2. **Plucking** results in regrowth in 1 month.
   3. **Bleaching** with hydrogen peroxide may improve appearance.
   4. **Depilatories** commonly contain thioglycolates, which chemically degrade hair, but may rarely cause severe dermal reactions.
   5. **Waxing,** actually mass plucking, is painful and may result in scarring.
   6. **Electrolysis** is painful, time-consuming, and expensive. If not performed with competence, scarring may occur. A galvanic low-voltage current is slower but safer than short-wave diathermy. Electrolysis is the **only method of treatment that removes unwanted hair permanently,** but in patients with severe hirsutism it should probably be used with a form of systemic therapy.
   7. **Eflornithine** is a topical cream. It is postulated that it irreversibly inhibits the activity of skin ornithine decarboxylase.

References

1. Azziz R, et al. 21-Hydroxylase deficiency in female hyperandrogenism: screening and diagnosis. *J Clin Endocrinol Metab* 1989;69:577.
2. Barnes R, et al. The polycystic ovary syndrome: pathogenesis and treatment. *Ann Intern Med* 1989;110:386.
3. Barth JH, et al. Spironolactone is an effective and well tolerated systemic antiandrogen therapy for hirsute women. *J Clin Endocrinol Metab* 1989;68:966.
4. Barth JH. Hirsute women: should they be investigated? *J Clin Pathol* 1992;45:188.
5. Committee on Technical Bulletins, American College of Obstetricians and Gynecologists. Evaluation and treatment of hirsute women (ACOG Tech Bull No. 203; March 1995). *Compendium of Selected Publications* 2001:439–444.
6. Cusan L, et al. Comparison of flutamide and spironolactone in the treatment of hirsutism: a randomized controlled trial. *Fertil Steril* 1994;61:281.
7. Leshin M. Southwestern Internal Medicine Conference: hirsutism. *Am J Med Sci* 1987;294:369.
8. Lincoln SR. Androgen excess disorders. In: Cowan BD, Seifer DB, eds. *Clinical reproductive medicine.* Philadelphia: Lippincott-Raven, 1997:95–101.
9. Loy R, et al. Evaluation and therapy of polycystic ovarian syndrome. *Endocrinol Metab Clin North Am* 1988;17:785.
10. Pasquali R, et al. Clinical and hormonal characteristics of obese amenorrheic hyperandrogenic women before and after weight loss. *J Clin Endocrinol Metab* 1989;68:173.
11. Precis V. *An update in obstetrics and gynecology.* Washington, DC: ACOG, 1994.
12. Rittmaster RS, et al. The role of adrenal hyperandrogenism, insulin resistance, and obesity in the pathogenesis of polycystic ovarian syndrome. *J Clin Endocrinol Metab* 1993;76:1295.
13. Sawaya ME, et al. The antiandrogens: when and how should they be used. *Dermatol Clin* 1993;11:65.

22. CONTRACEPTION

Arthur F. Levit

The contraceptive user has an array of methods from which to choose. **Appropriate considerations** include the user's age, need for concomitant protection against sexually transmitted infections, future plans for childbearing, health status, pattern of sexual activity, and feeling about method options. **Method safety and efficiency are usually the two issues of greatest concern** for users and clinicians. **The morbidity for any methods of contraception is low.**

The important trends in ensuring the **safest possible use of contraception** include the following:

1. Use of **low-dose oral contraceptive products** (i.e., ≤35 µg of estrogen, low-potency progestin).
2. **Use of long-lasting progestins** when estrogen may not be safely used.
3. **Proper patient selection** for the **intrauterine device** (IUD).
4. Use of **barrier methods** to **decrease** risk of **sexually transmitted disease (STD), HIV,** and **hepatitis B virus** transmission are sometimes used in addition to other contraceptives.
5. Careful **counseling concerning sterilization** including counseling the partner on the safety of vasectomy.
6. Use of emergency contraception (EC): **postcoital.**
7. **Early recognition and diagnosis of pregnancy and ectopic pregnancy.**

Two groups who need special consideration when discussing contraceptive choices are adolescents and women older than 35. The U.S. teen pregnancy rate exceeds that of other Western countries by up to 50%, and over half of these pregnancies are aborted. Peer pressure, feelings of invincibility, misinformation, fear about hormonal contraception, and fear of discovery by parents all contribute to an ever-increasing teen pregnancy rate. Teens are more likely to be nonmonogamous and are at risk for STDs, HIV, and hepatitis B transmission. Adolescents are at high risk for ineffective contraception.

Women older than 35 also have a large unintended pregnancy rate and between 40 and 50 have the second highest rate of abortion (second only to girls younger than 15). Misinformation and persistence of old ideas regarding hormonal contraception have previously limited the choices. Reanalysis of old data and recent evidence on the lower dose oral contraception confirm that **"the pill" is a reasonable option for healthy nonsmokers older than 35 and even until menopause** (5). The risk of **cardiovascular disease** is **highest** in women who **smoke** and in those who have **predisposing factors** (i.e., **hypertension or diabetes**). The **estrogen component** of the **combination** oral contraceptive pill (OCP) is associated with **increased risks** of **thrombophlebitis** and **pulmonary embolism,** but when taken alone, as in the **"minipill,"** the **progestin compounds do not increase these risks** (13). Although fertility diminishes in the 40s, women should continue to use contraception until follicle-stimulating hormone (FSH) levels are elevated, signaling an irreversible decline in ovarian function.

Although there are many different contraceptives, there is no perfect method. Each choice involves some degree of responsibility and compromise on the part of the patient. Failure rates of all the methods discussed in the following are listed in Table 22.1.

I. **Oral contraceptives** are the **second most commonly used method overall** and the **most common method for patients younger than 30.** The pill has undergone substantial changes since its development in the 1950s. Most important is the reduction in the amount of estrogen. Initially, pills contained 40 to 80 µg of ethinyl estradiol, whereas today 30 to 35 µg is the standard. This

This chapter is a revision of the third edition chapter by Lesley R. Levine.

Table 22.1. Percentage of women experiencing an unintended pregnancy
during the first year of typical use and the first year of perfect use and the
percentage continuing use at the end of the first year, United States

% of women experiencing an unintended pregnancy within the first year of use

Method	Typical use	Perfect use	% of women continuing use at one year
Chance	85	85	—
Spermicides	26	6	40
Periodic Abstinence	25	63	—
Calendar	9	—	—
Ovulation method	3	—	—
Symptothermal	2	—	—
Postovulation	1	—	—
Withdrawal	19	4	—
Cap			
Parous women	40	26	42
Nulliparous women	20	9	56
Sponge			
Parous women	40	20	42
Nulliparous women	20	9	56
Diaphragm	20	6	56
Condom			
Female (reality)	21	5	56
Male	14	3	61
Pill			
Progestin only	5	0.5	71
Combined	0.1	—	—
IUD			
Progesterone T	2.0	1.5	81
Copper T 380A	0.8	0.6	78
LNg20	0.1	0.1	81
Depo-Provera	0.3	0.3	70
Norplant (6 capsules)	0.05	0.05	88
Female sterilization	0.5	0.5	100
Male sterilization	0.15	0.10	100

Emergency contraceptive pills: treatment initiated within 72 hours after unprotected intercourse reduces the risk of pregnancy by at least 75%.
Lactational amenorrhea method (LAM): LAM is a highly effective, *temporary* method of contraception.
From: Updated from Trussell et al.

reduction of estrogen almost eliminates concern about cardiovascular risk in healthy nonsmoking women. Cardiovascular risk seems to be related to the thrombotic effect of estrogen, which is dose-related. At 35 μg the risk is not any higher than the baseline risk of a healthy woman. Figure 22.1 is a chart on relative potency of estrogens and progestins in currently available oral contraceptives.

A. **Types of pills**
  1. **Combined pills** when used perfectly have a very low failure rate of approximately 0.1% to 3.0%. They provide a daily dose of estrogen and progestin for 21 days in a 28-day cycle. Almost all pills today are comparable in efficacy, side effects, and complications.
      a. **Estrogen** acts by **inhibiting FSH production** and **decreasing follicle development** thereby limiting ovulation. It also may prevent **implantation** and **potentiates** the **effects** of **progestins.** Estrogen also **stabilizes** the **endometrium.**
      b. **Progestins inhibit luteinizing hormone (LH)** release and, therefore, can interfere with ovulation. The **endometrium** atrophies, the **cervical mucus** becomes thick and hostile to sperm, and the **fallopian tubes** have decreased motility. Bleeding occurs when the estrogen and progestin are withdrawn, usually during the last 7 days of the 28-day cycle.
          (1) There are **several different progestins used in oral contraceptives.**
              (a) They are of **varying potency** but in each formulation **potency** is **compensated** by the **dosage.**
              (b) Progestins have an androgenic pharmacology and **may affect lipid levels adversely;** however, clinically this is rarely a problem.
              (c) Of the progestins, **norethynodrel** may produce **estrogenic effects,** and **norethindrone acetate** and **norgestrel** may produce **antiestrogenic or androgenic effects** or both. There had been some concern that the so-called newer progestins (gestodene, desogestrel, and norgestimate) present in third generation OCPs may incur higher thromboembolic risks. However, more recent **data** does **not support** this hypothesis (14).
          (2) **Multiphasic preparations** contain varying daily dosages of estrogen and progestin. Theoretically, this decreases the progestin dose and androgenic effects. Clinically, however, there is very little difference between the monophasic and multiphasic preparations.
  2. The **minipill** contains progestin only and is taken **continuously** at the **same time of day** and with **no cyclic interruption** for maximum effectiveness. The preparation's main effects are on the endometrium, cervix, and fallopian tubes.
      a. **Failure rates of the minipill** when it is used correctly are **only slightly higher** than combination pills, **0.5% to 3.0%.**
      b. It causes anovulation in only 40% to 60% of users.
      c. Since the minipill has no estrogen, it is **recommended** for **women** who have a **contraindication to the combined pill** (see section I.C.).
      d. Minipills are often well tolerated by women who experience side effects, such as headaches, when using combined pills.
      e. It is likely that some noncontraceptive benefits of pills, such as protection against pelvic inflammatory disease (PID), are mediated by progestin.
B. **Contraindications and risk factors.** Certain systemic conditions contraindicate the use of the pill.
  1. Women with **absolute contraindication** should **never** be given the pill.

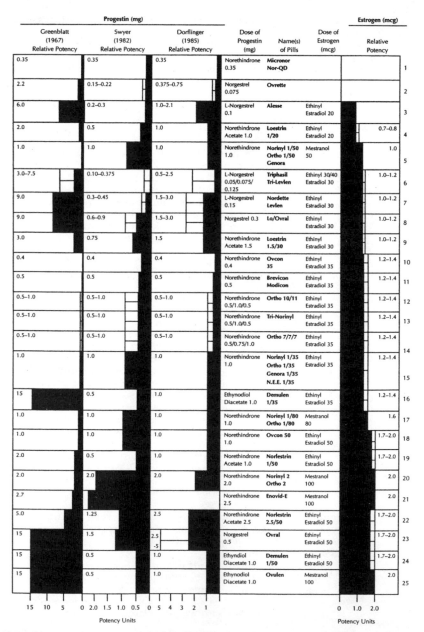

FIG. 22.1. Relative potency of estrogens and progestins in currently available oral contraceptives reflecting the debate about the strength of the progestins. (From Hatcher R, et al. *Contraceptive technology,* 17th rev ed. New York: Ardent Media, 1998, with permission [Sources: Dorflinger, 1985; Greenblatt, 1967; Swyer, 1982; Heinen].)

2. For those with **strong relative contraindications, risk** and **benefits** should be **weighed** carefully.
3. Table 22.2 lists contraindications for combined pills.
C. **Evaluation issues.** When discussing options with the patient, it is important to determine whether or not she has any of the risk factors found in Table 22.2. It is also important to discuss **lifestyle issues, noncontraceptive benefits, side effects,** and **severe complications.** Recent evidence has confirmed that combined oral contraceptives are extremely safe. Some authors have suggested that pills should be available over-the-counter without a prescription.
   1. **Noncontraceptive benefits.** The pill offers many benefits other than contraception and is used in the treatment of several clinical conditions. The following is a summary of these benefits:
      a. **Decreased menstrual flow, dysmenorrhea,** and **anemia.**
      b. **Decreased fibrocystic changes** of the breast with prolonged use.
      c. **Decreased risk of PID,** although the **risk** of **cervicitis may be increased.**
      d. **Decreased acne.**
      e. **Decreased ovarian** and **endometrial cancer** risks. The risk of **breast cancer** may be slightly increased but tumors, when found, tend to be diagnosed earlier and are of a less aggressive type (5).

Table 22.2. Contraindications to use of combined oral contraceptive pills

---

ABSOLUTE CONTRAINDICATIONS
Thrombophlebitis or thromboembolic disorder (or history thereof) [a]
Cerebrovascular accident (or history thereof)
Coronary artery or ischemic heart disease (or history thereof)
Known or suspected estrogen-dependent neoplasia (or history thereof)
Known or suspected estrogen-dependent neoplasia (or history thereof)
Pregnancy
Markedly impaired liver function [b]
Undiagnosed abnormal vaginal bleeding
Smoker over the age of 35

RELATIVE CONTRAINDICATIONS
Vascular headaches
Uncontrolled hypertension [c]
Major surgery requiring immobilization of the lower extremities
Current medications that would interfere with the absorption or metabolism of the pill (i.e., rifampin, seizure medications)
Diabetes mellitus [d]
Sickle cell disease (SS) or sickle C disease (SC)
Active gallbladder disease
Congenital hyperbilirubinemia (Gilbert's disease)
Intestinal malabsorption
Term pregnancy within past 3–4 weeks
Obstructive jaundice during pregnancy
Lactation
Family history of hyperlipidemia, thromboembolic or cardiovascular disease

---

[a] A history of the thrombotic complication secondary to surgery or trauma may not be considered an absolute contraindication.
[b] If this is a temporary and correctable condition, it may not be an absolute contraindication.
[c] If a woman is successfully treated for hypertension, the pill may be considered.
[d] Diabetes may increase the cardiovascular risk minimally but the benefit of the pill may outweigh this risk. Previous gestational diabetes should not be considered a contraindication.
Source: Adapted from Hatcher RA, et al. *Contraceptive technology: international edition.* Atlanta, GA: Printed Matter, 1990, with permission.

      f. Decreased risk of ovarian cysts, although this may not be as true with the low-dose pills.

      g. Decreased risk of rheumatoid arthritis.

      h. Fewer ectopic pregnancies and abortions owing to its contraceptive effectiveness.

   2. Lifestyle and other issues.

      a. It must be stressed that pills do **not** provide protection from STDs, HIV, or hepatitis B transmission. Patients who are **not mutually monogamous** should be encouraged to also **use** a **barrier method with the pill.**

      b. Family history should be explored to determine if occult risk factors exist (Table 22.2).

      c. Discussions with patients will reveal fears and misinformation that the clinician can correct.

      d. A good understanding of the pill's benefits, risks, and method of use will increase compliance and effectiveness.

D. How to determine correct dosage and type. The axiom for determining pill dosage is to use the **lowest dosage that provides effective protection from pregnancy.**

   1. Most women should be prescribed a 35-µg or less estrogen pill.

      a. These pills contain the more potent ethinyl estradiol and may not have a markedly lower estrogenic effect than do pills containing 50 µg of mestranol.

      b. Spotting or failure to have withdrawal bleeding are common problems associated with use of low-dose pills. Patients should be warned of these problems and advised that they often spontaneously resolve after three cycles.

   2. Pills containing more than 50 µg estrogen (80 or 100 µg) are for the most part unavailable now. Pills containing 50 µg estrogen may occasionally be appropriate for women with severe acne, dysfunctional bleeding, or endometriosis.

   3. Progestin-only pills may be the initial pill choice for postpartum or nursing mothers, women older than 30 to 35 years, or women who have vascular headaches.

   4. The minipill is also a good choice for women who do not tolerate combined pills or for those who develop relative contraindications to the use of combined pills.

E. Instructions

   1. Clinicians.

      a. A thorough history including the foregoing risk factors, lifestyles, and considerations must be obtained.

      b. A thorough examination including blood pressure, breast examination, Papanicolaou (Pap) smear and pelvic examination is done.

      c. Be sure that every pill user is aware of the **pill danger signs (see later discussion).**

      d. New users may benefit from an **initial follow-up visit** at 3 months to check blood pressure and review problems. Most users who discontinue use do so because of side effects. Thus, it is very important to **emphasize** that most of these side effects **resolve spontaneously** within the first 3 months of use (15).

      e. Thereafter, annual examinations and Pap smears are appropriate.

      f. For women older than 35 who may have risk factors, a blood sugar concentration and lipid panel should be checked. Healthy women with no family history do not need these tests.

      g. Documentation of counseling and examination findings is essential.

      h. It is important that the patient fully understands the method of taking the pill, the side effects, and the severe complications. She should know when and whom to call with any questions.

2. Patients.

    a. Every pill user should memorize the **five pill danger signs.** The first letter of each symptom spells the acronym **ACHES:**

        *A*bdominal pain.

        Chest pain or shortness of breath.

        *H*eadaches.

        *E*ye problems, such as blurred vision, flashing lights, or blindness.

        *S*evere leg pain.

    b. A pill user who develops a **breast lump,** notices **growth or change in a mole,** develops **liver disease** or **jaundice,** or becomes **depressed** should contact her clinician.

    c. Pill users should know how to report problems to the clinician and know what to do if they experience bleeding, skip a period, or forget to take one or more pills.

    d. A new pill user should start the first pack of pills within the first 5 days of menses.

        (1) Most can start on a Sunday, which makes it easy to remember and relegates menses to the weekdays.

        (2) If she cannot start within the first 5 days, a backup method for the first full cycle should be used.

        (3) Starting a package beyond the first 6 to 7 days may **increase the failure rate.**

        (4) In adolescents with a negative pregnancy test, an immediate start may be helpful to prevent forgetfulness. A backup method must be used for the first cycle.

    e. Patients should **take** one pill a day at about the same time of day.

F. Sequelae. Pill hormones **affect virtually every organ system,** and about 40% of users notice **side effects or noncontraceptive benefits. Severe complications are rare.**

    1. Complications and side effects. The major complications of pills are **cardiovascular.** These, however, are **primarily limited to women older than 35 who smoke or have a history of other cardiovascular problems or diabetes.**

        a. Life-threatening complications:

            (1) Thrombophlebitis.

            (2) Deep pelvic vein thrombosis.

            (3) Pulmonary embolism.

            (4) Arterial thromboembolic events resulting in cerebrovascular accident or myocardial infarction.

            (5) Hepatic adenomas. These may regress after discontinuation of the pill.

        b. Serious side effects include:

            (1) Hypertension.

            (2) Gallbladder disease.

            (3) Vascular headache.

            (4) Depression.

        c. Other minor side effects, which usually **improve with time,** include:

            (1) Nausea.

            (2) Weight gain.

            (3) Breast tenderness.

            (4) Breakthrough bleeding.

            (5) Decreased libido.

            (6) Women who develop **acne** may want to discontinue use or change to formulations with lower androgen-potency progestins. Orthotricycline has been approved to treat acne.

        d. Higher rates of cervical neoplasia (dysplasia, carcinoma in situ, and invasive carcinoma) have been reported for pill users. Whether this is an effect of the pill or of lifestyle is unclear. The pill can be continued with **very careful follow-up.**

        2. **Pill effects on subsequent fertility.**

           a. Resumption of ovulation is usually within the first 14 to 21 days of discontinuing the pill.

           b. The **pregnancy rate** in the first 3 months lags behind that of users of other methods. However, within a year the rates are relatively the same.

               (1) There is no indication that infertility is increased by the pill.

               (2) Older data indicate that the higher dose pill may have caused a pregnancy rate lag of up to 42 months.

        3. **Noncontraceptive benefits.** Use of the pill is associated with a **decreased incidence of PID, ovarian and endometrial cancer, ectopic pregnancy, iron-deficiency anemia, rheumatoid arthritis, ovarian functional cysts, benign breast lumps, dysmenorrhea,** and **acne** (3).

    G. **Clinical dilemmas.** Optimal management of pill problems involves numerous clinical dilemmas.

        1. **Forgotten pills.**

           a. A woman who **forgets to take one pill** should double up the next day.

           b. If two pills are missed, she should double up for 2 days **and** use a backup method of birth control until the next menstrual period.

           c. If three or more pills are missed, the user should start a new pack of pills **and** use a second method of contraception as well.

           d. If she is a Sunday starter, she may continue the pills until Sunday and **then** start a new package.

        2. **Breakthrough bleeding** is a **common** occurrence in the **first 3 months** of starting the pill. If breakthrough bleeding persists beyond that time, a different formulation may be tried **or** a small amount of estrogen may be added in the first 7 days of the cycle (1.25 mg of conjugated estrogens or 1 mg of estradiol).

        3. **Skipped periods or amenorrhea.** The pill's effect on the endometrium is dominated by progestin and causes atrophy. Amenorrhea may be a response to continued progestin stimulation.

           a. If the patient takes the pills regularly and she is **not** concerned about the lack of a "withdrawal period," nothing need be done. It may be advisable to check a pregnancy test, if there is any doubt about whether the pills are taken correctly.

           b. If the patient is concerned, a period may be induced by adding estrogen, 1.25 mg of conjugated estrogens or 1 mg of estradiol for 21 days of the cycle. This can be done for one or two cycles to thicken the endometrial lining.

           c. Alternatively, a patient may be switched to an oral contraceptive with a lower progestin potency.

        4. **Development of vascular headaches, hypertension, or cholestasis are reasons to discontinue the pill.**

        5. **Development of cervical dysplasia** is not a reason to discontinue the pill. **Pap smear** or **colposcopy surveillance** is necessary. These patients may be at risk for other STDs, HIV, and hepatitis B transmission and should be counseled to use a barrier method as well as the pill.

    H. **Special considerations**

        1. **Adolescents** may benefit in many ways by using the pill.

           a. Cycles are regulated, are less painful, and have decreased blood loss.

           b. There is less risk for PID, although the pill does nothing to mitigate against STDs, HIV, and hepatitis B transmission.

           c. Adolescents who are not mutually monogamous should use a barrier method in addition to the pill.

        2. **Women older than 35** who are perimenopausal benefit from pill use.

           a. The pill will regulate cycles.

           b. There is increased bone density and less risk of rheumatoid arthritis.

      c. It is an extremely effective method of birth control that should not be denied simply because of age.

      d. **"Morning-after pill"** (see section IX.). **Minipills** may be given to women who have relative contraindications to the combination pills. It must be taken every day at the same time. If a pill is missed, a backup method must be used.

   4. **Postpartum** and **breast-feeding** women also need effective protection.

      a. **Combination pills** can be started after 3 weeks if **postpartum** and **not breast-feeding.**

      b. A patient exclusively breast-feeding may start the minipill 6 weeks postpartum.

      c. **Combination** pills are **not recommended** in women who are **breast-feeding** because estrogen can decrease the amount and quality of breast milk.

II. Injectable combination contraceptive

   A. Lunelle, a combination of medroxyprogesterone acetate and estradiol cypionate, has received Food and Drug Administration (FDA) approval as a monthly injectable contraceptive. In comparison to the oral combination pill, **contraceptive effectiveness is very high** since the problem of forgetting pills is eliminated. In an initial study over the course of 1 year, there were no pregnancies in 782 women.

   B. **Side effects** are expected to be similar to that of the OCP. There seems to be higher rates of irregular bleeding during the initial months of use when compared with corresponding rates in OCP users.

   C. Compared with long-acting progestins, **return to fertility** after discontinuation of this method is **more rapid.** Ovulation can occur as early as 6 weeks after the last injection. **For this reason it is also important to receive follow-up injections within 5 days of the prescribed 28-day injection schedule.**

III. Long-acting progestin contraceptives. Since 1992, long-acting injectable forms of progestins have been approved in the United States. Medroxyprogesterone acetate (Depo-Provera) has been used around the world for more than a decade. Levonorgestrel implants (Norplant system), silastic capsules that release progestin for up to 5 years, were approved in 1990. The mechanisms of action for these forms of progestin are the same as with the combined pill and the minipill. Progestin interferes with endometrial growth, cervical mucus production, and possibly fallopian tube transport. It may suppress LH surge and prevent ovulation but this is not consistent. About one third to one half of cycles are ovulatory. Effectiveness has been shown to be excellent, exceeding even that of sterilization in one large study.

   A. **Types of progestins**

      1. **Norplant system** is six silastic subdermal capsules that contain levonorgestrel.

         a. Each capsule is 34 mm long and 2.4 mm in diameter. The levonorgestrel is very stable and is released over a period of 5 years. During the first year, 80 μg/day is released, which is comparable with the minipill and is about 50% of the progestin in the combined pills. Gradually, the release decreases to 30 to 40 μg/day. At 5 years, the amount released is not enough to provide adequate protection.

         b. **Very obese women** may have relatively lower serum levels and, therefore, **less contraceptive efficacy.**

         c. A modification of the Norplant system (Norplant II) has only two subdermal capsules. This product is currently undergoing trials.

      2. **Depo-Provera** is the depot form of medroxyprogesterone acetate. It is given as an injection of 150 mg every 3 months. The contraceptive effects may last up to 4 months.

   B. **Failure rate.** The failure rates for either method are extremely low, from 0.2% to 0.3% in the first year. Most of the "failures" were in women who were pregnant at the time of insertion or injection. The Norplant failure rate increases with time until at 5 years it is as high as 1.1%.

C. Contraindications and risk factors are fewer than with the combined pills.
  1. These methods may be safely used in women who may have contra-indications to the combined pills (i.e., estrogen; Table 22.2).
  2. Theoretically, there are concerns with progestins' effects on lipid levels. However, studies do not show a significant change in lipids (5) or carbohydrate metabolism.
D. Evaluation and counseling considerations. Long-acting progestins have noncontraceptive benefits similar to those of the pill (see section I.E.), except that there is no protection from ovarian cysts. In fact, ovarian cysts can occur more frequently.
E. Complications and side effects
  1. Early animal research with Depo-Provera suggested increased breast tumors in beagle dogs. Worldwide use and many years of follow-up have alleviated fears of this severe complication. **A multinational study** showed a **slightly increased risk ratio of 1.2** in **women younger than 35 only** in the **first 4 years of use. Risks were not increased** in women who had used this **method longer than 5 years.**
  2. **Serious side effects are rare.** However, many side effects are such nuisances that patients discontinue use.
    a. The **most common side effect** is **irregular bleeding** from the lack of estrogen's stabilizing influence on the endometrium.
    b. **Bleeding patterns are unpredictable.**
    c. **Amenorrhea** can occur.
  3. **Other side effects** include:
    a. **Headaches.**
    b. **Nausea.**
    c. **Weight gain.**
    d. **Acne.**
    e. **Ovarian cysts.**
    f. **Hyperpigmentation** over the **Norplant site.**
    g. **Depression, which can be severe, more so with Depo-Provera than with Norplant implants.**
  4. **Other considerations.**
    a. This method does **not interrupt** sex for contraception.
    b. It provides **no protection** against **STDs, HIV,** or **hepatitis B** transmission.
    c. Long-acting progestins are not as accessible as other methods. Norplant requires an appointment to have it inserted and removed.
    d. In some cases it is costly because it involves a procedure charge.
    e. **Depo-Provera must be given every 3 months** so **patients must remember** (or be reminded) to return regularly for injections.
    f. There are **no long-term effects** on **fertility.** Most women ovulate in the first month after discontinuing this method. However, medium-range delays in ovulation (up to 9 months) can occur with Depo-Provera.
F. Instructions
  1. Clinicians should discuss all of the foregoing considerations with the patient (see sections III.B.–E.).
    a. Some practitioners recommend a **trial of a minipill before** committing to the **injection** or **Norplant system.**
    b. It is ideal to **begin** the progestin **within** the **first 7 days of menses.**
    c. A **pregnancy test** is recommended before administering the first dose of Depo-Provera or inserting the Norplant.
    d. The Norplant insertion procedure is not difficult and takes about 15 to 20 minutes. Wyeth-Ayerst can be contacted for training materials.

       e. Removal of Norplant can take **longer** and may be **complicated** by an initial irregular placement or by a fracture of the silastic capsule.

    2. Patients should be **aware** of **possible side effects** and may want to **keep track of bleeding.**

    3. Patients should call in with any **change** in the **bleeding pattern** since a **pregnancy test** may be indicated.

G. Clinical dilemmas

    1. If spotting or irregular bleeding continues, the patient may be treated with

        a. Ibuprofen (Motrin), 800 mg PO tid for 5 days.

        b. Conjugated estrogens, 1.25 mg PO or **estradiol,** 1 mg PO every day for 7 days.

        c. Ethinyl estradiol, 20 μg PO every day for 25 days.

        d. Methyltestosterone with conjugated estrogens **(Premarin),** 2.5 mg every day for 25 days.

        e. Some clinicians use **low-dose birth control pills** such as ethinyl estradiol-norethindrone (Ovcon 35) for one cycle.

        f. If **all** of the foregoing **methods fail** and the woman **wishes** to **continue** treatment, then a **hysteroscopy** and a **D & C** can be done to rule out intrauterine pathology.

        g. A **barrier method should be used with any estrogen-only method of treatment as it may decrease the effectiveness of the progestins** by thinning cervical mucus.

    2. If a patient develops **amenorrhea,** a **pregnancy test** should be obtained. The patient can be reassured that the method is still effective even without a period.

    3. It is important to **remember** that **many patients still ovulate while taking progestins.** If there is any change in a regular pattern of bleeding, a **pregnancy test** is **advised.**

    4. Headaches, severe acne, and **depression** may be indications for discontinuing this method.

H. Special considerations

    1. Both Depo-Provera and Norplant may be used by **lactating** women.

    2. Adolescents and women older than 35 may be well suited to one of these methods for the same reasons as those discussed for the combined pills (see section I.E.).

    3. Mentally disabled patients may particularly benefit from this method.

IV. IUDs have been used since the beginning of the twentieth century. This is a popular method of birth control worldwide but less so in the United States. With proper patient selection and counseling, products could be used more often. IUDs are believed to inhibit pregnancy by producing a local inflammatory response in the endometrium. This hostile environment is thought to be spermicidal and there is theoretical evidence that tubal motility is affected. It is important to realize that IUDs are thought to be **contraceptive not abortifacient. Failure rates** of any IUDs are **low.** The Progestasert fails between 2% and 3% of the time, whereas the failure rate for the CuT 380A is between 0.5% and 0.8%.

A. Types of IUDs

    1. Nonmedicated IUDs are **no longer available** in the United States but some **women still** have them. Among the more common types are the **Lippes Loop** and the **Saf-T-Coil.** These types of IUDs **work indefinitely** and there is **no need to remove** and replace them.

    2. Copper T-380A (ParaGard) is a copper-containing device in a T-shape, 36 mm long by 32 mm wide. It is currently **approved** for up to **10 years** of use.

    3. Progestasert contains progesterone that is released locally, has progestin (atrophic) effects on the endometrium, and affects the cervical mucus. This particular progestin IUD must be **replaced every year.**

    4. **Mirena** is a new levonorgestrel-releasing IUD that has received FDA approval. This IUD can be used for **up to 5 years.**
B. **Contraindications and risk factors**
    1. **PID** and **pregnancy** are **absolute contraindications** for use of an IUD.
        a. The risk of developing PID for the first time while using an IUD is dependent on the sexual activity of the woman and her partner.
        b. A woman in a **mutually** monogamous relationship will have little increased risk of developing PID while using the IUD.
    2. A previous ectopic pregnancy is no longer considered an absolute contraindication.
        a. The **newer copper IUDs protect against ectopic as well as intrauterine pregnancy.**
        b. The **Progestasert** offers **less protection** against ectopic pregnancy.
        c. Experimental **levonorgestrel IUDs** offer good **protection against ectopic pregnancies,** probably by interfering with ovulation.
    3. Table 22.3 provides a **complete list** of contraindications.
C. **Counseling considerations. The manufacturers of IUDs have developed extensive consent forms that the provider should review with the patient.**
    1. The **best candidate** for an IUD is a **multiparous** (proven fertility) woman involved in a **mutually monogamous** relationship.

Table 22.3. Possible contraindications to use of intrauterine devices (IUDs)

ABSOLUTE CONTRAINDICATIONS
Active, recent, or recurrent pelvic infection (acute or subacute)
Pregnancy (known or suspected)

RELATIVE CONTRAINDICATIONS
Undiagnosed, irregular, or abnormal uterine bleeding
Risk factors for pelvic inflammatory disease
    Postpartum endometritis
    Infection following an abortion that occurred in the past 3 months
    Purulent cervicitis, until controlled
    Impaired response to infection (diabetes, steroid treatment)
    Recurrent history of gonorrhea
    High risk for a sexually transmitted disease, including multiple sexual partners or
        a partner who has multiple sexual partners
Risk factors for exposure to the human immunodeficiency virus (HIV)
Cervical or uterine malignancy (known or suspected), including unresolved Pap smear
Impaired coagulation response (idiopathic thrombocytopenic purpura, anticoagulant
    therapy, etc.)
Valvular heart disease, which may make the patient susceptible to subacute bacterial
    endocarditis (may need prophylactic antibiotics)
Uterine anomalies
Myomas
Menstrual disorders such as severe dysmenorrhea, severe menorrhagia,
    or endometriosis
Anemia
History of impaired fertility in a woman who desires a future pregnancy
History of fainting
Allergy to copper or diagnosed Wilson's disease is a contraindication for the use of
    the Cooper T-380A IUD

Note: It may be possible to use an IUD, with Progestasert or levonorgestrel, in women with some of the above conditions.
From: Adapted from Hatcher RA, et al. *Contraceptive technology: international edition.* Atlanta, GA: Printed Matter, 1990, with permission.

2. As with the pill, it must be stressed that this method provides **no protection against STDs, HIV, or hepatitis B transmission.**
3. Wearing an **IUD** and contracting an STD can lead to **severe PID** and **possibly abscesses.**
4. **Selecting the type of IUD.** Most patients will prefer to have the longer lasting CuT 380A (ParaGard).
   a. Progestasert may decrease the severity of dysmenorrhea and anemia in some women.
   b. Mirena has the same benefits as Progestasert, with the additional **advantage** of needing replacement only **once in 5 years** instead of yearly.
5. **Risks** at the time of **insertion** include **perforation** and **infection.** There is about a 5% expulsion rate.
6. Patients should expect some cramping and discomfort for a few months.
7. There can also be **heavy menses, spotting, or** an **increase** in **vaginal discharge.**
   a. These symptoms can be **treated** with standard doses of **nonsteroidal antiinflammatory** drugs.
   b. Approximately 10% of patients will discontinue this method because of these problems.
8. Return of fertility is as rapid as with barrier methods. The endometrial cavity returns to normal almost immediately after removing the IUD.

D. **Instructions**
   1. **Clinicians** should be well skilled in how to insert the different types of IUDs.
      a. It is best to insert the IUD during menses or just after an abortion. This is not a strict rule as long as **pregnancy** has been **completely ruled out.**
      b. If there is a suspicion of STDs, **cultures** need to be **taken** and **results obtained prior to inserting** the IUD.
      c. **Perform a bimanual examination** to determine size and position of the uterus.
      d. Grasp the anterior lip of the cervix with a tenaculum and **sound the uterus** slowly and gently.
      e. **Load the IUD into the inserter barrel** and with slow steady traction on the tenaculum **slide the IUD inserter barrel into the uterus.**
      f. **Gently remove the inserter, being careful not to tug the IUD string.**
      g. **Clip the strings** about 3 to 5 cm from the os. Leaving them longer initially allows for some retraction over the next several days as the IUD becomes seated within the uterine cavity. If the strings are cut too short, the partner may feel them.
      h. **Paracervical injection of 10 to 20 mL of 0.5% lidocaine** provides an effective anesthetic block for difficult or painful insertion. However, a paracervical block is usually not needed for insertion.
      i. Since the **risk of perforation** is **greatest** at the **time of insertion,** patients should **return** in **2 to 3 weeks** to have the placement checked and to rule out expulsion or perforation. At this return visit, preferably after a menses, the string length can be cut shorter if needed.
   2. **Patients.** Be sure each patient **knows how to check for her IUD strings** and does so regularly. If the strings are absent or if a period is missed, the patient should contact the clinician.
      a. A **second method of birth control** is recommended during the first 3 months after insertion.
      b. Each user **should know what type of IUD she has and when her IUD should be replaced.**

      c. Most important, she should **memorize the IUD danger signs.** The first letter of each sign spells the acronym **PAINS.**
      Period late or missing.
      Abdominal pain.
      Increased temperature.
      Noticeable discharge.
      Spotting.

E. Sequelae. Potential IUD complications are listed **in order of decreasing severity.**

  1. Infection is the cause of most IUD-associated hospitalizations and deaths. IUD users are two to eight times more likely to require hospitalization for PID than women using no contraception. Infection rates are highest among women at high risk for PID, including young women with multiple sexual partners in areas where STD rates are high.

    a. IUD **infection** can occur **without any obvious sign of systemic sepsis and without fever.** Symptoms, such as abnormal discharge, bleeding, or pelvic pain, should be treated as infection until proven otherwise.

    b. Because fertility impairment can be a consequence, IUD infection warrants immediate aggressive management.

  2. Uterine perforation, embedment, or cervical perforation can occur silently (with no symptoms) and may be discovered when IUD removal is attempted or when unintended pregnancy occurs. Symptoms may include pain, bleeding, and disappearance of IUD strings.

    a. Ultrasound is often helpful in determining the location of an IUD but may not be accurate for a woman with large fibroids.

    b. Cervical perforation may occur as an IUD is being expelled.

    c. The **Dalkon Shield** is not visible on x-ray films. Although it has been off the market since the 1980s, a few women may still have it.

  3. Pregnancy. Whenever pregnancy occurs in an IUD user, **the probability of ectopic pregnancy must be carefully evaluated.** Although IUD use does not cause ectopic pregnancy, the IUD's effectiveness in preventing conception with ectopic implantation is lower than its effectiveness in preventing intrauterine pregnancy.

    a. If pregnancy occurs, the **IUD should be removed when** the **string is still visible.**

      (1) If the string is not visible, patients should be counseled that there is a **50% spontaneous abortion rate** and elective termination may be offered.

      (2) Ectopic pregnancy should always be considered and ruled out by ultrasound or D & C, if appropriate.

  4. Lost IUD strings are a common complaint. In most cases the string may be seen inside the cervical canal. Narrow forceps can be used to probe the cervical canal in an attempt to bring the strings into view.

    a. Consider **pregnancy** if the strings are not visible on careful examination. If pregnancy is ruled out, then a search must be made for the IUD.

    b. Ultrasound will be able to determine if it is inside the cavity or if it has eroded into the myometrium.

      (1) IUDs that are totally inside the cavity may be left in place.

      (2) In many places worldwide, IUDs are routinely placed **without strings.**

    c. If ultrasound is unable to identify the IUD, a three-way x-ray of the abdomen should be obtained to ensure that it is not floating in the abdominal cavity.

    d. If the IUD is in the **abdominal cavity,** the patient should be referred for **laparoscopic removal.**

    e. If the IUD is not seen on x-ray examination, most likely it was expelled without the patient's awareness. **Remember that the Dalkon Shield is not visible on x-ray films.**

5. **Spotting and bleeding** may vary depending on the type of IUD. Unusual spotting or cramping may represent **pregnancy** or **mild infection** and should **always be considered prior to any treatment.**
   a. The **progestin-type** IUDs generally lead to **hypomenorrhea,** but long-time use can cause atrophy and irregular spotting.
   b. **Copper IUDs** are more likely to cause **irregular spotting** and **cramping than are progestin-containing ones.** Nonsteroidal antiinflammatory drugs can decrease these problems:
6. **Difficult removal of an IUD.** Removal of the IUD during menses is generally easy. An IUD should be removed with gentle traction on the string.
   a. In older IUDs, the string may pull off or the IUD may not move from its position, indicating that it may be partially embedded.
   b. A narrow packing forceps may be used to grab the end of the **IUD.**
      (1) Sometimes, a paracervical block and cervical dilation may be necessary.
      (2) If this is unsuccessful, an IUD hook may be used inside the cavity.
      (3) A "Novak" curette, used for endometrial biopsies, is useful because of the serrations at the end of the curette.
      (4) The patient should be referred for hysteroscopic removal when other methods have failed.
7. **IUD expulsion.** Between 5% and 20% of users expel the IUD within the first year of use.
   a. Expulsion or partial expulsion is **often entirely asymptomatic. Symptoms** may include the following:
      (1) **Unusual vaginal discharge.**
      (2) **Cramping or pain.**
      (3) **Spotting.**
      (4) **Dyspareunia.**
      (5) **Lengthening of the IUD strings.**
      (6) **Feeling the plastic of the IUD.**
      (7) **Noting the passage of the IUD from the vagina.**
   b. **Replacement** of an IUD can be done in one office visit. **Preprocedural** antibiotic coverage, such as doxycycline 200 mg PO, may be used. Although a recent study showed no benefit to the use of prophylactic antibiotics in reducing pelvic infection rates in new IUD placements (18).
8. **Cramping and pain should not be accepted as normal consequences of IUD use. The possibility of ectopic pregnancy or infection must be carefully evaluated.** Increased menstrual cramping or intermittent cramping can occur, especially with larger IUDs.

F. **Special considerations**
   1. **Postcoital contraception.** Insertion of a copper IUD within 5 days after unprotected intercourse provides effective postcoital contraception. This approach to morning-after treatment is logical only for women who wish to continue using the IUD as a method of contraception and who have **no contraindications.**
      a. It is contraindicated in nulliparas, adolescents, and rape victims.
      b. All of the previously discussed contraindications and risk factors must be considered (see section IV.B.).
      c. Effectiveness has been reported to be >99%.
      d. Newer, very effective, hormonal methods of postcoital or emergency contraception (EC) have been approved for safe and effective use by the FDA. These approaches make IUD insertion for this indication less attractive. (See section IX.)
      e. The IUD may be an ideal method for the **perimenopausal patient** who has completed her family and does not want to risk another pregnancy.

G. Clinical dilemmas. Most of the problems arising with an IUD in place can be mimicked by pregnancy. Therefore, **always consider pregnancy.**

 1. Infection, especially PID, can occur in users of IUDs and may develop serious sequelae.
    a. Be sure that the patient does not have an ectopic pregnancy.
    b. Any patient with a suspicion of PID should be treated immediately and probably hospitalized.
    c. Frank PID must treated with antibiotics.
    d. After the first dose is given, the IUD should then be removed.
    e. An ultrasound should be obtained, if an abscess cannot be ruled out on clinical examination.
    f. If the infection seems to be limited to the cervix (i.e., cervicitis, asymptomatic positive *Chlamydia* or gonorrhea culture), it can be treated without removing the IUD and with very **close follow-up.**
    g. Following an episode of PID, a woman should wait at least 3 months (preferably 1 year) for insertion of another IUD.
    h. If future fertility is a goal, then should be avoided.
 2. **Uterine or cervical perforation.**
    a. **When partial cervical perforation occurs,** the IUD can usually be removed by using alligator forceps to push the device back into the uterine cavity and then removing the IUD by grasping it with forceps or pulling gently on the string.
    b. **In a nonpregnant woman,** an IUD located outside the uterus **(intraperitoneal)** usually can be removed through a laparoscope.
 3. **Management of pregnancy.** Obtain a serum pregnancy test to exclude ectopic or intrauterine pregnancy for any IUD user who has missed one or more periods. If **pregnancy is intrauterine, the IUD should be removed** because of the high risk (50%) of spontaneous abortion and, often, of associated infections. **IUD removal reduces but does not eliminate the possibility of miscarriage.**
    a. **If the strings cannot be seen or located** in the cervical os, IUD removal cannot be attempted and therapeutic abortion should be considered.
    b. If a woman decides to **continue a pregnancy with an IUD in place,** she should be warned about the **50% risk** of spontaneous abortion and should be educated about signs of infection.
    c. **Ectopic pregnancy** should **always** be considered and **ruled out** by ultrasound or D & C, if appropriate.
    d. Most of the IUD-associated deaths have been the result of rapidly progressive infection with incomplete spontaneous abortion.
 4. **Management of lengthening string.**
    a. When an IUD is partially expelled, in many cases the string descends through the cervix and appears longer. The possibility of **expulsion must be excluded before other causes are considered. Pelvic sonography and examination of the endocervical canal with a sterile swab can assist in this determination.**
    b. The string can also lengthen if, after insertion, part of the string remained in the uterine cavity and the clinician cut the string based on the segment visible in the canal.
 5. **Indications for IUD removal.**
    a. **Pregnancy, pelvic infection, and partial expulsion are indications for immediate IUD removal.**
    b. Removal is also indicated when **persistent pain** is a problem, **excessive bleeding** causes a drop of 5% or more in hematocrit, or the patient requests removal.
    c. An IUD **can be removed at any time in the menstrual cycle.** If the patient has had midcycle intercourse and the IUD is removed immediately thereafter, there may be some **reduction in IUD efficacy for that cycle.**

V. Barrier methods. Although possibly more cumbersome than the methods already discussed, barrier methods, specifically condoms, have assumed new importance in this age of the potentially life-threatening STD—HIV—as well as other problematic STDs such as hepatitis B, HPV (human papillomavirus), HSV (herpes simplex virus), *Chlamydia,* and gonorrhea. It is important to explain to sexually active couples that prevention **does require** different or supplementary measures in conjunction with pregnancy prevention.

  A. Diaphragm. The diaphragm acts as a barrier and serves as a receptacle to hold **spermicide** against the cervical os. Diaphragms are ineffective unless used with spermicide. **Failure rates** are related to the motivation of the patient and range from **6% to 18%.** There are several types of diaphragms and familiarity with them will help the practitioner recommend the appropriate one to the patient.

  1. **Types of diaphragms.** Each diaphragm is available in size increments of 5 mm.
    a. **Arcing-spring rim.** This diaphragm provides the **sturdiest of spring strengths;** the rim arcs can be folded, thus facilitating insertion for some women. Available sizes range from 55 to 95 mm.
      (1) Two arcing-spring products, Koro-Flex and Bendex, **fold at only two points** along the rim.
      (2) The Ortho product, All-Flex, **folds at any point,** although it is less sturdy than the other two.
    b. **Flat-spring rim.** This diaphragm has a thin rim, with gentle spring strength. The rim folds flat for insertion and is available in sizes 55 to 95. It is slightly harder than others to place correctly, but comfortable once placed behind the pubic bone.
    c. **Coil-spring rim.** The coil-spring diaphragm has firm spring strength and is available in sizes 50 to 95. It folds flat for insertion and can also be used with an introducer.
    d. **Wide-seal rim.** This diaphragm has an **arcing-spring or a coil-spring rim with an additional soft flange along the inner edge to create a seal with the vaginal mucosa.** It is available through Milex Products in sizes 65 to 85.
  2. **Contraindications and risk factors** include the following:
    a. **Allergy to latex or spermicide.**
    b. **Recurrent urinary tract infection.**
    c. **Introital or pelvic pain.**
    d. **Active lesions** that interfere with comfortable fitting or insertion.
    e. **History of toxic shock syndrome** (TSS) or **colonization with** *Staphylococcus aureus.*
    f. **Lack of medical staff to fit and instruct** adequately on diaphragm use.
    g. **Inability of the patient to master correct insertion or removal.**
    h. **Anatomic abnormalities.** Diminished vaginal muscle tone, previous obstetric laceration, uterine prolapse, cystocele, rectocele, extreme and fixed retroversion, vaginal fistula, and vaginal septum may make **diaphragm fitting or use impossible.**
    i. **Fitting may not be accurate for a woman who has had a full-term delivery in the past 6 weeks.**
  3. **How to determine correct size and fit.** Select the **largest rim size that is comfortable** for the user. Since **vaginal depth increases during sexual arousal, a diaphragm that is too small may slip out of place.** On the other hand, a diaphragm that is too **large** may **cause discomfort** or **recurrent** urinary infection.
    a. The anterior **rim should tuck just behind the symphysis pubis and the posterior portion of the rim resides snugly in the posterior vaginal fornix.**

    b. The **diaphragms** or **rings used** for fitting should be **washed with soap and water and then immersed in a 70% alcohol solution for 20 minutes** after each use.

    c. Many clinicians rely primarily on the arcing-**spring diaphragm** since it **fits most women and is easy to insert.** The arcing-spring diaphragm is also useful for a woman with a long and firm cervix.

    d. The **coil-spring or flat-spring diaphragm** may provide a comfortable fit for a woman who has firm vaginal tone, who finds the arcing spring uncomfortable, or who has had problems with recurrent urinary infections.

4. Instructions.

    a. Clinicians.

        (1) Be sure each user is **able to insert and remove her diaphragm** and **can verify correct position** by palpating her cervix.

            (a) Have her practice placement and removal while in the office.

            (b) Ensure that she is comfortable with the method and answer any questions.

        (2) The **importance of spermicide and consistent use** should be stressed. Spermicide must be used with initial coitus and **replenished with subsequent acts without removal of the diaphragm.**

        (3) Each patient should also be aware that TSS could occur with diaphragm use if not removed within 24 hours.

    b. Patients.

        (1) **Apply 1 tablespoon of spermicide cream or gel** to the inner dome of the diaphragm and along the rim.

        (2) If the diaphragm is placed in the vagina **more than 6 hours before intercourse, another applicator** full of spermicide should be inserted.

        (3) **Insert the diaphragm by pushing the rim downward and toward the back wall of the vagina.** The rim should fit just behind the pubic bone and should reach back behind the cervix.

        (4) Always check to make certain the diaphragm is covering the cervix.

        (5) **Leave the diaphragm in place for at least 6 hours after intercourse.** If you have **intercourse again** during the 6-hour time, **insert an applicator full of spermicide, but do not remove the diaphragm.**

        (6) **Remove the diaphragm any time after 6 hours, wash it with soap and water, and let it dry.** It can then be reinserted with new spermicide or stored in its case until again needed.

        (7) **Avoid leaving the diaphragm in place any longer than 24 hours,** but **do** keep to the 6-hour minimum time.

        (8) **Do not use talcum or perfumed powder or any petroleum products** (e.g., Vaseline) on your diaphragm.

        (9) If you experience danger signs of possible **TSS** while using the diaphragm, contact your clinician immediately. The danger signs are:

            (a) **Fever of 100°F or more.**

            (b) **Diarrhea and vomiting.**

            (c) **Muscle aches.**

            (d) **Rash** (like sunburn).

    c. Diaphragm size should be **reassessed** after **childbirth,** or when approximately **10%** of body **weight** is **gained** or lost.

    d. See Table 22.4 for rules of use with vaginal barrier methods.

Table 22.4. Vaginal barrier methods—rules for use

	Diaphragm	Cap	Sponge	Female condom
Pelvic exam required for fitting	Yes	Yes	No	No
Spermicide needed	Yes	Yes	Yes	No
Spermicide supplies needed for insertion	Yes	Yes	No	No
Additional spermicide needed for repeated intercourse	Yes	No	No	No
Supplies needed to add spermicide after initial insertion	Yes	No	No	No
Equipment needed for storage after use	Yes	Yes	No	No
Can be used during menses	Yes	No	No	Yes
Duration of protection after insertion	6 hours	48 hours	24 hours	8 hours
Longest wear recommended	24 hours	48 hours	30 hours	8 hours

5. **Sequelae.**
   a. **Side effects.** Overall, the **diaphragm** is a **very safe** method of contraception.
   (1) **TSS is the most serious potential problem, but is very rare.** A handful of TSS cases, however, have been reported in association with prolonged diaphragm placement. These cases did not arise during menses as is more typical for TSS. Any patient who experiences TSS danger signs must be evaluated promptly, which includes diaphragm removal, vaginal culture for *S. aureus,* and prompt antibiotic treatment when indicated.
   (2) **Other problems** that can occur with diaphragm use include
      (a) **See section on spermicides discussed in C, below.**
      (b) **Recurrent cystitis.**
         (i) The size of the diaphragm should be checked.
         (ii) If size is not the problem, the patient should be counseled to void prior to and after intercourse.
         (iii) In some cases an antibiotic may be given prophylactically [i.e., nitrofurantoin (Macrodantin), 50 mg PO, or sulfamethoxazole-trimethoprim (Bactrim or Septra), PO after coitus].

          (c) Allergic reactions to latex or spermicide. If the reaction is to the spermicide, try different brands. It may, in fact, be a reaction to perfume or other additives.

          (d) Irritation from spermicide.

          (e) Foul-smelling vaginal discharge when a diaphragm is left in place too long.

          (f) Recurrent candidiasis if the diaphragm is not thoroughly cleaned out and dried after use.

          (g) Pelvic discomfort from rim pressure.

          (h) Patient or **partner discomfort.** There are many ways this may manifest itself. There has to be a level of comfort in the relationship to incorporate the use of barrier methods. Furthermore, some patients may have physical discomfort with the diaphragm. If it is too small, the partner may notice it as well as it will move around in the vagina during coitus.

     b. Noncontraceptive benefits. Use of a diaphragm and spermicide may provide **significant protection against STDs.** Their use is associated with a **decreased risk of developing cervical dysplasia.**

B. Cervical cap. The soft, thimble-shaped cup **fits over the cervix and is held in place by suction.** Pregnancy is prevented through the cap's action as a barrier over the cervix and by its ability to hold spermicide in place. The reported failure rate is similar to that of the diaphragm. Manufactured and long used in England, the Prentif cap was approved by the FDA for use in the United States in 1988.

   1. The **cervical cap** has a deep dome with a groove inside the firm rim to aid suction and it is available in four sizes, ranging from 22- to 31-mm internal rim diameter.

   2. Contraindications and risk factors are the same as for the diaphragm (see section V.A.2.), with the following **exceptions:**

     a. Cap use is **contraindicated** for a **woman** who has **Pap** smear evidence of **HPV infection, cervical intraepithelial neoplasia,** or **cervical dysplasia.**

     b. Cap use should **not** be **initiated** if the woman has **acute PID, acute cervicitis,** or **vaginal infection** or has **undergone cervical biopsy** or **cryosurgery within** the past 6 to 12 weeks.

     c. The cap should **not be used** during the **first 6 weeks after full-term delivery,** when **vaginal bleeding** is **occurring** after spontaneous or induced **abortion,** or during normal **menses.**

   3. How to determine correct size and fit. Because of variations in normal anatomy and the limited number of cap sizes available, **it is not possible to fit every patient satisfactorily.** Only about 50% of women can use this method successfully.

     a. The cap must fit snugly over the cervix and remains by suction.

     b. The cap dome should be deep enough so that it does not rest on the cervical os.

     c. The cap should not be easily dislodged with a fingertip.

     d. The cap user should check carefully for cap dislodgment after intercourse.

   4. Instructions are the **same** as for the **diaphragm** (see section V.A.4.), with the **following exceptions:**

     a. Spermicide is not necessary. If used, it should fill the dome of the cap one third full. Using spermicide may prolong the wearing time.

     b. The cap should be left in place at least 6 hours after intercourse but can be in for up to 36 hours.

   5. Sequelae.

     a. Little is documented concerning possible side effects or complications of the cervical cap.

(1) Reports have noted **vaginal lacerations** and **abrasions** caused by the Vimule cap (not currently available in the United States) and **abnormal thickening of the vaginal mucosa,** possibly a reaction to chronic irritation (2).

(2) Other researchers have expressed concerns about **pelvic infection,** acute **cervicitis,** and **abnormal Pap smears** possibly linked to cap use.

  b. **Failures** occur when the **cap** is **dislodged during intercourse.**

  c. Any **noncontraceptive benefits are likely to be similar to those afforded by diaphragm use** (see section V.A.5.b.).

C. **Spermicides and the contraceptive sponge.** Spermicidal contraceptives consist of **two components:** an **inert substance,** such as foam, gel, cream, or in the case of the sponge **(currently unavailable),** polyurethane; and a **spermicidal agent (non-oxynol 9). Spermicides immobilize and kill sperm.** In addition, the sponge provides a barrier between the sperm and the cervical os and traps the sperm within the sponge. The typical failure rates are 21% to 28%.

  Although **contraceptive sponges have been discontinued,** they **may** again **become available. Spermicidal agents are often used in combination with condoms to provide an extremely effective method** of contraception, with a failure rate possibly lower than 1:100 woman-years. In the United States, the active spermicidal agent for products is non-oxynol 9. This is a surface-active substance that destroys cell membranes of sperm. Currently, controversy exists as to the practical effectiveness of non-oxynol 9 in destroying many organisms that cause STDs. **In the laboratory,** the chemical is lethal to organisms that cause gonorrhea, genital herpes, syphilis, trichomonas, and HIV. However, the evidence that non-oxynol 9 decreases STD risks (including HIV) in human studies has been mixed (16,19). There is even some concern that **frequent** non-oxynol 9 use can irritate the mucosa of the vagina and skin of the vulva, possibly increasing susceptibility to HIV. Also, cystitis (discussed later) may be increased by non-oxynol 9 use, which allows for intravaginal proliferation of *Eschericia coli,* which is a frequent cause of cystitis (5).

  1. **Type of spermicidal method.** All methods are available **without prescription.**

    a. **Foam.** Used alone, there is a wide disparity between perfect-use effectiveness and actual-use effectiveness. **Common mistakes** include inconsistent or **careless use,** using **too little foam, failing to shake the container** vigorously enough, **not placing** the **foam high enough** in the vagina, and **douching too soon after intercourse.**

    b. **Cream and gel.** When **used alone, these are slightly less effective** than other spermicides. **Cream products have better dispersion** to cover the cervix and vagina than do gels. Cream and gel are often used in conjunction with the diaphragm or cervical cap.

    c. **Suppositories and tablets** dissolve over a period of 10 to 30 minutes after placement in the vagina but **retain their full effectiveness for less than 1 hour.** Mistakes arise from not allowing the tablet or suppository to dissolve, failing to remove the wrapper, placing the spermicide incorrectly, or having intercourse after the fully effective interval.

    d. **Contraceptive sponge.** In the future, this method may again become available. The polyurethane sponge incorporates 1 g of nonoxynol-9. Approximately 200 mg of spermicide is released during the initial 24 hours of use. It has a concave dimple on one side that fits over the cervix and a woven loop to facilitate removal.

  2. **Contraindications and risk factors.**

    a. **Contraindications** to spermicide use **include allergy** to the active ingredient or base or **physical inability to insert or use** the product correctly.

      b. Additional contraindications specific to sponge use include:
        (1) Anatomic abnormalities such as uterine prolapse, rectocele, cystocele, extreme uterine retroflexion, or vaginal septum when they interfere with placement or retention of the sponge.
        (2) History of TSS or vaginal colonization with *S. aureus*.
      c. Prevention against STDs, HIV, and hepatitis B transmission is **less ensured** when these methods are used alone.
   3. Instructions. Different formulations of spermicides have different effective times. Most must be placed within 1 hour of intercourse. The length of time protection lasts varies from 1 to 8 hours.
      a. Correct use of a spermicide entails following package instructions carefully:
        (1) Removing the wrapper from tablets or suppositories.
        (2) Filling the applicator completely with foam, cream, or gel.
        (3) Placing the spermicide as close to the cervix as possible.
        (4) Applying additional spermicide for each act of intercourse.
        (5) Inserting the spermicide before intercourse.
        (6) Not douching for at least 6 hours after intercourse.
      b. The sponge.
        (1) Correct use requires moistening the sponge with clean water, placing it over the cervix, and leaving it in place for at least 8 hours after intercourse.
        (2) The sponge **should not be worn for longer than 24 hours.**
        (3) Each user should learn the **danger signs** of TSS and know how to contact her clinician if these signs occur. TSS symptoms include high fever, rash, diarrhea, vomiting, and muscle aches.
   4. Sequelae.
      a. Spermicides.
        (1) Possible complications of spermicide use include irritation, allergic reaction, and failure of suppository or tablet to melt or foam.
        (2) Noncontraceptive benefits include decreased incidence of gonorrhea and trichomoniasis, augmented vaginal lubrication, and possibly some protection against cervical neoplasia.
      b. Contraceptive sponge.
        (1) Sponge use involves the possible **complications of spermicide** listed in section V.C.4.a.(1).
        (2) Some users also experience **dryness of the vagina and difficulty with removal or tearing of the sponge.**
        (3) It is **not known whether or not sponge use increases the risk of TSS.**
        (4) Noncontraceptive benefits of the sponge include those listed for spermicides [see section V.C.4.a.(2)] as well as absorption of vaginal secretions and ejaculate.
   5. Clinical dilemma. When spermicide users experience an **allergic reaction,** the offending agent is often the perfume or base, although it may be the active spermicidal ingredient. **Recommend a nonperfumed spermicide.** Check the ingredients of the problem product and consider recommending one containing different ingredients.
D. Condoms. Mechanical **barriers to cover the penis** during intercourse have been used for hundreds of years. Synthetic condoms were developed after 1840. The popularity of condoms has made this the third most commonly used contraceptive method in the United States. Reported failure rates range from 2 to 12 pregnancies per 100 woman-years.
   1. Types of condoms.
      a. Most condoms are made of latex. About 1% are made from lamb cecum ("natural" skin condoms). Newer polyurethane (plastic) condoms are available and are also useful for those with latex allergy.

    b. Condoms are available **lubricated** or **nonlubricated, straight** or **tapered,** and **with or without reservoir tip.** Some condoms have **external ribbing.**

    c. **Latex and plastic** condoms **can prevent** transmission of all STDs, including the viral ones (HIV, HPV, HSV, hepatitis B), but **natural or lambskin do not prevent** transmission of viral STDs.

    d. When protection against transmission of HIV is a consideration, latex condoms in conjunction with spermicide use are recommended. Skin condoms (natural) are more porous than latex, and small particles such as HIV may traverse the intact condom barrier.

    e. See Table 22.5 and Table 22.6 for a consumer's guide to condoms.

Table 22.5. A sample of the variety of condoms available to the consumer. This table is not all-inclusive.

Manufacturer	Condom types				Features available[a]	Examples of brands
	Latex	Natural skin	Plastic			
			Male	Female		
Ansell Public Sector	X	—	—	—	a,b,c,d,e,g,i,j	Kiss of Mint, Lifestyles, Prime, Rough-Rider
Carter-Wallace, Inc.	X	X	—	—	a,b,c,f,h	Trojan, Trojan-Enz, Trogan Magnum, Class Act, *Naturalamb*
Durex Consumer Products	X	X	X	—	a,b,c,d,e,h	Avanti, Circle Cloin, *Fourex*, Ramses, Saxon, Sheik
Female Health Co.	—	—	—	X	a,e	Reality Female Condom
Mayer Laboratories	X	—	—	—	a,b,c,e,f,h	Kimono, MAXX, P.S., Sensation
Okamoto U.S.A., Inc.	X	—	—	—	a,b,c,e,h	Beyond Seven, Crown
Sagami, Inc.	X	—	—	—	a,b,e	Excalibur, Sagami Type E, Vis-à-vis

Note: Natural skin condoms are italicized; plastic condoms are underlined.

[a] Feature codes: a, lubricated; b, reservoir end; c, spermicidal lubricant; d, thick (>0.10 mm); e, thin (<0.05 mm); f, wide (>2.2 in.); g, narrow (<2.0 in.); h, long (>7.5 in.); i, short (<6.5 in.); j, scented.

From: Hatcher RA, et al. *Contraceptive technology,* 17TH ed. New York: Irvington, 1998:341, with permission.

Table 22.6. Resource guide for condoms available in the United States

Manufacturer name	Institutional sales phone number	Latex	Natural skin	Plastic Male	Plastic Female	Features available[a]	Examples of brands
Ansell Public Sector	1-800-327-8659 www.lifestyles.com	X				a, b, c, d, e, g, i, j	Kiss of Mint, Lifestyles, Prime, Rough-Rider
Carter-Wallace, Inc.	1-800-828-9032 www.trojancondoms.com	X	X			a, b, c, f, h	Trojan, Trojan-Enz, Trojan Magnum, Class Act, *Naturalamb*
Durex Consumer Products	1-888-266-3660 www.durex.com	X	X	X		a, b, c, d, e, h	Avanti, Circle Coin, *Fourex* Ramses, Saxon, Sheik
Female Health Company	1-800-274-6601				X	a, e	Reality female condom
Mayer Laboratories	1-800-426-6366 www.MayerLabs.com	X				a, b, c, e, f, h	Kimono, MAXX, P.S., Sensation
Okamoto U.S.A., Inc.	1-800-283-7546	X				a, b, c, e, h	Beyond Seven, Crown
Sagami Inc.	1-800-551-1888	X				a, b, e	Excalibur, Sagami Type E, Vis-à-vis

Note: Natural skin condoms are italicized; plastic condoms are underlined.
[a] Feature codes: a, lubricated; b, reservoir end; c, spermicidal lubricant; d, thick ($\geq$ .10 mm); e, thin ($\leq$ .05 mm); f, wide ($\geq$ 2.2 in.); g, narrow ($\leq$ 2.0 in.); h, long ($\geq$ 7.5 in.); i, short ($\leq$ 6.5 in.); j, scented.
From: U.S. Condom Manufacturers (1997), with permission.

    f. Female condoms are available. These are pouches of plastic that line the vagina and cover the cervix.

2. Contraindications and risk factors.

    a. Allergy to latex is a contraindication. Natural or plastic condoms can still be used.

    b. Some men report **difficulty maintaining an erection** when using condoms, although others find that condom use is helpful for this.

3. Instructions. A new condom must be used for every act of intercourse and placed on the penis before any vaginal entry.

    a. Patients should be instructed to place the condom on the erect penis before the penis touches the partner.

    b. The end of the condom should extend beyond the tip of the penis and air should be removed to form a small receptacle.

    c. Lubricants should be water-based only. Oil-based lubricants can **weaken** the condom.

    d. After intercourse, the penis should be withdrawn while it is still erect, taking care to keep the bottom of the condom from coming off the base of the penis.

    e. Jewelry, fingernails, and sex toys may tear the condom.

    f. Average breaking rates for latex condoms are 1% to 2% and are **greater for plastic,** up to 7%. If breakage occurs, concomitant use of spermicides substantially decreases the risk of pregnancy.

    g. Condoms should be **stored** in a cool, dry place and should **not** be reused.

    h. Petroleum jelly can cause a condom to deteriorate.

    i. Couples using condoms need to know about morning-after hormonal treatment.

4. Sequelae.

    a. Complications.

        (1) The condom may **reduce sensitivity** of the glans penis. In some cases, use of the natural skin condoms may help.

        (2) Some users **object to interruption in lovemaking** to place the condom on the penis.

        (3) Very rarely, an **allergic reaction** to latex or lubricant can occur.

    b. Noncontraceptive benefits. Condom use is **one of the few opportunities for men to play an active role in contraception.**

        (1) Condoms greatly **reduce the transmission of STDs, hepatitis B,** and **HIV** and **diminish the likelihood of cervical cancer.**

        (2) Condoms may also be of **help in treatment of premature ejaculation** and in **preventing exposure to ejaculate** for a woman who is allergic to her partner's semen or develops antibodies that cause infertility.

VI. Fertility awareness is also called natural family planning. The various methods include **rhythm, basal body temperature (BBT), Billings** (mucus) **method,** and the **symptothermal methods.** All these methods require periodic abstinence with unsafe days determined by physiologic changes that occur during a woman's menstrual cycle. Women who are well educated concerning their cyclic changes, have regular menses, are disciplined, and are willing to cope with possible pregnancy may have good success with fertility awareness. Some users choose to monitor several cyclic changes or combine fertility awareness with alternative contraceptive methods or both.

    Failure rates range from 2% to 35%, depending on the method used and on whether alternative birth control was employed. Best success is reported for couples who abstain throughout the preovulatory phase and do not have intercourse until the fourth day after ovulation is clearly documented. **Most failures occur because of intercourse during "early safe" days,** when ovulation occurs a few days earlier than anticipated. **Temperature and mucus changes do not predict ovulation accurately enough to avoid this problem.**

VII. Sterilization is the **most commonly used method of birth control** in the United States. The pregnancy rates are 0.2 to 0.4 for tubal ligation and 0.15 for vasectomy per 100 woman-years. For the purpose of decision making about sterilization, these procedures **should be considered irreversible.**

A. Types of sterilization

1. Vasectomy.

a. This operation for men is a **simple and safe procedure that prevents sperm passage by blocking the vas deferens.** The clinician can ligate the vas deferens through a **small incision of the scrotum.**

b. Reversal is moderately successful. Depending on the type of vasectomy performed and the time interval to vasovasostomy, vasectomy reversal procedures can result in clinical success up to 50% of the time. Success diminishes if the vasectomy was performed over 10 years ago.

2. Tubal ligation. The fallopian tube can be blocked by **ligation, coagulation,** or **mechanical occlusion** with clips, bands, or rings. Tubal reanastomosis is generally less successful than is vasovasostomy and will be recommended only if a substantial portion of undamaged fallopian tube is available for repair. Reversal rates as high as 50%, however, have been reported for reanastomosis after clip ligation or surgical ligation with minimal damage. This rate is much lower when electrocautery has been used. The types of tubal ligation include the following:

a. Abdominal approach. More than 100 variations of abdominal tubal ligation have been developed. Two of the most commonly used methods are laparoscopy and minilaparotomy. Both procedures can be performed under local or general anesthesia.

(1) For **laparoscopy,** one or two 1-in. incisions may be required, one for the laparoscope and one through which the tubes are grasped with forceps for coagulation or clip applications.

(2) For **minilaparotomy,** a 2- to 3-cm incision approximately 3 cm above the symphysis pubis allows the surgeon to grasp the fallopian tube for ligation. Minilaparotomy is **most feasible for patients with minimal abdominal wall fat.**

b. Vaginal approach. The fallopian tubes can be approached by **vaginal culdotomy or rarely by culdoscopy.** Because of **high complication rates,** the advantages of an unobtrusive scar and rapid recovery are less attractive.

3. Hysterectomy. At one time, hysterectomy was the most common method of sterilization. This approach may be considered for women who are likely to require later hysterectomy because of known gynecologic disease but **should not be a routine recommendation.** Hysterectomy mortality is 10 to 100 times higher than that of tubal ligation, and the **associated morbidity as well as cost in money and time is much greater.**

B. Contraindications and risk factors

1. Ambivalence is a strict contraindication. Only a patient who wishes to **terminate fertility** should undergo sterilization. In reaching a decision, the possible impact of divorce or family tragedy should be considered. Remarriage is the most common reason cited for requesting reversal.

2. A patient who is **obese,** has **cardiovascular disease,** or has a **serious medical condition** that might increase anesthesia or surgery risks should be encouraged to consider **alternative methods** of fertility control.

C. Counseling. Every patient must understand that sterilization surgery is **not 100% effective** and that pregnancy can occur in rare cases. Because of the permanent and completely elective nature of sterilization surgery, **informed choice and informed consent are crucial.** The mnemonic **BRAIDED** has been developed for the essential components of informed consent counseling.

Benefits: It is effective and convenient.

Risk: Risk of method including consequences of method failure.

Alternatives: The patient must be informed about possible alternatives, including advantages and disadvantages of each.

Inquiries: Any questions the patient may have should be answered fully by the clinician.

Decision: The patient must feel free to decide against the proposed method, without implied pressure or coercion.

Explanation: The procedure planned must be explained in specific detail.

Documentation: Information provided to the patient should be entered in the medical record, along with a written consent form signed by the patient.

D. **Sequelae**

1. **Male sterilization.**
    a. Vasectomy is a **very safe procedure.** Complications are generally minor and short term. Swelling, discoloration, and discomfort are common during the first few days after surgery.
        (1) More **significant,** but **uncommon, complications** are **hematoma, granuloma, epididymitis,** and **wound infection.**
        (2) One half to two thirds of men **develop sperm antibodies after vasectomy,** but the possible significance of this is unknown.
    b. Approximately **0.4%** of **vasectomy procedures fail to terminate fertility.** In most cases, failure is evident within a few weeks, as postoperative semen shows continuing sperm release.
        (1) Sperm counts should be obtained after 20 ejaculations **and** a repeat sperm count done at 2 months.
        (2) Approximately 10% will need to repeat the sperm count 1 to 2 months later to ensure that the count has decreased.
        (3) It is recommended that all men have a repeat sperm count 6 months after the vasectomy.
        (4) A backup method of contraception should be used until the semen no longer shows sperm release.

2. **Female sterilization.** Tubal ligation is also extremely safe. The greatest risk is in the type of anesthesia used with general anesthesia having the highest risk.
    a. **Complications of tubal ligation** could involve damage to one or both ovaries or to the ovarian blood supply, and this could **cause menstrual disturbance or a change in the hormonal milieu.** Whether such problems can be linked to uncomplicated tubal ligation, however, has been an issue of controversy. Long-term follow-up in large case-control studies have found **menstrual disturbances equally as frequent among controls as among sterilization cases.**
        (1) Complications occur in fewer than 2% to 3% of women undergoing minilaparotomy and include infection, hematoma, uterine perforation, and bladder injury.
        (2) **Complications** are also **rare** with **laparoscopy.** The procedure can cause mesosalpingeal tear, bowel burn, uterine perforation, or hemorrhage.
        (3) **Vaginal tubal ligation** complication rates are approximately twice as high as those for laparoscopy or minilaparotomy, with infection and hemorrhage accounting for most of the problems.
    b. **Tubal ligation failure rates depend on the specific surgical method used.**
        (1) Following laparoscopy, approximately 0.25% of patients experience failure. Ectopic pregnancy and pregnancy already established at the time of the surgery are the most common.
        (2) Postpartum tubal ligation, sterilization at the time of caesarean section delivery, and abdominal ligation by the Pomeroy method have somewhat **higher failure rates.**

VIII. Abortion. Approximately 1.6 million abortions are performed annually in the United States; more than 90% are performed early in **pregnancy using vacuum aspiration.** Although the **complication rate for abortion is as low as, or lower than, any other method of fertility control,** very few women choose it as a primary fertility control method. Patient acceptance of effective contraception is extremely high at the time of unintended pregnancy, so birth control information and supplies are an important part of clinical management. Early identification and confirmation of pregnancy are also crucial tasks for all family-planning clinicians.

With the marked increase in ectopic pregnancy rate, early pregnancy identification can be lifesaving. Early confirmation also permits optimal initiation of prenatal precautions and care and early termination if abortion is the patient's decision. Abortion risks are lowest at approximately 7 to 8 weeks gestation and double for every 2-week delay thereafter. See Chapter 24 for more in-depth discussion.

IX. Postcoital or EC has been mentioned in other sections. Practitioners need to be more aware of this option and feel comfortable using it. Patients need to be counseled that it is available as a backup if one of the foregoing methods is not used correctly (i.e., a failed condom). EC **prevents** ≈ 75% of expected pregnancies, probably closer to 95% when used within 24 hours of intercourse. In a recent review article about EC, Glasier thoroughly discusses the mode of action of these hormonal techniques and states, "The prevention of pregnancy before implantation is contraception and **not** abortion") (12). There is considerable current advocacy to make EC available without prescription in the United States. Evidence exists that this approach could reduce the unwanted pregnancy rate without risk to the users (17). There are two methods of postcoital contraception, **hormonal** and the **IUD.**

   A. There are **two main hormonal** approaches to EC using either combination estrogen and progestin OCPs or progestin-only contraceptive pills. Together these are referred to as emergency contraceptive pills (ECPs). In 1997 the FDA declared the **combination method of ECP use both safe and effective** for use in pregnancy prevention. Previously studied, but not currently used, methods include danazol (an antigonadotropin) and high-dose estrogen-only regimens. It may be that antiprogesterone, mifepristone (RU-486), will be used for postcoital contraception. Effective contraception must be used within 72 hours of unprotected sex.

   1. Combination estrogen and progestin methods include a large number of easily available formulations.

   a. In **all cases two doses** are **required,** the first within 72 hours of intercourse, the second 12 hours after the first dose.

   b. All use **ethinyl estradiol 100 to 120 mcg and levonorgestrel 0.50 to 0.60 mg per dose.** This is convenient because many conventional OCPs contain appropriate dosages of these hormones when taken in multiples.

   c. For example, Ovral contains 50 mcg ethinyl estradiol **and** 0.25 mg levonorgestrel. Thus, taking **two** Ovral pills 12 hours apart provides the correct dose of ECPs.

   d. Similarly, Lo/Ovral contains 30 mcg ethinyl estradiol **and** 0.15 mg levonorgestrel. Thus, **four** Lo/Ovral pills per each dose provides the correct dose.

   e. One commercially available product, Preven, contains four tablets each containing 50 mcg of ethinyl estradiol **and** 0.25 mg levonorgestrel.

   2. Progestin-only method. Currently, only one such method is commercially available; "Plan B," which contains a single pill containing 0.75 mg of levonorgestrel, is taken within 72 hours of intercourse. This method was shown in a large multinational trial to be as effective as the combination estrogen and progestin regimen and may be preferred because of its **low incidence of nausea and ease of single dosing.**

3. The most common side effect of ECPs is nausea. Using combination pills, the incidence of nausea is 30% to 50% and approximately 20% have emesis. These rates drop by more than half with the progestin-only method. If vomiting does occur within 3 hours of either dose, some feel it should be repeated with an antiemetic.

4. Although the ECPs may slightly alter the expected menstrual interval, patients should expect to see their menses by 21 days after treatment. If the pregnancy ensues, the patient should be counseled appropriately concerning an undesired pregnancy. If she opts to continue the pregnancy, there is no evidence of teratogenic effects.

5. IUD placement within 5 days of conception can successfully prevent pregnancy with failure rates of less than 1%. The contraindications, side effects, and complications are discussed in section IV.B.

X. **Future possibilities** of safer, more reliable, and easily used contraception are limited by research financing. Some ideas that are currently under investigation include: Norplant II (two subdermal capsules), biodegradable capsules, injectable microspheres of progestins, IUDs with levonorgestrel for longer effectiveness, and progestin vaginal rings. The GnRH agonists may prove useful for male or female contraception.

References

1. Barrier methods. *Popul Rep* 1984;[H]:7.
2. Bernstein GS, et al. Studies of cervical caps: I. Vaginal lesions associated with use of the Vimule cap. *Contraception* 1982;26:443.
3. Division of Reproductive Health, Centers for Disease Control. Oral contraceptive use and the risk of endometrial cancer. *JAMA* 1983;249:1596.
4. Food and Drug Administration. *FDA Drug Bull* 1984;14:2.
5. Hatcher R, et al. *Contraceptive technology,* 17th rev ed. New York: Ardent Media, 1998:416.
6. Ory HW. The noncontraceptive health benefits from oral contraceptive use. *Fam Plann Perspect* 1982;14:182.
7. Pike MD, et al. Breast cancer in young women and use of oral contraceptives: possible modifying effect of formulation and age at use. *Lancet* 1983;2:926.
8. Vassey M, et al. Neoplasia of the cervix uteri and contraception: a possible adverse effect of the pill. *Lancet* 1983;2:930.
9. White MK, et al. Intrauterine device termination rates and the menstrual cycle day of insertion. *Obstet Gynecol* 1980;55:220.
10. Yuzpe A, Smith P, Rademaker AA. Multi-center clinical investigation employing ethinyl estradiol combined with DL norgestrel as a post-coital contraceptive agent. *Fertil Steril* 1982;37:508.
11. Cox S, et al. *Contraception.* Monograph of the APGO Educational Series on Women's Health Issues. Feb. 1999.
12. Glasier A. Emergency postcoital contraception. *N Engl J Med* 1997;337;1058.
13. McCann M. Progestin-only oral contraception: a comprehensive review. *Contraception* 1994;[Suppl 50]:S1–S195.
14. Farmer RD, Lawrenson RA. Oral contraceptives and venous thromboembolic disease: the findings from database studies in the United Kingdom and Germany. *Am J Obstet Gynecol* 1998;179(3S)[Suppl]:78S–86S.
15. Rosenberg M, Waugh M. Oral contraceptive discontinuation: a prospective evaluation of frequency and reasons. *Am J Obstet Gynecol* 1998;179:577–582.
16. Roddy RE, et al. A controlled trial of nonoxynol 9 film to reduce male-to-female transmission of sexually transmitted diseases. *N Engl J Med* 1998;339:504–510.
17. Glasier A, Baird D. The effects of self-administering emergency contraception. *N Engl J Med* 1998;339:1–4.
18. Walsh T, et al. Randomised controlled trial of prophylactic antibiotics before insertion of intrauterine devices. *Lancet* 1998;351:1005–1008.
19. Cook R, Rosenberg M. Do spermicides containing nonoxynol-9 prevent sexually transmitted infections?: a meta-analysis. *Sex Transm Dis* 1998;25:144–150.

23. INFERTILITY

Michael J. Murray

Infertility affects approximately 15% of all couples. The number of people seeking medical attention for this problem appears to be on the rise in the United States (1). This trend is believed to be related to women postponing childbearing in lieu of career development, to readily available contraceptive methods, and to an awareness of advances in assisted reproductive technologies.

Infertility is defined as the inability to attain pregnancy after 1 year of regular, unprotected intercourse since 85% of couples will conceive within this timeframe. This definition should not preclude the earlier evaluation and counseling of a couple or woman wishing to start a family when there are obvious factors known to be associated with reproductive dysfunction such as oligomenorrhea, amenorrhea, tubal disease, endometriosis, uterine pathology, or for a woman 35 years of age or older.

A complete gynecologic and medical history combined with a focused physical examination will often elicit common causes of infertility and guide the evaluation. In addition, the initial consultation provides an opportunity for preconception counseling and instructions to optimize the chances for conception. Since **the incidence of male factor and female factor infertility are similar, the assessment of both partners should begin simultaneously** (Table 23.1).

An algorithm guideline for infertility evaluation including history, physical, investigative procedures, and treatment is provided in Fig. 23.1. The initial evaluation may consist of the history, physical examination, and investigative procedures being simultaneously ordered and performed.

I. **History.** Primary infertility refers to a patient who has never conceived; whereas, secondary infertility implies at least one previous pregnancy. Primary infertility potentially is more ominous than secondary infertility. The following items need to be included in the history and may suggest potential infertility problems.

   A. **Obstetrical.** Gravidity, parity, pregnancy outcomes, and complications, i.e., repeated spontaneous abortions (SABs), operative deliveries, TABS. How long was pregnancy attempted before conception occurred? Were fertility treatments necessary to conceive? Was the delivery spontaneous or operative?

   B. **Gynecologic.** Age at menarche, menstrual cycle length, duration of flow, severity of dysmenorrhea, contraceptive methods, previous pelvic infections, and abnormal Papanicolaou (Pap) smears and subsequent treatment may alert the clinician to an etiology of infertility.

   1. **Oligomenorrhea and amenorrhea:** Infrequent or absent menses signifies infrequent or absent ovulation. Women who **do not experience regular, cyclic menses** with typical **moliminal signs** (such as breast tenderness, abdominal bloating, and menstrual cramps) **often mistake** episodes of **anovulatory, dysfunctional uterine bleeding (DUB)** for a **menstrual period.**

   2. **Abnormal uterine bleeding** occurs during one of the four following circumstances (with decreasing frequency).

      a. **Pregnancy.**

      b. **Hormonal dysfunction** (e.g., DUB).

      c. **Anatomical.** History of problems such as intracavitary leiomyoma, endometrial polyp, endometritis, cervical lesion, cervicitis, or neoplasia may suggest an anatomical cause for infertility.

      d. **Bleeding dyscrasia** such as von Willebrand's factor deficiency.

This is a revision of the third edition chapter by Frederick W. Hanson.

Table 23.1. Causes of infertility

Factor	% of cases
Ovary factor	25%
Tubal and pelvic factor	25%
Uterine factor	<5%
Cervical factor	<5%
Male factor	30%
Unexplained infertility	15%

3. **Dysmenorrhea** that is worsening or begins just prior to the onset of menstrual bleeding raises the question of endometriosis.
4. **Hormonal contraceptive** methods such as Depo-Provera may prevent ovulation up to 18 months **after** the last dose. Discontinuation of oral contraceptive pills may result in some **delay** of normal menstrual cycles, but usually less than 3 months.
5. **Pelvic infections may** cause tubal disease (see section IV.).
6. **Abnormal Pap smears** are often treated with cryotherapy, a LEEP, or a cold knife cone biopsy. Each of these procedures has the **potential** to destroy cervical mucous glands and consequently impair fertility.

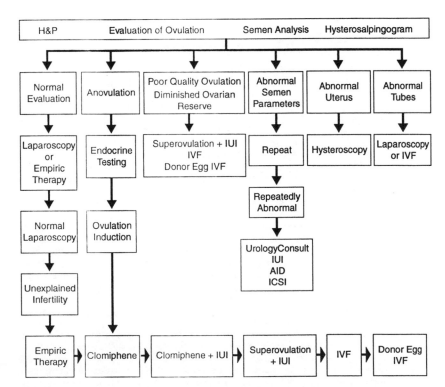

FIG. 23.1. Algorithm guideline for infertility evaluation.

  C. Sexual
    1. Timing is everything. It is reasonable to expect a couple to conceive after 1 year of unprotected intercourse if their **coital frequency averages at least twice per week.** However, if twice per week means only Fridays and Saturdays, this average may not hold true.
    2. Regular douching and most lubricants have a spermicidal effect.
    3. Deep dyspareunia can be a sign of pelvic pathology.
  D. Surgical. Previous abdominal or pelvic surgery often leads to pelvic adhesions, particularly after a ruptured appendix. A previous D & C with a perioperative pelvic infection increases the risk of acquiring **Asherman's syndrome** (intrauterine adhesions).
  E. Medical
    1. Patients with **endocrinologic disorders** (i.e., hypothyroidism, diabetes mellitus) may have concomitant **ovarian dysfunction.**
    2. Many **psychotropic medications** work by altering relative levels of central nervous system (CNS) neurotransmitters, which may interfere with CNS regulation of the hypothalamic-pituitary-ovarian axis and thus ovulatory function.
    3. Chronic disease, such as renal insufficiency, can cause reproductive dysfunction.
    4. A review of systems should focus on hirsutism, galactorrhea, symptoms of thyroid disease, and excessive weight gain or loss.
  F. Male. Factors pertinent in the male partner's history include:
    1. Any previous pregnancies that he has fathered.
    2. Pelvic surgery (such as vasectomy, vasovasotomy, herniorrhaphy, or orchiopexy).
    3. Exposure to environmental toxins including tobacco and excessive ethanol.
    4. Testicular trauma.
    5. History of sexually transmitted diseases.
II. Physical examination
  A. Female examination
    1. Height and weight. Women with a body mass index at either the lower or upper extremes often have ovulatory dysfunction.
    2. Skin. Hirsutism is a clinical indicator of relative hyperandrogenism. The combination of hirsutism and oligomenorrhea or amenorrhea essentially confirms the diagnosis of **polycystic ovary syndrome (PCOS). Acanthosis nigricans** is often a sign of hyperinsulinemia, which may cause or exacerbate chronic anovulation seen with PCOS.
    3. Thyroid. Thyroid enlargement or nodularity is a sign of thyroid disease, which is an uncommon, but easily treatable cause of ovulatory dysfunction.
    4. Abdomen and pelvis. A large pelvic mass may represent a leiomyomatous uterus, an ovarian neoplasm, or other pathology.
    5. Uterus, cervix, and vagina. Müllerian anomalies are found in approximately 0.1% of the general population, 1% of women with infertility, and 10% of women with recurrent pregnancy loss. Pelvic pain may indicate endometriosis or infection. Nodularity palpated in the posterior cul-de-sac is always abnormal and highly suggestive of endometriosis. Abnormalities of the cervix (and uterine cavity) may result from *in utero* exposure to diethylstilbestrol (DES), which was banned in the United States in 1971. A cervicitis may be the only sign of an occult infection higher in the reproductive tract.
    6. Adnexa. An adnexal mass or tenderness can be due to an endometrioma, hydrosalpinx, infection, or neoplasia.
  B. Male examination of the genitalia is usually not necessary unless the semen analysis is repeatedly abnormal. A urologist with expertise in male fertility usually performs the examination and the focus is on normal tes-

ticular volume and location, the presence of the vas deferens, and the absence of a varicocele (a varicose vein in the scrotum).

III. **Preconception counseling.** Patients preparing to start a family with or without infertility will benefit from brief preconception counseling.

    A. **Social history.** Primary smoking and second hand smoke both decrease the time until conception and have a negative impact on fetal outcome (2,3). Women who abuse alcohol or other drugs should be "clean and sober" prior to initiating fertility treatments.

    B. **Family history.** If the patient has a relative with a congenital anomaly or is from an ethnic group known to be at high risk for a specific inheritable disorder, genetic counseling and testing should be offered.

    C. **Advanced maternal age (AMA)** refers to all women who will deliver at or beyond the age of 35 years. Women of AMA should be informed that they are

        1. More likely to experience infertility.

        2. More likely to experience a SAB.

        3. At a higher risk of having a child with a birth defect due to a chromosomal abnormality.

        These three factors are attributed to the increase in oocyte aneuploidy that occurs with the aging ovary (Table 23.2).

    D. **Immunizations** should be updated as necessary.

    E. **Prenatal vitamins** or **folic acid** 400 mcg daily should be initiated prior to conception.

    F. **Medications** that the patient is currently taking should be scrutinized and, if possible, discontinued or switched to formulations that are safe in pregnancy.

    G. **Optimizing coital timing.** At the end of the initial visit couples can be instructed on how to use a urinary luteinizing hormone (uLH) surge predictor kit, commonly referred to as an ovulation predictor kit.

IV. **Ovary factor** infertility accounts for 25% of all causes of infertility for couples. Many women identified with ovary factor infertility will have PCOS. Other than pregnancy, proof of ovulation can only be ensured by recovery of the ovum outside of the ovary. Such proof requires surgery during ovulation and is impractical. Therefore indirect ovulation detection methods that provide presumptive evidence are accepted.

    A. **Ovulation detection methods**

        1. **Menstrual history** is often all that is required. A well-documented clinical diagnosis of oligomenorrhea or amenorrhea warrants therapy without further testing. Conversely, while clinical symptoms of ovulation such as **mittelschmerz** (midcycle discomfort associated with ovulation) and **moliminal** signs are reassuring, more objective data are necessary to confirm ovulation.

        2. **Basal body temperature (BBT)** charting is inexpensive and can be useful to retrospectively confirm regular ovulatory cycles as indicated by a sustained rise in temperature above baseline for at least 11 days. The rise in temperature coincides with increased circulating progesterone

Table 23.2. The effect of maternal age on reproduction

Maternal age	Infertility	Spontaneous abortion	Chromosomal abnormality
20	7%	7%	0.2%
25	9%	20%	0.2%
30	15%	21%	0.3%
35	22%	29%	0.5%
40	29%	60%	1.5%

Modified from references 4–7.

secreted from the corpus luteum. However, BBT charting has significant limitations because the temperature rise occurs 1 to 2 days **after** ovulation and some ovulatory women have monophasic BBT patterns (8).

3. **Serum progesterone** levels greater than $3^{ng}/_{mL}$ infer that ovulation has occurred (9). However, progesterone levels above $10^{ng}/_{mL}$ may be associated with greater reproductive potential (10). Because progesterone peaks during the midluteal phase, the best time to assay progesterone levels are 7 to 10 days after ovulation. The timing of the midluteal progesterone level should be based on objective data such as a BBT chart or an ovulation predictor kit and not arbitrarily assessed on cycle day 21 or 23. For example, a woman who has a 35-day menstrual cycle is likely to ovulate on cycle day 21 and her progesterone level on the day of ovulation will invariably be < $10^{ng}/_{mL}$. This only **suggests** that the patient received **poor instructions not** poor luteal phase function.

4. **Urinary luteinizing hormone** detection kits are the most cost-effective means to prospectively predict ovulation in spontaneously cycling women. These kits are available over the counter and are commonly known as **ovulation predictor kits.** Because the LH surge may only last 36 hours, it is important to **test at the same time each day.** Depending on the sensitivity and accuracy of a particular kit (not all ovulation predictor kits are created equal), detection of LH in the urine provides patients with a convenient signal of the day of and just prior to ovulation, which are the days that conception is most likely (11).

5. **Endometrial biopsy** has been used to confirm ovulation by looking for distinct histologic changes in the endometrium that occur only after the proper sequence of exposure to estradiol then progesterone (12). This test is relatively expensive and debate continues as to its relevancy in the evaluation and treatment of infertility patients (13).

6. **Serial ultrasound** measurements of ovarian follicle growth and collapse provide good presumptive evidence of ovulation (14) but this method is expensive, time-consuming, and rarely necessary.

B. **Quality of ovulation** and measurements of **fertility potential** have been created in an attempt to evaluate the effectiveness or probability of success with or without various treatment regimens. Although the only true measure of egg quality is the delivery of a healthy child, several indirect measures of ovarian function are often useful in counseling patients when they are considering treatment options. For example, if a preliminary test suggests that the probability of having a live birth is <5%, the patient may not want to spend $10,000 on fertility treatments for such poor odds of success.

1. **Serum progesterone** levels <$10^{ng}/_{mL}$, when appropriately timed (see section IV.A.3.), may indicate ovulatory dysfunction and warrant treatment with clomiphene (see section V.A.2.). When patients are receiving clomiphene citrate as treatment, progesterone levels >$15^{ng}/_{mL}$ are desirable (15). Serum progesterone levels can vary widely during the day and are worth repeating when low and timed appropriately.

2. **Day 3 follicle-stimulating hormone (FSH)** levels along with serum **estradiol** have been used to estimate fertility potential, also called **ovarian reserve.** (16). In simplistic terms, high FSH levels indicate that the brain is working harder in an attempt to stimulate egg production. An elevated day 3 FSH is a sign of **diminished ovarian reserve,** which suggests poor pregnancy rates for a woman with **any** form of fertility treatment that relies on the use of her own eggs. The actual level of FSH that is considered high depends mainly on the assay methodology. In laboratories that use an automated chemiluminescence system, an FSH >$10^{mIU}/_{mL}$ usually signifies diminished ovarian reserve. It should be noted that a **low FSH** level does **not imply** an increased likelihood of pregnancy. For example, a 40-year-old woman with a day 3 FSH of $4^{mIU}/_{mL}$ has the same low chances of pregnancy as any other 40-year-old woman.

3. **Clomiphene citrate challenge test (CCCT)** is an extension of the day 3 FSH level. Day 3 FSH and estradiol levels are obtained. Clomiphene citrate 100 mg is administered on cycle days 5 to 9 and the FSH level is repeated on day 10. The prognostic results are based upon the highest (worst) FSH value. The CCCT is felt to be more sensitive than a day 3 FSH since up to 40% women with a normal day 3 FSH will have an elevated day 10 FSH (17).

V. **Tubal and pelvic infertility factor** account for approximately 25% of all causes encountered in the evaluation of couples. Common etiologies of tubal and/or peritoneal disease are *Chlamydia trachomatis* or *Neisseria gonorrhoeae* salpingitis, PID, tuboovarian abscess (TOA), endometriosis, prior ectopic pregnancy, peritonitis (especially ruptured appendicitis), and surgery of the pelvis or abdomen.

A prognostic distinction is made between genital tract infections and adhesive disease originating in the peritoneal cavity. Postoperative adhesions are more likely to cause external blockage of the fallopian tubes that **often** can be entirely **corrected** by a careful surgeon.

However, PID can cause both external obstruction as well as destruction of the cilia and mucosal folds inside the tube, which are necessary for moving the fertilized egg (embryo) from the ampullary portion of the tube into the uterine cavity. When the intratubal cilia are damaged from an episode of salpingitis, the incidence of a tubal pregnancy significantly increases. Similarly, after the first, second, and third bout of PID, the incidence of infertility increases 12%, 25%, and 50%, respectively (18).

Several tests are available to evaluate tubal patency. Accurate diagnosis and effective treatment of tubal obstruction often requires more than one of the following techniques (19).

A. **Hysterosalpingogram (HSG).** HSG provides radiographic images of the uterus and fallopian tubes. The HSG is a 5- to 10-minute procedure using minimally invasive fluoroscopic procedure with little more than oral nonsteroidal antiinflammatory agents for analgesia. **The HSG is one of the preliminary tests necessary for virtually all patients.** Antibiotic prophylaxis should be administered when warranted (20).

B. **Laparoscopy** is an outpatient surgery that usually requires general anesthesia **and has the advantage over other diagnostic techniques in that treatment of abnormalities can be rendered at the time they are discovered.** Laparoscopy with **chromopertubation** (instillation of dilute blue dye through the fallopian tubes) is often necessary to further delineate abnormalities seen during HSG, detect **pelvic and adnexal adhesions** that may not be evident with HSG, and often is the only method to definitively diagnose **endometriosis** (see Chapter 16).

VI. **Uterine factors** are relatively uncommon causes of infertility and are more often associated with **recurrent early pregnancy loss** (see section II.A.5.). Congenital uterine factors include müllerian anomalies (e.g., uterine septum) and a small, T-shaped uterine cavity associated with *in utero* DES exposure. Acquired uterine lesions that may reduce fertility include intracavitary leiomyomas (21), endometrial polyps, and Asherman's syndrome. Several methods are available to evaluate the uterine cavity.

C. **HSG** (see section V.A.).

D. **Sonohysterography** combines transvaginal sonography during the instillation of sterile saline into the uterine cavity. This method effectively detects uterine pathology but rarely provides information regarding tubal status.

E. **Hysteroscopy** is regarded as the definitive method to evaluate the uterine cavity and can be performed in the office setting or at the time laparoscopy is planned. Hysteroscopy is often necessary to delineate abnormalities seen with HSG and when intrauterine abnormalities are found, it is the preferred method of treatment.

VII. Cervical factors are rarely identified as the sole or principal cause of infertility (19). A cervical factor is believed to be present when the cervical mucus does not become thin and watery in the periovulatory interval and/or when sperm cannot pass through the cervix into the uterus and tubes. The most agreed upon **treatment** for cervical factor infertility is intrauterine insemination (IUI), which bypasses the cervix (see section X.C.1.). In the contemporary treatment of infertility, IUI is quickly added to the therapeutic regimen for other reasons such as suspected male factor infertility or empirically for unexplained infertility. Therefore many infertility specialists omit the methods discussed later that evaluate cervical mucus-sperm interaction. If cervicitis is detected upon speculum examination, therapy is warranted.

Postcoital testing (PCT) involves sampling the cervical mucous several hours after coitus during or immediately prior to ovulation. A PCT is declared normal when 5 to 10 progressively motile sperm are seen per high-power microscopic field. However, PCT is considered to lack validity (22) and does not effect pregnancy rates (23).

VIII. Male infertility factor accounts for **30%** or more of **all causes** encountered in the evaluation of couples. Therefore **evaluation of the male partner should begin at the same time as the female partner.** Invasive or expensive diagnostic procedures or therapies for female infertility should **not** be pursued until the male has been evaluated. It is common for couples to have **both** male and female factors contributing to their subfertility.

A. **Semen analysis (SA) is absolutely necessary for the evaluation of all couples.** If the SA is normal then testing for male factor infertility is usually considered complete. The ejaculate should be collected via masturbation into a sterile specimen cup after 2 to 5 days of abstinence, kept near body temperature, and examined by an experienced andrologist **within an hour** after collection. Normal parameters for the SA are as follows (24):
   Volume: >2.0 mL.
   Sperm concentration: >20 million/mL.
   Motility: >50% with forward progression.
   Morphology: >30% normal forms.
   White blood cells: = 14% normal forms (Tygerberg/Kruger strict criteria) <1 million/mL.
   Other semen parameters are often evaluated such as viscosity and sperm agglutination, which if consistently abnormal are an indication for further evaluation or treatment. Every man is permitted a bad sperm day.
   If the initial SA has abnormal parameters, it should be repeated. Since sperm production requires approximately 74 days, events negatively impacting the SA such as fever or trauma may not be evident until weeks later. Consequently, the repeat semen analysis should be postponed for 2½ months. Male factor subinfertility is **seldom diagnosed** on the basis of **one** SA, whereas values for sperm concentration, motility and morphology can be used to classify men as subfertile. None of these parameters are diagnostic of absolute infertility (26).

B. **Antisperm antibodies (ASAb)** bound to sperm in a man's ejaculate can prevent sperm from migrating up the female genital tract or penetrating an oocyte. ASAb are suggested when there is a significant amount of sperm agglutination seen on SA. ASAb are common **after vasectomy reversal** (27). The treatments range from attempting to suppress the male immune system prior to the female partner's ovulation usually combined with IUI, to *in vitro* fertilization and intracytoplasmic sperm injection (IVF/ICSI) (see section IX.C.).

C. **Urologic evaluation** by a urologist that specializes in male infertility is warranted when two, or ideally three, SA results are abnormal. Although most causes of male factor infertility are idiopathic, there are several known conditions that are worth ruling out.
   1. A **varicocele** (varicose vein in the scrotum) will often produce SA parameters that are all somewhat low. Diagnosis of a varicocele is usually

made by genital examination. A small varicocele discovered only by ultrasound is of doubtful significance. Surgical ligation of a large varicocele improves male factor infertility in about 40% of cases and probably improves pregnancy rates (28).

2. Other known causes of male infertility less commonly seen include:
   a. Congenital bilateral absence of the vas deferens, usually with cystic fibrosis, presenting as **azospermia (no sperm in the ejaculate).**
   b. Klinefelter's, Kartagener's, or Kallman's syndrome.
   c. Secondary hypothalamic-pituitary insufficiency from surgery or brain tumors.
   d. Infections such as mumps orchitis or prostatitis.
   e. Testicular failure.
   f. Damage from previous genital surgery.
   g. Chemotherapy.
   h. Excessive alcohol, tobacco, or drug use.
   i. Exposure to some environmental toxins.
   j. Mechanical trauma from long-distance cycling can decrease sperm motility, however, other forms of endurance exercise do not seem to impair SA parameters (29).

   Although there is a widely held belief that boxer shorts can improve fertility, wearing polyester briefs, which increase scrotal temperature, seem to have little impact on SA parameters (30).

IX. **Unexplained infertility** accounts for **15%** of **all causes** encountered in the evaluation of couples. The diagnosis is made **after** all male and female testing, including laparoscopy, has been completed. The typical approach for the treatment of unexplained infertility follows a progression of empiric therapies with progressively higher success rates and costs (Table 23.3).

X. **Treatment** is targeted at the underlying identified etiology. More aggressive therapies are pursued when less expensive, less invasive, and less risky options fail to cause pregnancy after 3 to 4 cycles. A couple's decision to pursue more therapy is based on **time** (how long is the history of infertility and how old is the female partner); **emotion** (how aggressive or risky do they want to be and what is their level of frustration); and **finances** (what does their insurance carrier cover, if anything, because IVF is cost prohibitive for many couples).

   A. **Ovulation induction** is indicated for women with oligomenorrhea or anovulation. The primary cause of anovulation dictates the proper pharmacologic agent.
      1. Anovulation caused by hyperprolactinemia, severe hypothyroidism, or hyperinsulinemia may be treated with bromocriptine, levothyroxine, or metformin, respectively (31).
      2. **Clomiphene citrate** (Clomid, Serophene) is used to treat oligomenorrheic or anovulatory women, most commonly resulting from **PCOS.**

Table 23.3. Empiric therapy for unexplained infertility (maternal age < 35 years)

Therapy	Approximate pregnancy rate/cycle	Approximate cost/cycle
Observation	4%	$0
IUI	5%	$350
Clomiphene	7%	$20
Clomiphene + IUI	9%	$370
Superovulation + IUI	18%	$ 2,000
IVF	40–50%	$12,000

IUI, intrauterine insemination; IVF, *in vitro* fertilization.

Clomiphene is often prescribed to couples as empiric therapy to increase the odds of pregnancy, theoretically by improving the "quality" of ovulation and/or correcting any subtle causes of ovulatory dysfunction.

a. Clomiphene is a selective estrogen receptor modulator that primarily works through the hypothalamus to increase pituitary secretion of FSH that in turn stimulates ovulation.

b. The typical starting dose is 50 mg on cycle days 5 to 9. Ovulation may occur anywhere between cycle days 12 to 20 (usually day 16 or 17). Patients are encouraged to use an uLH kit starting on cycle day 12 to optimally time coitus or insemination. If ovulation does not occur by cycle day 20 **and the patient is using the uLH kit properly** (see section IV.A.4.), she can be administered a progestational agent to induce a withdrawal bleed. The process is then restarted by increasing the clomiphene dose by 50 mg. An ovulatory ultrasound or a serum midluteal progesterone level is often helpful to confirm adequate ovulation during the first cycle. In general a patient's response to clomiphene will be consistent from cycle to cycle.

c. If a woman does not ovulate with clomiphene 150 mg on cycle days 5 to 9, this agent is unlikely to induce ovulation and other options should be considered. However, some women will ovulate on doses of clomiphene up to 250 mg. **If pregnancy does not occur by sixth ovulatory cycle with clomiphene, an alternative therapy should be pursued.**

d. The most serious side effect resulting from clomiphene therapy is multiple gestation (rarely more than twins), which occurs in <10% of pregnancies. Some other side effects include hot flushes, emotional instability, abdominal bloating, nausea, ovarian cysts, and rarely ovarian hyperstimulation syndrome. If a painful or large cyst is present, clomiphene therapy should be **withheld.**

e. When clomiphene **fails to induce ovulation,** the next therapeutic option is usually ovulation induction with injectable gonadotropins. **Anovulatory women** with hypothalamic amenorrhea, by definition, have hypothalamic-pituitary dysfunction and thus rarely respond to clomiphene. These women usually respond very well to gonadotropin therapy.

B. **Controlled ovarian hyperstimulation (COH),** also known as superovulation, is indicated for patients with unexplained infertility, diminished ovarian reserve, failure to conceive with clomiphene, "ovulatory dysfunction" associated with endometriosis or AMA, and other more vague diagnoses. **The goal of COH is to create 4–6 mature eggs per cycle.** The theory is that the more eggs available in one cycle, the greater the chance that one of those eggs will fertilize, transport from the tube to the uterus, implant, continue to grow, and grow normally. This is in contradistinction from **ovulation induction** in young women with PCOS in whom the therapeutic goal is ovulation of **ONE egg per cycle.**

1. COH is accomplished with **injectable gonadotropin** (FSH or FSH/LH) therapy. Clomiphene increases endogenous production of FSH, gonadotropin injections are FSH. Thus gonadotropins bypass the hypothalamus-pituitary and directly expose the ovaries to more FSH than the pituitary can make in one cycle.

2. **COH/IUI** requires intense monitoring to avoid multiple gestation (risk ≈ 25% per cycle) and ovarian hyperstimulation syndrome (risk <5% per cycle). Once pregnancy is achieved, early ultrasound is performed to verify gestation number and location. Ectopic pregnancy is more common with both clomiphene and gonadotropin therapy due to multiple eggs released. **COH** is often combined with IUI since the pregnancy rates nearly double with this dual therapy (Table 23.3) (33).

C. Male factor. Pharmacologic therapy for male factor infertility rarely works, therefore treatment is limited to surgical correction of anatomic abnormalities (see section VIII.C.), IUI, ICSI, or donor sperm.

  1. **IUI** with husband's or donor sperm has become one of the principal modalities in contemporary infertility management (34).
    a. Ejaculate is collected in the same manner as is done for the SA.
    b. Ejaculate is then washed of prostaglandins, WBCs, bacteria, and nonmotile sperm, which would normally be filtered by the cervical mucus during coitus.
    c. Sperm is then concentrated either by centrifugation or a swim-up technique.
    d. A narrow plastic catheter is used to deposit washed, concentrated sperm directly into the uterine cavity.
    e. Pregnancy rates are low when total motile sperm (sperm concentration × motility) are <10 million/mL and rare if <1 million/mL (35,36).
    f. Unwashed semen should not be injected directly into the uterine cavity.
  2. **ICSI** is a microscopic technique that involves capturing one sperm and injecting it directly into one mature oocyte. ICSI can only be performed in conjunction with IVF. **The combination of IVF with ICSI has virtually eliminated male factor infertility.**
  3. **Sperm extraction** techniques such as **microsurgical epididymal sperm aspiration** or **open testicular biopsy** can often successfully retrieve sperm when **azospermia** is apparent on SA.
  4. **Artificial insemination with donor sperm (AID)** is a commonly used option for couples with severe male factor infertility and for single women. AID IUI is slightly more expensive than using husband donor IUI and far less expensive than IVF/ICSI.

D. Surgery is warranted when an anatomic abnormality is identified. However pregnancy rates with IVF, which is far less invasive, are beginning to equal or surpass pregnancy rates with traditional surgical therapy. Interestingly, insurance carriers are more likely to include infertility surgery as a benefit than IVF.

E. IVF was initially used when a woman's tubes were damaged beyond the point of surgical correction (37). In addition to **tubal and pelvic factor** infertility, the indications for IVF **now include** the same as those for COH/IUI. As the success rates with IVF improve every year, some experts argue that IVF is becoming more cost-effective than many other forms of therapy (Table 23.3). There are several steps to the IVF process:

  1. **Stimulation** of egg production begins with a protocol involving higher doses of gonadotropins than used for conventional COH to essentially recruit as many eggs as possible.
  2. **Egg retrieval** is performed a few hours prior to ovulation under ultrasound guidance.
  3. **Fertilization** occurs in a laboratory (*in vitro*) under controlled conditions. Usually approximately 100,000 sperm are incubated per mature egg or if indicated, ICSI is performed.

F. Embryo transfer involves placing fertilized eggs (called embryos) back into the uterine cavity 2 to 5 days after *in vitro* incubation.

XI. Sources of information for clinicians and patients
American Society for Reproductive Medicine. http://www.asrm.org

The Society of Assisted Reproduction and Centers for Disease Control. http://www.cdc.gov/nccdphp/drh/art.htm

Resolve: The National Infertility Association. http://www.resolve.org

References
  1. Stephen EH, Chandra A. Updated projections of infertility in the United States: 1995–2025. *Fertil Steril* 1998;70:30.

2. Augood C, Duckitt K, Templeton AA. Smoking and female infertility: a systematic review and meta-analysis. *Hum Reprod* 1998;13:1532.
3. Hull MGR, North K, Taylor H, et al. Delayed conception and active and passive smoking. *Fertil Steril* 2000;74:725.
4. Menken J, Trussell J, Larsen U. Age and infertility. *Science* 1986;233:1389.
5. Stein ZA. A woman's age: childbearing and child rearing. *Am J Epidemiol* 1985; 121:327.
6. Hook EB. Rates of chromosome abnormalities at different maternal ages. *Obstet Gynecol* 1981;58:282.
7. Hook EB, Cross PK, Schreinemachers DM. Chromosomal abnormality rates at amniocentesis and in live-born infants. *JAMA* 1983;249:2034.
8. Luciano AA, Peluso J, Koch EI, et al. Temporal relationship and reliability of the clinical, hormonal, and ultrasonographic indices of ovulation in infertile women. *Obstet Gynecol* 1990;75:412.
9. Wathen NC, Perry L, Lilford RJ, et al. Interpretation of single progesterone measurement in diagnosis of anovulation and defective luteal phase: observations on analysis of the normal range. *BMJ (Clinical Research Ed)* 1984;288:7.
10. Jordan J, Craig K, Clifton DK, et al. Luteal phase defect: the sensitivity and specificity of diagnostic methods in common clinical use. *Fertil Steril* 1994;62:54.
11. Wilcox AJ, Weinberg CR, Baird DD. Timing of sexual intercourse in relation to ovulation: effects on the probability of conception, survival of the pregnancy, and sex of the baby. *N Engl J Med* 1995;333:1517.
12. Noyes RW, Hertig AW, Rock J. Dating the endometrial biopsy. *Fertil Steril* 1950;1:1.
13. Balasch J. Investigation of the infertile couple. *Hum Reprod* 2000;15:2251.
14. De Crespigny LC, O'Herlihy C, Robinson HP. Ultrasonic observation of the mechanism of human ovulation. *Am J Obstet Gynecol* 1981;139:636.
15. American College of Obstetricians and Gynecologists (ACOG). *Infertility.* (ACOG technical bulletin no.125). Washington, DC: ACOG, 1989.
16. Scott RT Jr, Hofmann GE. Prognostic assessment of ovarian reserve. *Fertil Steril* 1995;63:1.
17. Scott RT, Leonardi MR, Hofmann GE, et al. A prospective evaluation of clomiphene citrate challenge test screening of the general infertility population. *Obstet Gynecol* 1993;82:539.
18. Westrom L. Incidence, prevalence, and trends of acute pelvic inflammatory disease and its consequences in industrialized countries. *Am J Obstet Gynecol* 1980; 138:880.
19. American Society for Reproductive Medicine (ASRM). *A practice committee report: optimal evaluation of the infertile female.* Birmingham, AL: ASRM, 2000.
20. Pittaway DE, Winfield AC, Maxson W, et al. Prevention of acute pelvic inflammatory disease after hysterosalpingography: efficacy of doxycycline prophylaxis. *Am J Obstet Gynecol* 1983;147:623.
21. Farhi J, Ashkenazi J, Feldberg D, et al. Effect of uterine leiomyomata on the results of in-vitro fertilization treatment. *Hum Reprod* 1995;10:2576.
22. Griffith CS, Grimes DA. The validity of the postcoital test. *Am J Obstet Gynecol* 1990;162:615.
23. Oei SG, Helmerhorst FM, Bloemenkamp KW, et al. Effectiveness of the postcoital test: randomised controlled trial. *BMJ* 1998;317:502.
24. *WHO laboratory manual for the examination of human semen and semen-cervical mucous interaction,* 4th ed. Cambridge: Cambridge University Press, 1999.
25. Van Waart J, Kruger TF, Lombard CJ, et al. Predictive value of normal sperm morphology in intrauterine insemination (IUI): a structured literature review. *Hum Reprod Update* 2001;7:495–500.
26. Guzick DS, Carson SA, Coutifaris C, et al. Efficacy of superovulation and intrauterine insemination in the treatment of infertility. National Cooperative Reproductive Medicine Network. *N Engl J Med* 1999;340:177–83.
27. Meinertz H, Linnet L, Fogh-Andersen P, et al. Antisperm antibodies and fertility after vasovasostomy: a follow-up study of 216 men. *Fertil Steril* 1990;54:315.

28. Madgar I, Weissenberg R, Lunenfeld B, et al. Controlled trial of high spermatic vein ligation for varicocele in infertile men. *Fertil Steril* 1995;63:120.
29. Lucia A, Chicharro JL, Perez M, et al. Reproductive function in male endurance athletes: sperm analysis and hormonal profile. *J Appl Physiol* 1996;81:2627.
30. Wang C, McDonald V, Leung A, et al. Effect of increased scrotal temperature on sperm production in normal men. *Fertil Steril* 1997;68:334.
31. Speroff L, Glass R, Kase N. *Clinical gynecologic endocrinology and infertility,* 6th ed. Philadelphia: Lippincott Williams & Wilkins, 1999.
32. Opsahl MS, Robins ED, O'Connor DM, et al. Characteristics of gonadotropin response, follicular development, and endometrial growth and maturation across consecutive cycles of clomiphene citrate treatment. *Fertil Steril* 1996;66:533.
33. Guzick DS, Carson SA, Coutifaris C, et al. Efficacy of superovulation and intrauterine insemination in the treatment of infertility. National cooperative reproductive medicine network. *N Engl J Med* 1999;340:177.
34. Hammond MG, Talbert LM. Therapeutic insemination. In: Seibel MM, ed. *Infertility: a comprehensive text,* 2nd ed. Stanford, CT: Appleton & Lange, 1997:309.
35. Nulsen JC, Walsh S, Dumez S, et al. A randomized and longitudinal study of human menopausal gonadotropin with intrauterine insemination in the treatment of infertility. *Obstet Gynecol* 1993;82:780.
36. Van Voorhis BJ, Sparks AE, Allen BD, et al. Cost-effectiveness of infertility treatments: a cohort study. *Fertil Steril* 1997;67:830.
37. Steptoe PC, Edwards RG. Birth after the reimplantation of a human embryo. *Lancet* 1978;2:366.

24. ABORTION

Victor Chan and Maureen Park

Worldwide, abortion is probably the oldest and most prevalent method of fertility control. In the United States, nearly 1.4 million abortions are performed each year. Abortion became legal in the United States in 1973, making the **decision to terminate a pregnancy a matter between the pregnant woman and her physician.** As no contraceptive is 100% effective, unintended pregnancy is inevitable. Since 1973, several court cases have considered issues that would limit this decision but the basic tenet has been upheld.

Availability of abortion provides a choice for the woman who has an unwanted pregnancy. Moreover, legal abortion has greatly reduced the incidence of illegal abortion and its consequences of extremely high rates of complications, including death. Legal abortion is **among the safest of all fertility control methods,** with a mortality rate of 0.6 per 100,000 abortions. In comparison, the U.S. mortality resulting from complications of pregnancy and childbirth (excluding ectopic pregnancy and induced and spontaneous abortion) was 6.5 per 100,000 births. Thus, the mortality risk associated with pregnancy and childbirth is approximately ten times that associated with induced abortion (1). This chapter does not address the legal issues surrounding abortion, which will vary from state to state.

I. **Reasons for abortion.** The reasons a woman obtains an abortion vary, depending on **her reproductive life plan or current circumstances.** A clinician should consider including in the discussion **issues of mental, emotional, or physical well-being** with a woman seeking an abortion. **Fetal reasons** for abortion may include anomalies or other problems detected prenatally or an untoward environmental exposure to x-rays, infection, or medication (e.g., Accutane, Vasotec). **Maternal medical indications** for abortion include pregnancy with an intrauterine device (IUD) *in utero,* an incomplete abortion (either spontaneous or illegal), severe maternal cardiac or respiratory disease, or other conditions that jeopardize the life of the mother.

II. **Counseling the woman.** Since the abortion issue is one of serious religious and philosophic debate, **health care providers must recognize their own feelings** when counseling a woman. Referral of clients is one way to overcome this dilemma for some providers.

   Objectivity, education, and empathy are the hallmarks of good patient counseling. Objectivity includes counseling the woman to make her own decision, providing her with access to alternatives should she desire them, and providing an open discussion. Education involves a review of the woman's current life situation and her plans for the future as well as information about the abortion procedure; its safety, risks, and follow-up instructions; and a description of the contraceptive methods available for her to use after the abortion. **Every woman should understand that, in general, the earlier an abortion is performed, the safer the abortion is** (see section IV.E. for exceptions). Empathy requires supporting the woman and her decision whatever it may be and discussing her feelings about the pregnancy, the abortion, and her relationship with her partner. The woman must be able to change her mind and further discuss her options at any time prior to the abortion procedure.

III. **Confirming the diagnosis of pregnancy. Early and accurate pregnancy determination is essential.** Determination of pregnancy is made by history, physical examination, laboratory testing, radiologic imaging, and recognition of possible problems in the interpretation of tests.

This is a revision of the third edition chapter by Gary K. Stewart and Sara Peterson.

A. **History and symptoms**
   1. The **menstrual period is missed or abnormal in character,** and the woman is likely to experience **breast tenderness and nipple sensitivity, fatigue, nausea, and other signs of pregnancy.**
   2. **Ectopic pregnancy** often presents with vaginal bleeding or spotting and lower abdominal pain (often unilateral).
B. **Physical examination.** In early pregnancy, the **cervix and uterus are softened, the cervicouterine angle is blurred, and the uterus may be enlarged. If the uterine size does not correlate** with the duration of amenorrhea, then consider possibilities such as an incorrect date of last menstrual period (LMP), ectopic pregnancy, twin gestation, incomplete or missed spontaneous abortion, uterine anomaly, or molar pregnancy. Although a number of physical signs are associated with pregnancy, confirmation of a normal intrauterine pregnancy appropriate for elective abortion must include either a laboratory test for human chorionic gonadotropin (hCG) or ultrasound.
C. **Investigative procedures**
   1. **Pregnancy tests** detect hCG, a hormone produced by the pregnancy as early as 11 days after ovulation, or 3 days before anticipated menses.
      a. **Types of pregnancy tests.**
         (1) **Immunometric tests** use urine and correctly diagnose positive pregnancy results in 98% of women within 7 days after implantation (4).
         (2) **Quantitative beta-hCG radioimmunoassay (RIA)** tests can detect pregnancy within 7 days after fertilization. RIA requires use of radioisotopes and therefore, is appropriate for hospitals and large clinics (10).
         (3) **Agglutination inhibition slide** tests detect pregnancy when the gestation is between 6 and 16 weeks. These are inexpensive and simple tests to perform (10).
         (4) **Home pregnancy testing** is a popular option for many women because of privacy, anonymity, and convenience.
      b. **Problems in interpretation.**
         (1) **Laboratory errors occur,** such as specimen mix-up and incorrect performance of test procedures.
         (2) The provider **must understand that the sensitivity of the pregnancy test increases with increasing gestational age** to properly interpret the clinical significance of a negative result or the possibility of a false-positive test.
         (3) The **test is conducted too early** to detect the elevation of hCG levels.
         (4) The **patient has potentially interfering conditions** affecting blood and urine such as a recent pregnancy, an hCG-secreting tumor, lipemia, proteinuria, hematuria, or other reasons for serum or urine turbidity.
         (5) Of great concern are the **problems associated with abnormal pregnancies.** Ectopic pregnancy, spontaneous or missed abortion, malignancy, and trophoblastic disease can produce misleading pregnancy test results.
   2. **Ultrasound** can determine the location and gestational age of the pregnancy in addition to anatomical abnormalities, such as leiomyomata.
      a. Doppler ultrasound can reliably detect fetal heart tones at 10 weeks gestational age.
      b. A transvaginal ultrasound should detect a gestational sac at hCG levels higher than 1180 mIU/mL.
      c. Abdominal ultrasound can reliably detect an intrauterine pregnancy at hCG levels higher than 6500 mIU/mL.
      d. **Transvaginal ultrasound is more sensitive than transabdominal ultrasound in detecting early pregnancies.**

IV. Abortion procedure
A. Preabortion procedure
1. **History.** Prior to abortion, the clinician should obtain the following information:
   a. **A complete contraceptive history.**
   b. **A complete review of prior pregnancies.**
   c. **A review of prior trauma and surgeries to the uterus or cervix such as conization or cesarean section.**
   d. **Any history of known uterine abnormalities,** such as myoma or bicornuate uterus.
   e. **An accurate determination of LMP.**
   f. **A review of systems including drug use and any medication allergies.**
2. **Physical examination.** The preoperative examination must include **bimanual palpation of the pelvis** to determine uterine size and angulation and whether an **adnexal mass** is present. The corpus luteum of pregnancy is a normal cystic structure commonly persisting **up to 10 weeks gestational age.**
3. **Investigative procedures.**
   a. Routine studies should include a **hemoglobin or hematocrit count, an Rh determination** (Rh-negative women should receive Rh immunoglobulin), **gonorrhea and chlamydial screening, and a pregnancy test.** Tests for **HIV** and **hepatitis B surface antigen** (HBsAg) should also be offered.
   b. **Ultrasound dating.** Some clinicians use transvaginal or transabdominal ultrasound to more **accurately estimate gestational age.**
B. Surgical abortion techniques. Local anesthesia offers the advantage of decreased risks for serious anesthetic complications. The following commonly used **surgical abortion techniques are listed in order of increasing risk:**
1. **Vacuum curettage** is the **safest** of all techniques and is **performed through 13 weeks gestation.** It is simple and can be done **using local anesthesia in an office setting.** Manual and electrically powered vacuum aspirators are available in the United States.
   a. The cervical **os can be dilated** with instruments; laminaria, a dried and compressed hydrophilic seaweed; or hydrophilic dilator. **The laminaria or hydrophilic dilator** is inserted 4 to 12 hours before the abortion procedure. Laminaria comes in three different sizes. The size and quantity used are dependent on the woman and her response to it.
   b. The products of conception are **evacuated using negative pressure from a vacuum curette.**
   c. **A complete evacuation can be confirmed with careful use of sharp curettage, a review of the tissue obtained, and/or a postprocedure ultrasound.**
   d. **Dilation and curettage** (D & C) uses a sharp metal curette as **opposed to a vacuum curette** to terminate a pregnancy. D & C **without** vacuum aspiration **has a higher rate of retained products of conception and subsequent infection.**
2. **Dilation and evacuation** (D & E) is generally performed during the **second trimester** (from 13 to 20 weeks gestation).
   a. Since the products of conception may be large, the **cervix is dilated with laminaria** and the procedure performed under **paracervical block or general anesthesia.**
   b. **Fetal-crushing instruments may be necessary to minimize trauma to the cervix.**
   c. Because of **increased safety, lower cost, and better acceptability,** D & E has reduced the number of intraamniotic methods performed (see section IV.C.).

   d. Routine use of methylergonovine maleate (Methergine) and oxytocin postoperatively vary with practitioner. These agents **may limit blood loss by increasing uterine contractility.**
   e. Real-time ultrasound can verify complete evacuation.
3. **Hysterotomy and hysterectomy.** These procedures are reserved for **unusual presentations** of gynecologic **conditions** and **complications.** The overall morbidity and mortality of these procedures have limited their use as abortion techniques.
   a. Hysterotomy is a small uterine incision similar to a cesarean section to remove the pregnancy.
   b. Hysterectomy may be necessary **if medically and/or surgically indicated for reasons other than the abortion.**
C. **Medical techniques. Medical abortion is the use of abortifacient medications to induce a miscarriage.** Since uterine instrumentation is rare, postabortal endometritis is rare with medical abortion. Medical abortion requires careful counseling and patient selection, reliable follow-up, and 24-hour access to surgical abortion services.
   1. **Early abortion. The earlier the gestational age, the higher the efficacy of medical abortion regimens.**
      a. Mifepristone (Mifeprex, also known as RU 486) is the first antiprogesterone agent specifically developed and marketed as an abortifacient. The U.S. Food and Drug Administration (FDA) approved its use as an abortifacient in October 2000. Mifepristone induces abortion by its antagonist action on progesterone receptors.
         (1) The current **recommended** treatment is for pregnancies of **less than 56 days of gestational age.**
         (2) The regimen is mifepristone 600 mg PO as a single dose (although large studies show that 200 mg may be equally effective) followed by misoprostol 400 mcg per vagina 2 days later.
         (3) The procedure is highly effective, with a success rate of 94% for gestations less than 49 days.
         (4) With RU 486, the efficacy is 94% with gestations less than 49 days and 80% with gestations between 50 and 56 days (15).
         (5) Approximately 2% to 10% of patients undergoing medical abortion require evacuation for incomplete abortions or continuing pregnancy (3).
         (6) In rare instances, excessive bleeding may require intervention.
         (7) Other **side effects of medical abortion include nausea, vomiting, diarrhea, and warmth or chills.**
      b. Methotrexate in combination with misoprostol has been used to induce abortion for women at less than 8 weeks gestation (6).
         (1) The efficacy of medical abortion with this combination compared to the efficacy of mifepristone and misoprostol are similar up to 57 days gestational age (2). For gestations **less** than 49 days, the efficacy of the **methotrexate regimen** is 90%. For gestations between 50 and 56 days, the efficacy is 82% (16).
         (2) The methotrexate and misoprostol regimen requires at least four clinic visits.
         (3) The regimen is methotrexate 50 mg/m$_2$ IM on day 1 **after confirming** early intrauterine pregnancy on **vaginal ultrasound,** followed by misoprostol 800 mcg vaginally on **day 3. Methotrexate** has been used to treat **early ectopic pregnancy** with success.
   2. **Second-trimester abortion.** A variety of **drugs administered intraamniotically can induce labor and terminate pregnancy.** Many practitioners recommend performing labor inductions in a hospital or facility equipped to manage complications.
      a. The concomitant use of laminaria reduces the risk of cervical laceration and also **decreases the time required for the abortion.**

b. After the patient empties her bladder, the clinician inserts a **spinal needle into the intrauterine cavity, withdrawing amniotic fluid** to ensure the needle has not entered the bloodstream.

c. The **drug is then infused into the amniotic fluid.**

    (1) Prostaglandin (PG) $F_{2\alpha}$ is used for **second-trimester abortion.** It has a rapid effect with a dose of 40 mg. A **small test dose of 5 mg is usually administered first** to test for adverse reactions.

        (a) Asthma is a contraindication to PG $F_{2\alpha}$.

        (b) PG $F_{2\alpha}$ is **expensive and may require a second infusion of PG $F_{2\alpha}$ or an adjuvant method.**

        (c) PG $F_{2\alpha}$ has a **higher risk of cervical laceration and delivery of a live fetus, causes more gastrointestinal symptoms, and costs more** than other methods.

    (2) Prostaglandin E_2. The effects of these 20-mg **vaginal suppositories** are similar to those of PG $F_{2\alpha}$. However, **PG E_2 has higher rates of gastrointestinal side effects and hyperthermia compared with PG $F_{2\alpha}$.**

    (3) Hypertonic saline. Since this procedure requires infusion of 150 to 250 mL of 20% to 25% saline solution, **the same amount of amniotic fluid must be removed beforehand.** Although inexpensive and readily available, the method has **several risks** including **disseminated intravascular coagulation** (DIC) in 1 in 750 patients; **myometrial necrosis** caused by extravasation; and if infused accidentally into the bloodstream, **hypernatremia, increased blood volume, and cerebral edema.**

    (4) Hypertonic urea. Because of a **high failure rate** as an abortifacient, this relatively safe drug is **generally used in combination with prostaglandins** to reduce the amount of prostaglandin required. About 80 g of urea dissolved in 200 mL water is infused intraamniotically.

d. Combination techniques using these medications require **careful medical monitoring** in a hospital and **often require a D & C** to remove any retained products.

3. Currently, **D & E procedures** predominate as the method of choice for **terminating third-trimester pregnancies** when indicated.

D. Postabortion procedures

    1. After surgical abortion, the **products of conception must be examined** to confirm complete uterine evacuation and exclude hydatidiform mole. In gestations between 6 to 9 weeks, fetal membranes and chorionic villi should be identifiable. In gestations 10 weeks and beyond, removal of all fetal parts should be verified.

    2. The patient must be instructed to notify the clinician if any of the **following danger signs** develop:

        a. Fever or chills.

        b. Muscle aches or tiredness.

        c. Abdominal pain, cramping, or backache.

        d. Tenderness to pressure on the abdomen.

        e. Prolonged or heavy bleeding.

        f. Foul-smelling vaginal discharge.

        g. Delay of 3 months or more in resuming menstrual periods.

    3. Remember that pregnancy test results may cause confusion after pregnancy termination. Since the hCG level gradually decreases, a pregnancy test may be positive even after complete evacuation. Generally, routine urine slide tests are negative by 7 days, and the serum assays are negative by 14 days.

E. Complications. The risks of the abortion procedure **increase with increasing gestational age** due to the need for more cervical dilation, the increased possibility of retained products, and subsequent bleeding and/or infection.

1. **Death.** A woman who has an abortion performed at **less than 9 weeks gestation has a 1 in 400,000 chance of dying. Between 9 and 12 weeks gestation, the risk** of abortion-related deaths is **four times higher;** and **between 13 and 16 weeks gestation, the risk is another four times higher. After 16 weeks** gestation, **death** occurs in **1 in 10,000 abortions.**

2. **Medical and surgical complications.**

   a. **Infections.** The **most common complication** is infection. Symptoms include **cramping, fever, discharge, bleeding, and pelvic pain.** The patient presenting with these symptoms must be evaluated for possible infection.

      (1) **Prevention.** Many abortion providers administer **prophylactic antibiotics** to their patients. When antibiotics are used, the choice is doxycycline, 200 mg PO prior to the procedure and 100 mg PO 12 hours later. The risk of infection is markedly **reduced** by **completely emptying the uterus and by treating vaginal or cervical infections before performing the abortion.**

      (2) **Treatment. Early diagnosis is the key** in preventing the more severe consequences of infection.

         (a) If the patient is **severely ill** or has an **infection that extends beyond the uterus** as in salpingitis or peritonitis, she should **be hospitalized and treated with intravenous antibiotics and fluids.** An ultrasound can assess for retained products or blood clots. A D & C should be done to remove any remaining products of conception. Once the patient is afebrile for at least 24 to 48 hours, she may be discharged with oral antibiotics.

         (b) If the infection is **mild and no obvious tissue remains in the uterus,** oral antibiotics should be administered and the patient placed at bedrest with close follow-up (see Chapter 5).

         (c) In patients who **do not exhibit satisfactory improvement** within 2 to 3 days, a **D & C, vacuum curettage, and/or hospitalization may be necessary.**

         (d) **A pelvic ultrasound** may help determine whether tissue is present in these patients with infection.

   b. **Retained products of conception.** Symptoms and signs include **pain, cramping or bleeding,** and an **enlarged, soft, and tender uterus.**

      (1) **Prevention. Evacuated tissue should be evaluated at the time of abortion** by weighing the tissue and visually inspecting it to confirm all fetal products have been removed.

      (2) **Diagnosis.** Infection must be ruled out. A pelvic examination followed by an ultrasound of the pelvis will show whether additional tissue or significant clots are present.

      (3) **Treatment.** The **retained tissue should be removed by vacuum aspiration or D & C.** The woman should receive **antibiotics** and possibly **methylergonovine,** 0.2 mg IM or PO initially then q6h PRN, **or other oxytocics** to expel remaining tissue and maintain firm uterine muscle tone.

   c. **Postabortal syndrome** is the accumulation of uterine blood clots after an abortion. After an early abortion, it occurs once in 200 to 300 cases. **Symptoms** of severe cramping pain often begin within a few hours **but may appear up to 5 days after the abortion.**

      (1) **Prevention.** Administration of **methylergonovine,** 0.2 mg IM or PO initially **then** q6h for six doses, may reduce the risk

of occurrence of blood clots. This drug is **contraindicated** in patients with **hypertension.**

   (2) Treatment [see section IV.E.2.b.(3)].

  d. Continuing pregnancy. Less than 0.3% of abortions fail to terminate the pregnancy. The problem **occurs most often when the abortion is performed before the seventh week of gestation without ultrasound confirmation of complete pregnancy evacuation.**

    (1) The reasons for this failure include **incomplete evacuation, twin pregnancies, ectopic pregnancy, or an anatomic abnormality of the uterus** (e.g., bicornuate uterus).

    (2) Symptoms include persisting symptoms of pregnancy such **as nausea, breast tenderness, fatigue, and increasing uterine enlargement.**

  e. Cervical or uterine trauma. Symptoms of **serious internal hemorrhage** include rapid pulse, weakness and faintness, and decreasing blood pressure that occurs as a **result of damage to large uterine blood vessels or uterine perforation.** Pain, vomiting, abdominal tenderness or rigidity, and decreased bowel sounds occur as a **result of damage to the intestines.**

    (1) Prevention. Placement of cervical laminaria and use of gentle techniques can reduce the risk of trauma. **Cervical dilation should keep pace with uterine contractions,** especially during late abortion induced with prostaglandins or with saline augmented with oxytocin.

    (2) Treatment.

      (a) Cervical trauma or less serious uterine damage can be managed by 24 hours of observation to make certain internal hemorrhage does not occur.

      (b) Most perforations or cervical tears close spontaneously and heal without treatment. Expectant management of known uterine perforations or cervical tears **requires** reliable observation and availability of medical resources.

      (c) Serious internal hemorrhage requires hospitalization.

  f. Bleeding is expected after abortion. It is **often scant or absent for the first 36 hours but increases as the endometrium loses hormonal support.** Moderate bleeding can then occur intermittently for as long as 3 weeks. The physician must **consider the potential for DIC** in patients undergoing a second-trimester abortion, including both the D & E and aminoinfused patients.

    (1) Prevention. Excessive bleeding can be prevented by using **local anesthetics, uterine contracting agents, and uterine massage. Prompt evacuation of the placenta** in second-trimester abortion is important.

    (2) Treatment. Bleeding that persists **longer than 4 weeks must be evaluated.** Retained products of conception or trauma to the cervix or uterus must be considered. Hemorrhage or other serious problems **may require hospitalization.**

  g. Anesthesia complications. Local anesthesia is safer than conscious sedation, which is safer than general anesthesia. Most second-trimester abortions are performed under conscious sedation or general anesthesia. **Anesthetic reactions** are among the **most common causes of death in first-trimester abortion patients.** Hyperventilation, drug reactions, and poorly trained clinical staff make these problems a real risk.

    (1) Prevention. By **intubating patients** with general anesthesia and **ensuring proper monitoring for cardiac arrhyth-**

mias, administration of general anesthesia should be safe. By **limiting the amount of the caine drug** (to <300 mg) **or using a less toxic local anesthetic** [i.e., chloroprocaine (Nesacaine)], this problem can be limited.

    (2) **Treatment. The most important treatment is prevention.** Immediate recognition and staff trained to deal with these problems are the key to limiting and managing anesthesia complications.

    h. **Long-term complications.** The **impact of abortion** (especially multiple abortions) on **subsequent fertility, spontaneous abortion, premature delivery, and low-birthweight infants remains in question.** Early first-trimester abortion, however, does not seem to contribute to any of these possible problems. A **more profound impact may result from the social, economic, and behavioral effects.**

V. Steps for preventing abortion complications. Abortions are safe procedures. Nonetheless, complications can occur, some of them serious. The **key is prevention** of complications. The following are important factors in the performance of safe abortions:

- **Pregnancy is in early stage.**
- **Patient is healthy.**
- **Clinician is well trained and experienced in abortion techniques.**
- **Uterus is not acutely anteverted or retroverted.**
- **Patient understands warning signs for potential problems.**
- **Prompt follow-up care is available on a 24-hour basis.**
- **Aspirated or curetted tissue is examined for possibility of molar or ectopic pregnancy.**
- **Ultrasound is available for guidance during a procedure or postprocedure confirmation of complete evacuation.**
- **Rh immunoglobulin is given to Rh-negative women.**
- **Patient does not have gonorrhea or chlamydial infection.**
- **Patient is not ambivalent about the abortion or can cope with her feelings.**
- **Abortion is complete (uterus is emptied).**
- **Local anesthesia is used.**

VI. Follow-up examination should be scheduled for **2 weeks after the abortion.** Bleeding and cramping may occur and may continue for 4 weeks. The next normal menstrual period should begin in 4 to 6 weeks. Since it is possible for a woman to become pregnant before she next menstruates, **she should be supplied with, and encouraged to use, contraception immediately after abortion.** She should **avoid intercourse for the first 2 weeks** following abortion. During that time, she **should not douche or use tampons.**

References

1. Paul M, Lichtenberg ES, Borgatta L, et al. *A clinician's guide to medical and surgical abortion.* Churchill Livingstone, 1999.
2. Kahn JG, Becker BJ, MacIsaa L, et al. The efficacy of medical abortion: a meta-analysis. *Contraception* 2000;61(1):29–40.
3. Kruse B, Peppema S, Creinin MD, et al. Management of side effects and complications in medical abortion. *Am J Obstet Gynecol* 2000;183[2 Suppl]:S65–S75.
4. Chard T. Pregnancy tests: a review. *Hum Reprod* 1992;7:701.
5. Creinin MD, Darney PD. Methotrexate and misoprostol for early abortion. *Contraception* 1993;48:339.
6. Hatcher RA, et al. Pregnancy testing and management of early pregnancy. *Contraceptive technology.* New York: Irvington, 1994.
7. Spitz IM, Bardin W, Benton L, et al. Early pregnancy termination with mifepristone and misoprostol in the United States. *N Engl J Med* 1998;338:1241–1247.
8. Creinin MD, Vittinghoff E, Keder L, et al. Methotrexate and misoprostol for early abortion: a multicenter trial. I. Safety and efficacy. *Contraception* 1996;53:321–327.

25. MENOPAUSE

Mary Ciotti and Rebecca King

The terms menopause and climacteric are commonly used interchangeably although, strictly speaking, **menopause** occurs when spontaneous menstruation ceases for 6 months to 1 year. At approximately 40 years, the frequency of ovulation decreases. This causes menstrual irregularities heralding the **climacteric** or **perimenopausal transition,** which encompasses the change from normal ovulatory cycles to cessation of menses (1).

The current average life expectancy of U.S. women is greater than 80 years. Since the mean age of menopause in the United States is 51 years, women spend approximately one third of their lives in the postmenopausal state. An understanding of the hormonal changes and sequelae of menopause is critical for those who wish to provide quality longitudinal health care for women.

I. **Physiology. The perimenopausal transition** represents the progressive loss of ovarian follicles with degeneration of granulosa and theca cells (1).
   A. **Estrogens** (1)
      1. **Estradiol** levels remain relatively stable **until** menopause
         a. The estradiol level dramatically **decreases** at menopause.
         b. Estradiol levels are **not predictive** of the **climacteric until actual menopause.**
      2. **Estrone accounts for most of the circulating estrogens in menopause.**
         a. **Estrone** results mainly from peripheral aromatization of circulating androstenedione.
         b. After menopause 85% of androstenedione comes from the adrenal gland.
   B. **Progesterone** is indicative of ovulation.
   C. **Androgens** (1)
      1. Total circulating **testosterone** is decreased after menopause (1).
      2. The **postmenopausal** ovary produces **more testosterone** than the premenopausal ovary.
      3. This relative increase in the testosterone to estrogen ratio may explain the slight virilization seen in some older women.
   D. **Gonadotropins** increase as a result of the absence of negative feedback of ovarian steroids and are elevated in menopause. However, they are often within normal limits in perimenopause (1).
      1. **Follicle-stimulating hormone** (FSH) **rises markedly,** reflecting the fall in estrogen levels.
      2. **Luteinizing hormone** rises moderately.
II. **Clinical findings**
   A. **Menstrual changes**
      1. Most women note a **gradual tapering** in both **amount** and **duration of flow.**
      2. A **minority** of women have **more frequent** and **heavier bleeding.**
      3. **Abrupt cessation** of menses is fairly rare.
      4. **Fertility** is reduced, however patients still need to be counseled regarding contraception.
   B. **Vasomotor instability** (hot flashes and night sweats)
      1. The classic symptom is the **hot flash,** which occurs in up to 85% of women, 80% of whom endure symptoms for over 1 year and some up to 5 years or more.

This chapter is a revision of the third edition chapter by Christine J. Chai.

   a. The symptom is described as a sensation of **intense warmth** in the **upper body** that **spreads to the face and neck,** sometimes is associated with palpitations and perspiration, and lasts a **few seconds to minutes.**

   b. The mechanism is not well understood but may result from hypothalamic alterations brought about by declining estrogen.

   c. Hot flashes may **precede menopause** by **months to years.**

   d. Hot flashes tend to be **common at night,** causing sleep disturbances.

C. Genitourinary changes

   1. **Atrophic vaginitis** can occur over time in women who are not receiving estrogen.

   a. The **vaginal mucosa** becomes **thin** and **pale,** causing **symptoms** of dryness, pruritus, and bleeding.

   b. **Intercourse** may be so difficult and uncomfortable that there can be secondary loss of libido.

   c. On **pelvic examination** after estrogen deprivation, the cervix may be flush with the vaginal vault. There may also be narrowing of the vaginal vault.

   2. The lining of the urethra and bladder trigone may become attenuated, leading to symptoms of **dysuria and frequency** without infection.

D. Somatic and nonspecific symptoms

   1. Other symptoms such as **fatigue, headache, apprehension,** and **mood swings** have been reported.

   2. Many postmenopausal women with hot flashes and night sweats **also experience** irritability, anxiety, nervousness, depression, fatigue, forgetfulness, and an inability to concentrate. These **same complaints are found** in those who suffer from **sleep deprivation** and **interrupted sleep.**

   3. Some women experience some level of **depression** at perimenopause due to hormonal shifts. It is more common to find depression in the perimenopause than after menopause.

   4. **Objective improvements of memory, insomnia, anxiety,** and **irritability** have been documented in postmenopausal women **receiving estrogen** in several drug trials (1,3).

E. Cardiovascular disease (2)

   1. **Cardiovascular disease** is the leading cause of death in U.S. women. Coronary heart disease is less prevalent in women than in men before the age of 55, but this difference decreases after this age. There is evidence to support the notion that loss of ovarian function increases the risk of coronary heart disease.

   2. **Lipids.**

   a. In animal studies, estrogens retard atherogenesis, decrease cholesterol deposition in vascular walls, and increase coronary blood flow and synthesis of vascular wall cyclooxygenase (2).

   b. **Estrogens raise levels of high-density lipoprotein** (HDL) and **decrease low-density lipoprotein-cholesterol** (LDL) (4).

   c. **Synthetic progestins** tend to have an **unfavorable effect** on lipids by **increasing LDL** and **decreasing HDL.** Although these changes could theoretically offset the apparent cardioprotective effects of estrogens, their clinical effects still remain unclear. **Oral micronized progesterone does not reduce the beneficial lipid effects of estrogens** (4).

   3. The results of observational studies have suggested **estrogen replacement therapy** (ERT) is associated with reduced cardiovascular risk (2). However, recent studies on women with **known** heart disease show an increase in mortality when starting hormone replacement therapy (HRT) (5). The Women's Health Initiative is currently in process. This is a 10-year trial to determine if ERT is an effective strategy for preventing heart disease in postmenopausal women.

F. Osteoporosis (see also Chapter 26)

1. **Osteoporosis** is the progressive reduction in bone mass that is seen after the fourth decade and accelerates after menopause.

   a. **One in three women** will sustain a **vertebral fracture** after 65 years.

   b. **One in three women** will suffer a **hip fracture** by age 90.

   (1) In addition to rising costs of care, hip fractures are associated with a 5% to 30% mortality rate.

   (2) Fifty percent of women experience decreased ability to walk after fracture (6).

2. **Trabecular bone** is affected earlier than cortical bone.

3. Most common fracture sites are the vertebrae, distal radius, and femoral neck.

4. **Risk factors** for developing **osteoporosis** include the following (6,7).

   a. Fair skin (Asian or Caucasian).

   b. Slight build.

   c. Family history of osteoporosis.

   d. Low-estrogen state, especially with early menopause or exercise-related amenorrhea.

   e. Cigarette smoking.

   f. High alcohol intake.

   g. Chronic liver or kidney disease.

   h. Sedentary lifestyle or immobilization.

   i. Treatment with glucocorticoids, heparin, or thyroid hormone.

   j. Excessive caffeine intake.

III. Diagnosis

A. History and physical examination

1. The diagnosis of **menopause or perimenopause** is generally a clinical diagnosis.

2. Complaints of **vasomotor instability** and findings that suggest **genitourinary atrophy, menstrual changes, or nonspecific somatic symptoms** should alert health care providers to consider **perimenopausal transition.**

3. If the history and clinical presentation are **inconclusive,** laboratory confirmation may be warranted. This may especially be true in posthysterectomy (ovaries intact) women when climacteric symptoms are vague and gradual.

B. Investigative procedures

1. **Serum FSH is elevated** >30 IU/L (1).

   a. This is the single **most important laboratory test** available.

   b. Large amounts of estrogen are needed to suppress postmenopausal FSH levels to the normal range. FSH levels **cannot** be used to clinically titer estrogen dosage.

2. **Serum estradiol** levels will be **decreased** (<20 pg/mL) at menopause. However, the level may be within normal range until then.

   a. Estradiol levels may be used to monitor estrogen therapy.

   b. Symptoms are the best indicator of adequate treatment.

3. **Endometrial biopsy** may be indicated in patients with greater than 6 months of irregular bleeding or those at increased risk for endometrial cancer or hyperplasia.

4. **Radiographic assessments of bone density.**

   a. Twenty percent to 25% of bone mineral content must be lost before osteoporosis is detected with routine x-ray films.

   b. **Bone densitometry** to assess rates of bone loss may be useful (6,7).

   (1) It is the preferred method of diagnosis.

   (2) Bone densitometry is useful in women at risk for osteoporosis and in those who cannot, or choose not to, take estrogen.

      (3) Z score is the standard deviation from the mean bone mineral density (BMD) of patient age.

      T-score based on BMD or normal young adult

      Normal T score greater than −1

      Low bone mass T score between −1 and −2.5

      Osteoporosis T score below −2.5 (7)

IV. Management of osteoporosis (see also Chapter 26)

  A. Patient education is indicated for all ages.

    1. Emphasis should be on prophylaxis, rather than treatment.

    2. Promotion of good health practices, such as adequate calcium intake, cessation of smoking, decreasing alcohol intake, and regular weight-bearing exercises, should be reinforced long before the menopause.

  B. Vitamin D is required for calcium absorption.

    1. Deficiencies can occur in some elderly patients owing to inadequate sun exposure, poor calcium intake, and decreased intestinal absorption of calcium.

    2. Adults need 400 IU per day, whereas **elderly patients need 800 IU per day** (6).

  C. Calcium

    1. Adequate calcium intake is most important during the years of skeletal growth (birth through adolescence).

    2. Postmenopausal women **not** receiving ERT require approximately **1,500 mg per day** of total calcium (6).

    3. Postmenopausal women **receiving** ERT require a total calcium intake of **1,000 mg per day.**

    4. For patients with inadequate dietary calcium intake, calcium supplementation is indicated.

      a. Calcium supplements should be taken in several small doses a day to avoid overloading the intestinal calcium absorption system (6).

      b. Calcium citrate is better absorbed but calcium carbonate is cheaper.

      c. Calcium supplementation, even with weight-bearing exercise, may not prevent osteoporosis (6).

  D. Estrogen will prevent **osteoporosis.**

    1. Estrogen acts by several mechanisms to reduce skeletal remodeling.

      a. Decreased bone resorption.

      b. Increased intestinal calcium absorption.

      c. Reduced renal calcium excretion.

    2. Studies have shown that estrogen arrests bone loss and reduces the incidence of fractures, even if treatment is begun later in life or after interruption of treatment (2,6).

    3. The goal is to use the lowest estrogen dose that is effective. Most studies indicate that CEE of 0.625 mg is effective. However, doses as low as 0.3 mg may preserve bone mass if calcium intake is adequate (8).

  E. Selective estrogen receptor modulators (SERMS) (7)

    1. Act as weak estrogen agonist, useful for the prevention of osteoporosis.

    2. Raloxifene reduces risk of vertebral fracture.

    3. Carries same risk of thrombotic events as ERT.

  F. Alendronate. Approved for osteoporosis prevention and therapy (see treatment)

  G. Treatment of established osteoporosis

    1. Calcitonin and alendronate are:

      a. Approved for osteoporosis therapy.

        (1) Alendronate is approved for both osteoporosis prevention and therapy.

        (2) Calcitonin is currently approved only for therapy of osteoporosis but not prevention.

        (3) Calcitonin does seem to decrease vertebral fractures but the effect on hip fractures is unclear.

      b. Will increase BMD and decrease fracture risk.

    2. Etidronate (7) is
      a. Approved in Canada but is currently only approved for treatment of Paget's disease in the United States.
      b. Typically given in 2-week cycles repeated every 3 months.

V. Hormone replacement therapy

  A. Indications

    1. Estrogen replacement is **indicated** for patients with **symptoms** or **physical findings** that are clearly the **result of estrogen deficiency and in whom absolute contraindications are not present** (see section V.B.).

    2. ERT is indicated in certain **asymptomatic women at high risk for osteoporosis** (see sec. II.F.4.).

    3. Estrogen therapy is **definitely indicated for women who have undergone premature menopause.**

    4. Estrogen may be considered **as a means of reducing atherosclerotic risk in certain postmenopausal women.** However, this indication is becoming more controversial (2,5,9).

  B. Contraindications (2)

    1. Absolute contraindications include:
      a. Unexplained vaginal bleeding.
      b. Active liver disease.
      c. Recent myocardial infarction.
      d. Recent or active vascular thrombosis, with or without emboli.
      e. History of estrogen-related thromboembolic disease.
      f. The use of estrogen in women with breast and/or endometrial carcinoma has been contraindicated in the past. It is still undergoing further evaluation. Oncologists will generally discuss the pathology test results and the current pros and cons of estrogen replacement with the cancer survivor. Potential risks and benefits must be carefully considered.

    2. Relative contraindications include:
      a. Migraine headaches.
      b. Thrombophlebitis.
      c. Active endometriosis.
      d. Gallbladder disease.
      e. Chronic impaired liver function.
      f. Poorly controlled hypertension.
      g. Acute intermittent porphyria.

  C. Risks of estrogen

    1. Endometrial carcinoma.
      a. Unopposed estrogen may lead to endometrial hyperplasia and, ultimately, adenocarcinoma of the endometrium.
        (1) There is a twofold to fourfold risk of developing endometrial cancer with the use of unopposed estrogen.
        (2) This incidence varies with duration and dosage of therapy.
      b. Addition of progestin to conjugated estrogen therapy significantly lowers the risk of hyperplasia and cancer (10).
        (1) Sequential addition of 5 to 10 mg of medroxyprogesterone for 12 to 14 days to cyclic estrogen virtually eliminates the risk of cancer (1).
        (2) Alternatively, 2.5 to 5 mg of medroxyprogesterone can be given daily.

    2. Breast cancer. Several studies have reported increases in relative risk with prolonged estrogen use (>10–15 years), but the increased risk identified has been twofold or less and often not statistically significant (2,11).

    3. Hypertension. Hormone replacement does not seem to cause the same increase in blood pressure as seen in oral contracep-

tive users. The potency of estrogen is much lower in ERT than in birth control pills (4).

4. **Thromboembolic disease.**
    a. **There is a twofold to fourfold increase in venous thromboembolism in users of HRT (12).**
    b. **Current or recent thrombosis or embolus is a contraindication to estrogen therapy.**
    c. **Transdermal estrogen avoids the first-pass effect of the liver, thereby theoretically reducing the risk of thromboembolic disease (1).**
5. **Gallbladder disease.** Estrogen therapy may double the risk for gallbladder disease.
6. Estrogens may cause nausea, headache, mood changes, and breast tenderness.

D. **Types of estrogens**
    1. **Oral.**
        a. All oral preparations are similar in effect and none has shown any particular advantage.
        b. Oral estrogens are subject to first-pass metabolism.
    2. **Transdermal.**
        a. Convenient for women who have undergone hysterectomy.
        b. Avoids first-pass effect.
        c. May not affect serum lipids as definitively as oral estrogens.
        d. Costly.
        e. Incidence of skin sensitivity.
    3. **Topical-vaginal.**
        a. Useful in alleviating symptoms of atrophic vaginitis.
        b. High doses (2–4 g daily) may have systemic effects.

E. **Progestins**
    1. Progestins are mainly used to reduce the risk of endometrial cancer.
    2. They may also be used to relieve hot flashes in patients unable to take estrogen.
    3. Adverse effects.
        a. Detrimental effects on serum lipids are dose-dependent and are not associated with micronized progesterone (4).
        b. Nuisance side effects include bloating, acne, weight gain, fluid retention, headache, mood changes, dysmenorrhea, and mastalgia.

VI. **Treatment regimens**
    A. **Before initiating therapy,** the following should be assessed:
        1. **History** and **physical examination** must include **blood pressure, breast** and **pelvic examination, Pap smear,** and **cholesterol level.**
        2. **Mammography** should be performed according to established guidelines.
        3. Routine endometrial biopsy is **not required unless** a history of abnormal bleeding is elicited.
    B. In women with an intact uterus, combination estrogen and progestin therapy is given (Table 25.1).
        1. **Cyclic or sequential therapy.**
            a. Cyclic or sequential therapy is the most commonly used initial HRT regimen since it allows for regular shedding of the endometrium and eventually for a more atrophic lining.
            b. The most commonly used regimen is oral estrogen given daily with an oral progestin given 10 to 12 days of the month.
                (1) The most commonly used oral estrogens are conjugated estrogen (Premarin) 0.625 mg, estradiol (Estrace) 0.5 to 1 mg, or a transdermal estrogen preparation.
                (2) These are commonly combined with medroxyprogesterone acetate (e.g., Provera), 10 mg for 10 to 12 days of the month or micronized progesterone 200 mg, 10 to 12 days per month.

Table 25.1. Estrogens and progestins available for treatment

ESTROGENS

Route	Type of estrogen	Dose	Brands
Oral	Conjugated equine estrogen	0.3–1.25 mg	Premarin
	Micronized estradiol	0.5, 1, 2 mg	Estrace
	Esterified estrogen	0.3, 0.625, 1.25, 2.5 mg	Menest, Estratab
	Ethinyl estradiol	0.02, .05, 0.5 mg	Estinyl
	Synthetic conjugated	0.625, 0.9	Cenestin
	Estropipate	0.625, 1.25, 2.5 mg	Ogen, Orthoest
Transdermal	Estradiol	0.05–0.1 mg (Change weekly)	Climera, Fempatch
		0.0375, 0.05, 0.075,0.01 (Change 2×/week)	Estraderm, Vivelle, Alora
Intravaginal	Conjugated Estrogen cream	0.5–2 g × 2 weeks then decrease dose	Premarin cream
	Estradiol cream	2–4 g × 2 weeks then decrease dose	Estrace cream
	Estradiol vaginal ring	Replace 3 months	Estring
	Estradiol vaginal tablet	1 tab qhs × 2 week then 1 tab 2×/week	Vagifem

PROGESTINS

Route	Progestin	Dose	Brands
Oral	Medroxypro-gesterone	10 mg 10–12 days of mo 2.5–5 mg daily	Provera, Cycrin, Amen, Curretab
	Micronized progesterone	200–300 mg 10–12 d/mo 100 mg daily	Prometrium
	Norithindrone acetate	1 mg daily 1.5 mg 10–12 d/mo	Aygestin

COMBINED THERAPY

Route	Estrogen/Progestin	Dose	Brands
Oral	Congutated estrogen/ medroxyproges-terone	0.625/2.5 mg 0.625/5 mg	Prempro
Transdermal	Estradiol/ norethindrone	0.05/0.14, 0.05/ 2.5 mg change 2×/week	Combipatch

   c. Patients will then have a withdrawal bleed after finishing the progestin.
   d. Use the **lowest dose** of estrogen needed to treat symptoms and prevent osteoporosis.
2. **Continuous therapy.**
   a. This can be given after the patient has been on sequential therapy without problems. If given as the first-line therapy there is often breakthrough bleeding that occurs at unpredictable times, necessitating endometrial biopsy.
   b. Estrogen, in doses sufficient to control symptoms, is given with Provera, 2.5 to 5 mg daily or micronized progesterone, 100 mg daily.
   c. Avoids withdrawal bleeding and is much simpler to use.
   d. Seventy-three percent to 95% amenorrhea can be achieved if patients can patiently stick with the regimen for at least 1 year (13).
   e. Avoids return of symptoms during the medication-free interval.
C. In women who have undergone **hysterectomy, estrogen** alone is given in **doses sufficient** to **prevent osteoporosis** and **control symptoms.**
D. **Management of problems**
   1. **Persistent vasomotor complaints.**
      a. If a patient is **still symptomatic after increasing the estrogen dose, obtain a serum estradiol level.**
      b. For patients taking generous amounts of estrogen yet still having low estradiol levels (<50 pg/mL), **consider another route of administration.** Women who **smoke,** who have **poor gastrointestinal absorption,** or those **who take medications that accelerate hepatic metabolism may receive lower than expected amounts of circulating estrogen** (14).
   2. **Withdrawal bleeding on continuous therapy (bleeding is expected on cyclic regimens).**
      a. **Add another 2.5 mg qd of Provera** to continuous regimen or increase to 200 mg micronized progesterone.
      b. **Reduce conjugated estrogen dose to 0.3 mg.** Since the long-term effectiveness of this lower estrogen dose is unknown, daily calcium intake should be 1,500 mg.
   3. **Adverse reactions to cyclic progestin.**
      a. **Reduce Provera** dose from 10 to 5 mg.
      b. Switch to **different types** of progestin.
         (1) Oral micronized progesterone, 200 mg qd.
         (2) Norethindrone (Micronor, Norlutin), 0.35 to 0.70 mg qd.
         (3) Norethindrone acetate (Norlutate), 5 mg qd.
      c. Switch to **continuous therapy.**
   4. **Unscheduled or heavy bleeding must be evaluated by endometrial biopsy.**
   5. **Decreased libido.**
      a. Rule out **atrophic vaginitis** and **psychosocial issues.**
      b. **Consider androgen treatment,** alone or in combination with estrogen (Estratest or Premarin with testosterone). Potential **concerns include masculinization** and **adverse effects on lipids.**
E. **Duration of therapy**
   1. HRT should be considered a long-term commitment.
   2. A prospective cohort derived from the Framingham Heart Study determined that at least 7 years of postmenopausal estrogen were required to have an effect on BMD. In addition, the authors concluded that very little benefit was gained in starting estrogen in women older than 75 (15).
F. **Nonestrogen treatment alternatives** (16) (see also Chapter 33)
   1. **Vasomotor symptoms.**
      a. Medroxyprogesterone acetate, 10 to 40 mg qd.
      b. Megestrol acetate (Megace), 20 to 80 mg qd.

      c. Clonidine (Catapres-TTS), 0.1 to 0.2 mg bid.
      d. Belladonna alkaloids (Bellergal-S) bid.
      e. Vitamin E 400 to 800 IU qd, herbs such as ginseng, and biofeedback.
   2. Vaginal atrophy symptoms may be alleviated with water-soluble vaginal lubricants.

References

1. Speroff L, Glass R, Kase N. *Clinical gynecologic endocrinology and infertility,* 5th ed, 1995.
2. American College of Obstetricians and Gynecologists (ACOG). *Hormone replacement therapy.* ACOG Technical Bulletin 247. Washington, DC: ACOG, May 1998.
3. Kampen DL, Sherwin BB. Estrogen use and verbal memory in healthy postmenopausal women. *Obstet Gynecol* 1994;83:979.
4. The Writing Group for the PEPI trial. Effects of estrogen or estrogen/progestin regimens on heart disease risk factors in postmenopausal women. *JAMA* 1995; 273:199–208.
5. Hulley S, Grady D, Bush T, et al. for the Heart and Estrogen/progestin Replacement Study (HERS) research group. Randomized trial of estrogen plus progestin for secondary prevention of coronary heart disease in postmenopausal women. *JAMA* 1998; 280:605–613.
6. American College of Obstetricians and Gynecologists. *Osteoporosis.* ACOG Technical Bulletin 246. Washington, DC: ACOG, April 1998.
7. *Postmenopausal osteoporosis—Strategies for prevention and treatment.* North American Menopause Society, February 2000.
8. Ettinger B, Genant HK, Cann CE. Postmenopausal bone loss is prevented by treatment with low dosage estrogen with calcium. *Am Intern Med* 1987;106:40.
9. Stampfer MJ, et al. Postmenopausal estrogen therapy and cardiovascular disease: ten-year follow-up from the nurses' health study. *N Engl J Med* 1991;325:756.
10. Woodruff JD, Pickar JH, for The Menopause Study Group. Incidence of endometrial hyperplasia in postmenopausal women taking conjugated estrogens (Premarin) with medroxyprogesterone acetate or conjugated estrogens alone. *Am J Obstet Gynecol* 1994;170:1213.
11. Colditz GA, Egan KM, Stampfer MJ. Hormone replacement therapy and risk of breast cancer: results from epidemiologic studies. *Am J Obstet Gynecol* 1993;168: 1473.
12. Daly E, Vessey MP, Hawkins MM, et al. Risk of venous thromboembolism in users of hormone replacement therapy. *Lancet* 1996;348:977–980.
13. Archer DF, Pickar JH, Bottiglioni F, for The Menopause Study Group. Bleeding patterns in postmenopausal women taking continuous combined or sequential regimens of conjugated estrogens with medroxyprogesterone acetate. *Obstet Gynecol* 1994;83:686.
14. Jones KP. Estrogens and progestins: what to use and how to use it. *Clin Obstet Gynecol* 1992;35:871.
15. Felson DT, et al. The effect of postmenopausal estrogen therapy on bone density in elderly women. *N Engl J Med* 1993;329:1141.
16. Miller KL. Alternatives to estrogen for menopausal symptoms. *Clin Obstet Gynecol* 1992;35:884.

26. OSTEOPOROSIS

Cheryl L. Lambing

Height loss, spinal deformity, and fragility are not inevitable consequences of growing old; rather, these features are symptoms of osteoporosis, a disorder characterized by low bone mass and heightened risk of fracture (1). Osteoporosis is the most common human bone disease. The cause of osteoporosis is multifactorial. Most often, osteoporosis is diagnosed after the first fracture (commonly a fragility fracture) has occurred. Osteoporosis affects more than 25 million people in the United States, 4 out of 5 of whom are women. The disease is responsible for more than 1.5 million fractures per year. Of those who experience hip fracture, 10% to 20% die, 25% of survivors are confined to long-term facilities, and 50% of survivors exhibit long-term loss of mobility (1).

I. **Definition(s)**
   A. No one definition encompasses its etiology, pathophysiology, diagnostic criteria, and treatment regimens. Two most commonly used definitions are as follows:
      1. The definition developed by the 1993 Consensus Development Conference on Osteoporosis best describes the clinical condition: A systemic skeletal disease characterized by low bone mass and microarchitectural deterioration of bone tissue, leading to bone fragility and an increased susceptibility to fracture (2).
      2. The World Health Organization (WHO) Working Group on Osteoporosis definition describes the diagnostic criteria set for postmenopausal women: bone mineral density (BMD) 2.5 standard deviations (SD) or more below the peak young normal mean (T-score) (3).
II. **Physiology**
   A. **Bone remodeling**
      1. In **normal skeletal remodeling,** bone resorption by osteoclasts is tightly coupled with subsequent bone deposition by osteoblasts. The resorptive phase of the remodeling cycle is rapid, occurring over weeks, whereas the bone-building phase of the cycle is much slower, occurring over months. If osteoblastic activity fails to keep pace with osteoclastic activity during each remodeling cycle, a net loss of bone mineral occurs.
      2. **Osteoporosis** may develop as a result of inadequate formation of bone and/or accelerated bone losses associated with increased age, because of age-related impairment of osteoblasts or their precursors, and because of decreased estrogen production.
      3. Osteoporosis represents loss of bone, both in actual bone lost and loss of structural "scaffolding" necessary for support. The disruption of the scaffolding weakens the bone support structure to a greater extent than the amount of bone lost.
   B. **Peak bone mass**
      1. Peak bone mass is defined as the maximal amount of bone that an individual will attain. Bone mass increases during childhood and adolescence and peaks between 20 and 30 years. Theoretically, each person is genetically programmed to reach an optimal peak bone mass under ideal conditions. The actual peak bone mass attained is influenced by age, gender, genetic factors, hormonal status, exercise, and calcium intake.
      2. Bone loss occurs during the normal aging process but is accelerated in women not treated with estrogens during the menopause.
      3. The higher the peak bone mass, the longer it may take for age-related and menopause-related bone losses to increase the risk of fracture. Adolescents with average nutritional calcium intakes **less than** 1,000 mg per day for boys and 850 mg per day for girls will probably **not reach optimal bone mass.**

4. Even with optimum peak bone mass, the rate of bone loss later in life strongly affects fracture risk. In the first 5 years after menopause, women lose bone at an annual rate of 1% to 5%.

C. Menopause
1. Cessation of ovarian function and a time of accelerated bone mass loss.
    a. One in three women will sustain a vertebral fracture after age 65.
    b. One in three women will suffer a hip fracture by age 90.

D. Risk factors. Table 26.1 lists risk factors.

III. Clinical presentation
A. Trabecular bone is affected more than cortical bone. The most common early osteoporotic fracture is vertebral.
B. Most common fracture sites are vertebrae, distal radius, and femoral neck.

IV. Diagnosis
A. **Bone mass assessment** appears to be the best method for detecting asymptomatic individuals at risk of fracture. Bone mass is assessed by measuring BMD. Standard radiography is not an acceptable method for determining early or mild bone loss. It may only be helpful for noting severe loss.

B. **Radiologic techniques**
1. **Bone mineral densitometry** is a useful technique for predicting the risk of fracture. BMD measurements are approved under Medicare guidelines.
2. Densitometry instruments.
    a. **Dual-energy x-ray absorptiometry (DXA)/peripheral DXA (pDXA): DXA generally denotes a central DXA measuring the spine and/or hip. It is currently the "gold standard" because it is the most precise and requires the lowest dose of radiation.**
    b. Single-energy x-ray absorptiometry.
    c. Radiographic absorptiometry of the phalanges.
    d. Quantitative computed tomography and peripheral quantitative computed tomography.
    e. Ultrasound of the calcaneus.

C. **Application and interpretation of densitometry (central DXA)**
1. **The Z-score** describes patient's bone mass compared with age and sex-matched mean, reported in SD from this curve (Fig. 26.1). This **cannot** be used to diagnose or confirm osteoporosis. It may be useful to determine secondary etiologies for bone loss.
2. **The T-score** describes the patient's bone mass compared with mean peak bone mass of a young adult reference population. This is reported in SD from this curve (Fig. 26.2). This is a **clinically relevant score** because it can be used to diagnose or confirm osteoporosis. BMD is the most important determinant of fracture risk and fracture risk approximately doubles for each SD by which this density is less than peak adult bone mass at age 20 to 45 years (Table 26.2).

D. **Indications for bone mass measurements**
1. Estrogen-deficient women (determine therapy).
2. Vertebral abnormalities or osteopenia on x-ray film (establish baseline bone loss).
3. Chronic corticosteroids (dose adjustments/determine therapy).
4. Asymptomatic primary hyperparathryoidism (determine therapy).
5. Treatment of established osteoporosis (assess interventions).
6. Table 26.3 lists BMD measurement guidelines and Table 26.4 discusses the Bone Mass Measurement Act.

E. **Densitometry conclusion.** Using the T-score number alone **does not predict who will develop fractures.** It can only predict risk. There is a wide overlap in bone densities of patients who suffer a fracture and those who do not. **Widespread screening is *not* standard of care and not recommended.** Fractures, however, do predict future fractures and these higher risk patients warrant BMD testing and intervention. For future assessment of intervention, central DXA is recommended.

Table 26.1. Risk factors for osteoporosis

Intrinsic risk factors (Non-modifiable)	Modifiable risk factors
Increasing age, female gender	Estrogen deficiency states
Caucasian or Asian ethnic background	Thin body habitus, low body weight
Personal history of low-trauma fracture	(<127 lbs)
Family history of osteoporosis-related fractures	Current cigarette smoking, excess alcohol and caffeine intake
Impaired eyesight despite adequate correction	Reduced calcium intake, dietary practices
Dementia and poor health/frailty	Sedentary lifestyle
	Falls (impaired eyesight, balance)
	Medications: corticosteroids, thyroid medications, anticonvulsants, heparin, cyclosporine
	Medical conditions: chronic renal failure, hyperparathyroidism, Cushing's, hyperthyroidism, hyperprolactinemia
	Poor health/frailty

Adapted from National Osteoporosis Foundation. *Physician's Guide to Prevention and Treatment of Osteoporosis*, 1998, 1999.

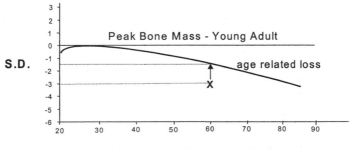

60-year old patient with Z-score= -1.5

FIG. 26.1. The Z-score. Based on the Bone Mineral Density (BMD) measured, a Z-score is calculated and reported in standard deviations (S.D.) above (positive) or below (negative) the age-matched and sex-matched mean age-related bone loss curve. Thus the individual 60-year-old female patient demonstrated here is compared to other 60-year-old females. A Z-score that is normal or falls on the curve is still consistent with age-related bone loss. However, this patient demonstrates 1.5 standard deviation below the curve, indicating that she may have further bone losses than predicted simply by age-related losses. A Z-score greater than −1.0 suggests that secondary causes of bone loss should be considered.

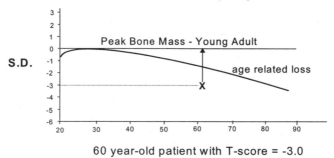

60 year-old patient with T-score = -3.0

FIG. 26.2. The T-score. Based on the Bone Mineral Density (BMD) measured, a T-score is calculated and reported in standard deviations (S.D.) above (positive) or below (negative) the sex-matched, peak bone mass (PBM) of the young adult reference population. That T-score along with the absolute BMD are the clinically relevant data that can be used to diagnose or confirm osteoporosis. The T-score and absolute BMD can be used to determine increases in BMD over time with intervention. This 60-year old patient has a calculated T-score of –3.0, which is consistent with osteoporosis.

    F. Biochemical markers
        1. Used as an index of bone remodeling and resorption. Biochemical markers cannot be used for the diagnosis of osteoporosis and they are not widely clinically used yet.
            a. Potential uses of biochemical markers: assess rate of bone turnover before beginning therapy and monitor effects of treatment.
            b. Limitations: provide no data about intensity or duration of bone loss, BMD, or fracture risk. Cannot be used for the diagnosis or confirmation of osteoporosis (too much variation in any population and within the individual patient).
V. Osteoporosis management
    A. Primary goal of osteoporosis management is prevention.
        1. Education and assessment of the osteoporosis risk.
        2. Achieve and maintain optimal bone mass via
            a. Diet (adequate nutrition and caloric intake).
            b. Calcium intake.

Table 26.2. Interpreting bone mass densitometry

Diagnostic Categories	T - Scores
Normal	Less than 1 S.D. below mean peak bone mass (PBM)
Osteopenia (low bone mass)	More than 1 S.D. but less than 2.5 S.D. below mean PBM
Osteoporosis	A value 2.5 S.D. or more below the mean PBM
Severe osteoporosis (established)	Osteoporosis with one or more fragility fractures

Table 26.3. National Osteoporosis Foundation guidelines for BMD measurement

- All postmenopausal women younger than 65 years and with ≥ 1 risk factor for fracture (other than menopause)
- All women aged 65 years or older
- Postmenopausal women with fracture
- Women considering therapy for osteoporosis (when BMD testing would facilitate the decision)
- Women taking a prolonged course of HRT
- Patient's taking glucocorticoid therapy for >2 months
- All patients at high risk for osteoporotic fracture

National Osteoporosis Foundation.
Physician's Guide to Prevention and Treatment of Osteoporosis, 1998, 1999.
(*Patients who might also benefit from BMD testing:* patients with height loss > 1½ inches)

        c. Weight-bearing exercise (walking, jogging, rowing, weight lifting, and bicycling).
        d. Use of hormone replacement therapy (HRT) (estrogen).
        e. Bisphosphonates and selective estrogen receptor modulators (SERMs) prevention indications.
    3. Avoid adverse influences.
        a. Smoking.
        b. Medications.
        c. Limit alcohol and caffeine consumption.
  B. Therapeutic approaches
    1. Therapy can be nonpharmacologic and/or pharmacologic.
    2. Goals of therapy.
        a. Increase or maintain bone mass.
        b. Stop or reverse bone loss by inhibiting bone resorption and/or stimulating bone formation.
        c. Reduce the incidence of osteoporotic fractures and resultant pain, deformity, disability, and mortality.
  C. Nonpharmacologic therapy and universal recommendations
    1. Adequate calcium and vitamin D intake.
    2. Regular weight-bearing exercise.
    3. Avoidance of tobacco and excessive alcohol.
    4. Adequate visual correction.
    5. Assessment and interventions to reduce risk of falls.
  D. Pharmacologic therapy. The National Osteoporosis Foundation **recommends initiating therapy to reduce fracture risk when BMD T-scores are:**

Table 26.4. BMMA (Bone Mass Measurement Act)–1998

Medicare reimbursement for FDA-approved BMD tests

QUALIFICATIONS
Estrogen deficient women at clinical risk for osteoporosis
Individuals being monitored to assess the response or efficacy of an approved osteoporosis drug therapy

CRITERIA FOR REIMBURSEMENT
BMD needs to be ordered by treating clinician
Testing once every 2 years
Any Medicare plan, including managed care

BMD, bone mineral density.

- Below −2.0 in women with no risk factors.
- Below −1.5 in women with risk factors.
- Women older than 70 years who have multiple risk factors (especially previous nonhip, nonspine fractures), even without BMD testing.

1. Calcium.
   a. Enhances bone formation.
   b. Helps maintain bone mass.
   c. Is best when obtained from dietary sources.
   d. Is adjunctive (not sole) therapy for osteoporosis.
      (1) Calcium and vitamin D may reduce fractures (up to 30%) but to a lesser degree than other pharmacologic agents (4,5).
      (2) Most clinical studies of osteoporosis therapy compare active treatment (e.g., estrogen, bisphosphonate, or calcitonin) with calcium and vitamin D, which would not be considered a placebo.
   e. Therapy.
      (1) Minimum 1,000 to 1,200 mg per day, diet should be supplemented to ensure adequate intake in adults.
      (2) In the event that no dietary calcium is ingested, then 1,500 mg per day is the recommended dose.

2. Vitamin D.
   a. Required for optimal calcium absorption.
   b. May aid bone formation and reduce fracture risk.
   c. Deficiencies often seen in older adults secondary to decreased sunlight exposure.
   d. Aging renders the kidney less able to convert vitamin D to its active form and the gastrointestinal (GI) tract more resistant to the actions of vitamin D.
   e. Minimum supplementation in multivitamins.
   f. Therapy. Optimal daily dose must be determined for each patient. Adults typically should receive 400 IU/day; older patients should receive 800 IU/day.

3. Estrogen replacement therapy.
   a. Inhibits bone resorption via high-affinity receptors, decreases urinary calcium loss, and increases intestinal calcium absorption.
   b. Epidemiologic and observational studies show reduction in the accelerated bone loss attributed to menopause.
   c. HRT is first-line therapy for prevention of osteoporosis and remains the gold standard.
   d. Observational studies indicate 50% fracture risk reduction.
   e. BMD increases approximately 2% to 8%.
   f. Therapy. Prevention: various options.
      (1) Conjugated estrogen (Premarin) 0.625 mg per day.
      (2) Micronized estradiol (Estrace) 1.0 mg.
      (3) Piperazine estrone sulfate (Ogen) 0.625 mg per day.
      (4) Transdermal estradiol (Estraderm) 0.05 mg per day.
      (5) Some studies show lower doses of estrogen (0.3 mg conjugated estrogen) when combined with calcium supplements may be effective for prevention of osteoporosis (6).

4. Bisphosphonates are absorbed onto newly synthesized bone matrix; bind strongly to hydroxyapatite crystals; prevent bone resorption via interference with the action of the bone-resorbing cell, the osteoclast; have high affinity for the target organ (bone); and are not taken up in significant quantities by any other organs. What is not taken up by bone is excreted unchanged in the urine. They have an extremely long half-life in bone and are not well absorbed from the GI tract, with absorption rates of 1% or less being common.
   a. Etidronate (Didronel, first-generation bisphosphonate) has been demonstrated to be beneficial in postmenopausal women with osteoporosis. A study of women over a 2- to 3-year treatment period showed increased bone mass and a reduction in fracture incidence.

       (1) A cyclic regimen is used secondary to concern for inhibition of bone formation and demineralization: Take 2 weeks then stop for 3 to 4 months. During the time off etidronate, only calcium and vitamin D are taken.

       (2) It is **not Food and Drug Administration (FDA) approved** for general therapy of osteoporosis although it has been widely used and studied in the United States for more than 5 years.

   b. Oral bisphosphonate is an acceptable first-line therapy for prevention and treatment of osteoporosis. It may be used as an **alternative to estrogen.** It is **not recommended as an alternative** to estrogen therapy in women with **normal bone mass unless risk factors are significant or the patient is intolerant of HRT.** It may be combined with HRT. It is a bone-specific drug that accumulates in bone over time. It is not associated with impairment in mineralization even at high doses. It is well-tolerated and GI side effects (epigastric or abdominal pain, nausea, diarrhea, or the development of erosions or ulcer) are most commonly reported.

   c. Alendronate (Fosamax, "second-generation" bisphosphonate).

       (1) FDA approved for prevention and treatment of osteoporosis.

       (2) Greater than 50% reduction in vertebral fractures and greater than 50% reduction in nonvertebral fractures with 5 years of use (7).

       (3) Increases BMD 2% to 8%.

       (4) Therapy.

          (a) The dosage is 10 mg per day on an empty stomach with 6 to 8 oz of water, 30 minutes before eating, drinking, or taking medicine. Patients should avoid supine position for 30 minutes to avoid increased risk of chemical esophagitis or gastric and duodenal ulcers. Intolerant patients may use 5 mg per day.

          (b) An alternative regimen is 70 mg 1 day per week. Prevention: 5 mg per day.

   d. Risedronate (Actonel, "third generation" bisphosphonate).

       (1) FDA approved for prevention and treatment of osteoporosis.

       (2) Potential advantages: possible reduction in adverse GI events and improved tolerability and increased potency; nevertheless, same dosing instructions as other available oral bisphosphonates.

       (3) Vertebral fracture risk reduction is approximately 50%.

       (4) Nonvertebral fracture risk reduction is approximately 36%.

       (5) Hip fracture risk reduction is approximately 40%.

       (6) Increased BMD 5% to 7% at spine and hip.

       (7) Therapy. Treatment and prevention: 5 mg per day.

5. Calcitonins.

   a. Inhibit bone resorption by inhibiting osteoclast function.

   b. FDA approved for therapy of postmenopausal (>5 years) osteoporosis.

   c. Efficacy data for calcitonin are weaker than for either HRT or bisphosphonates. Clinical trials indicate calcitonin may decrease osteoporotic vertebral fractures by approximately 36%; however, hip fracture data are limited (8,9).

   d. Increases spine BMD 1% over 5 years.

   e. Calcitonin is an alternative to HRT or bisphosphonate therapy in patients **unwilling** or **unable** to **tolerate either therapy.**

   f. Helpful for patients with acute osteoporotic vertebral fracture (short-term) secondary to potent analgesic properties (10).

   g. Therapy. Subcutaneous (SQ/IM) and intranasal dosage forms available. The **minimum effective dose has not** been **established;** however, 100 IU SQ/IM every other day may preserve vertebral BMD. The intranasal dose is one spray, 200 IU per day, alternating nostrils daily.

6. SERMs.
   a. Clinical response is based on differential tissue effects via binding to estrogen receptors, modeled after the antiestrogen prototype, tamoxifen.
   b. Potential advantages.
      (1) Improved serum lipid levels and reduced risk of cardiovascular disease (not proven).
      (2) Improved BMD and reduced risk of fracture.
      (3) Less impact on breast cancer than estrogen; less impact on uterine cancer than estrogen (except tamoxifen).
      (4) Maintenance of pelvic muscles and support structures (not proven).
      (5) Possible reduction in the risk of Alzheimer's disease (not proven).
   c. Potential disadvantages.
      (1) Increased incidence of thromboembolic events (especially in bedridden patients).
      (2) Exacerbation of hot flushes (cannot be used to treat menopausal symptoms).
7. Raloxifene (Evista).
   a. Action is via inhibition of bone resorption.
   b. FDA approved for postmenopausal osteoporosis prevention and treatment.
   c. Two-year data demonstrates approximately 40% reduction in the risk of vertebral fracture in patients with osteoporosis (MORE interim analysis). Hip fracture data is not available although data indicate reduced bone loss and increased BMD at the hip (11).
   d. Increases BMD approximately 3%.
   e. Therapy: 60 mg per day.
8. Agents to stimulate bone formation, unproved agents not FDA approved.
   a. Fluoride.
   b. Tamoxifen.
   c. Androgens.
   d. Parathyroid hormone.

VI. Corticosteroid-induced osteoporosis (CIO)

A. Glucocorticosteroids are the **most common cause** of **drug-related** (secondary) **osteoporosis** (12).
   1. Rapid bone loss occurs during the first 6 months of steroid use and continues with ongoing use.
   2. The majority of patients receiving long-term glucocorticoid therapy demonstrate reductions in BMD and 25% to 40% suffer osteoporotic fractures (13,14).
   3. Trabecular bone is affected to a greater degree than cortical bone, so the most common early fracture is vertebral.
   4. Patients with inflammatory conditions may have contributing factors for osteoporosis (concomitant drug therapy or the underlying condition; e.g., rheumatoid arthritis).

B. Pathophysiology
   1. Corticosteroids have a large impact on bone because of multiple effects on other organ systems.
      a. Inhibits vitamin D at the intestine and interferes with efficient calcium absorption.
      b. Affects the renal tubule and cause a calcium leak (reduced reabsorption of calcium, increased urinary calcium excretion).
      c. Inhibits gonadal function and may directly inhibit osteoblast function and recruitment so that new bone formation is inhibited.
   2. Secondary hyperparathyroid state, which leads to increased bone losses, may be induced in part as a result of the negative calcium balance.

C. **Assessment** and **treatment** of patients **requiring steroids**
1. **Obtain baseline** DXA (BMD) of the spine and hip (expect trabecular bone losses early and so many health care plans suggest a screening study of the spine only. However, sites may be discordant so both spine and hip should be assessed).
   a. Evaluate gonadal function; HRT for women or testosterone for men if deficient.
2. **Evaluate 24-hour urinary calcium excretion** and add calcium, vitamin D, or thiazide as needed to maintain adequate calcium balance.
3. **Add bisphosphonates or calcitonin if hormones are contraindicated** or bone loss continues on serial DXA.

VII. **Summary**
A. Osteoporosis affects a large and rapidly expanding portion of an aging U.S. population. Osteoporosis-associated fractures can cause pain, deformity, disability, and death.
B. Currently, HRT and the newer bisphosphonates are the first-line therapies based on clear evidence of increased bone mass and decreased fracture incidence.
1. **HRT is primarily for preventing osteoporosis** and **maintaining bone mass.**
2. **Bisphosphonates,** in particular, are for **therapy** in the **postmenopausal woman with osteoporosis** and are also **an alternative (preventive) in patients who cannot or should not take HRT or have increased risk and CIO.**
3. **SERMS** are an **alternative for patients who are not candidates for HRT** or a **bisphosphonate.**

Bibliography

American College of Rheumatology Task Force on Osteoporosis Guidelines. *Arthritis Rheum* 1996;39:1791–1801.

Black DM, et al. Randomized trial of effect of alendronate on risk of fracture in women with existing vertebral fractures. Fracture Intervention Trial Research Group. *Lancet* 1996;348:1535–1541.

Consensus Development Conference: Diagnosis, prophylaxis, and treatment of osteoporosis. *Am J Med* 1993;94:646–651.

Cumming RG, et al. Calcium for prevention of osteoporotic fractures in postmenopausal women. *J Bone Miner Res* 1997;12:1321–1329.

Davis MC, et al. Bone mineral loss in young women with amenorrhea. *Br Med J* 1990; 301:790–793.

Dawson-Hughes B, et al. A controlled trial of the effect of calcium supplementation on bone density in postmenopausal women. *N Engl J Med* 1990;323:878–883.

Dawson-Hughes B, et al. Effect of calcium and vitamin D supplementation on bone density in men and women over 65 years of age or older. *N Engl J Med* 1997;337:670–676.

Delmas PD, et al. Effects of raloxifene on bone mineral density, serum cholesterol concentrations, and uterine endometrium in postmenopausal women. *N Engl J Med* 1997;337:1641–1647.

Lukert BP, et al. Glucocorticoid-induced osteoporosis pathogenesis and management. *Ann Int Med* 1990;112:352–364.

Lyritis GP, et al. Analgesic effect of salmon calcitonin in osteoporotic vertebral fractures: a double-blind placebo-controlled clinical study. *Calcif Tissue Int* 1991;49:369–372.

National Osteoporosis Foundation. *Physician's guide to prevention and treatment of osteoporosis.* 1998.

Nelson DA, et al. Prevalence of osteoporosis in women referred for bone density testing: utility of multiple skeletal sites. *J Clin Densitometry* 1998;1:5–11.

Overgaard K, et al. Effect of calcitonin given intranasally on bone mass and fracture rates in established osteoporosis: a dose-response study. *BMJ* 1992;305:556–561.

Prince RL, et al. Prevention of postmenopausal osteoporosis: a comparative study of exercise, calcium supplementation, and hormone-replacement therapy. *N Engl J Med* 1991;325:1189–1195.

Pun KK, et al. Analgesic effect of intranasal salmon calcitonin in the treatment of osteoporotic vertebral fractures. *Clin Ther* 1989;11:205–209.

Ray NF, et al. Medial expenditure for the treatment of osteoporotic fractures in the United States in 1995: report from the National Osteoporosis Foundation. *J Bone Miner Res* 1997;12:24–35.

Sagg KG, et al. Low-dose long-term corticosteroid therapy in rheumatoid arthritis: an analysis of serious adverse events. *Am J Med* 1994;96:115–123.

Stock JL, et al. Calcitonin-salmon nasal spray reduces the incidence of new vertebral fractures in postmenopausal women: 3-year and 4-year interim results of the PROOF study. *J Bone Miner Res* 1997;12[Suppl]:S149.

References

1. National Osteoporosis Foundation. *Physician's Guide to Prevention and Treatment of Osteoporosis.* 1998.
   Nelson DA, et al. Prevalence of osteoporosis in women referred for bone density testing: utility of multiple skeletal sites. *J Clin Densitometry* 1998;1:5–11.
2. Consensus Development Conference: diagnosis, prophylaxis and treatment of osteoporosis. *Am J Med* 1993;94:646–651.
3. World Health Organization. Assessment of fracture risk and its application to screening for postmenopausal osteoporosis. Report of WHO Study Group. *World Health Organ Tech Rep Ser* 1994;843:1–129.
4. Dawson-Hughes B, et al. Effect of calcium and vitamin D supplementation on bone density in men and women over 65 years of age or older. *N Engl J Med* 1997;337:670–676.
5. Cumming RG, et al. Calcium for prevention of osteoporotic fractures in postmenopausal women. *J Bone Miner Res* 1997;12:1321–1329.
6. Ettinger B, Genant HK, Cann CE. Postmenopausal bone loss is prevented by treatment with low dosage estrogen with calcium. *Ann Intern Med* 1987;106:40.
7. Black DM, et al. Randomized trial of effect of alendronate on risk of fracture in women with existing vertebral fractures. Fracture Intervention Trial Research Group. *Lancet* 1996;348:1535–1541.
8. Stock JL, et al. Calcitonin-salmon nasal spray reduces the incidence of new vertebral fractures in postmenopausal women: 3-year and 4-year interim results of the PROOF study. *J Bone Miner Res* 1997;12[Suppl]:S149.
9. Overgaard K, et al. Effect of calcitonin given intranasally on bone mass and fracture rates in established osteoporosis: a dose-response study. *BMJ* 1992;305:556–561.
10. Lyritis GP, et al. Analgesic effect of salmon calcitonin in osteoporotic vertebral fractures: a double-blind placebo-controlled clinical study. *Calcif Tissue Int* 1991;49:369–372.
11. Delmas PD, et al. Effects of raloxifene on bone mineral density, serum cholesterol concentrations, and uterine endometrium in postmenopausal women. *N Engl J Med* 1997;337:1641–1647.
12. American College of Rheumatology Task Force on Osteoporosis Guidelines. *Arthritis Rheum* 1996;39:1791–1801.
13. Lukert BP, et al. Glucocorticoid-induced osteoporosis pathogenesis and management. *Ann Int Med* 1990;112:352–364.
14. Sagg KG, et al. Low dose long-term corticosteroid therapy in rheumatoid arthritis: an analysis of serious adverse events. *Am J Med* 1994;96:115–123.

27. EVALUATION OF SEXUAL DYSFUNCTION

Michel E. Rivlin

I. **Introduction.** Sexual desire is one of the three elements basic to being human, along with the body and the mind. The range of problems, including physical or emotional, that may affect sexual function is enormous. The general concept of a sexual dysfunction is **any impaired, incomplete, or abnormal functioning in the human sexual response.** The human sexual response includes the phases of desire, excitement, plateau, orgasm, and resolution.

A. **Incidence.** Data are incomplete but overall prevalence of sexual dysfunction is estimated to be about 15% to 30% of all women. Disorders of desire (libido) occur in about 31% of couples presenting to clinics, and arousal disorders occur in about 14% to 48% of couples in community studies. Orgasmic disorders are probably the most common, with primary anorgasmia in about 10% of women and secondary anorgasmia in from 65% to 80% in community studies.

B. **Physiology of the sexual response cycle. Dysfunctional problems** are divided into two categories: **disorders of desire (libido) and disorders of excitement and orgasm. Disorders of desire** tend to be a **neural phenomenon and disorders of excitement** tend to **involve** the **genital organs.**

  1. Sexual desire appears to be part of the brain system responsible for emotion and reproduction. There appears to be an excitatory center that is dopamine sensitive and is in balance with an inhibitory center that is serotonin sensitive.

    a. During the **excitement phase** there is **genital vascular engorgement and increased muscular tension.**

      (1) **Vasocongestion** results in vaginal lubrication and clitoral tumescence owing to fluid transudation.

      (2) This phase is primarily **parasympathetic** with **afferent fibers** from the **clitoris** and **labia** and **efferent fibers** from the **pelvic nerve.**

      (3) Marked **extragenital reactions include:**

        (a) Tachycardia.

        (b) Tachypnea.

        (c) Increased blood pressure.

        (d) Sex flush.

    b. In the orgasmic phase, uterine contractions occur and the pelvic muscles undergo a series of reflex clonic contractions.

      (1) **Orgasm** is primarily under **sympathetic control** with afferents from the labia and clitoris and efferents through the pelvic plexuses and the pudendal nerve to striated muscles.

      (2) The **spinal centers** involved are **T11** through **L2** for the **sympathetic nerves** and **S2** to **S4** for the **parasympathetic** and **pudendal nerves.**

    c. The sexual response **cycle ends** with the **phase** of **resolution.**

      (1) Women have no refractory period, may be multiorgasmic, and commonly reach orgasm slowly.

      (2) **Individual preference** seems to be the only difference between a vaginal or clitoral orgasm.

  2. **Physiologic factors that can influence sexual response.**

    a. **Pregnancy.** Frequency of sexual activity in pregnancy is reported to decrease during the first trimester, increase during the second, and markedly decrease during the third trimester. In general, although sexual interest may wax and wane during the pregnancy, the **desire**

275

for **affection, support,** and **physical closeness is increased** and is **vitally important.**

- **b. Age.** The aging process affects the entire body and **sexual desire** is among the **last** functions to **decline.** Men reach their sexual peaks in late adolescence, whereas female peaks are reached in the late 30s.
  - (1) **Postmenopausal changes** in the vagina include **epithelial atrophy, decreased lubrication, reduced elasticity,** and **outlet narrowing.**
  - (2) These changes may **increase susceptibility** to **vaginitis** and **dyspareunia.**
  - (3) All these **changes** may be **prevented** or **reversed,** to a major degree, by **estrogen replacement.**

C. Sexual history. Sexual function is as much a system as the cardiovascular or the gastrointestinal system. A clinician who does not include the sexual data in the general medical history with a new patient may be missing vital information in the database, which affects the diagnosis, the management, and the physical well-being of the patient.

Sexual problems play a role in many physical situations that present in medical practice, such as endocrine disorders, neurologic impairment, cardiovascular disorders, local genital pathology, the effects of surgical change, and side effects of medication particularly the central nervous system (CNS) depressants, anticholinergics, and antiadrenergics. **Psychological situations can also cause physical changes that result in sexual problems,** such as anxiety, depression, substance abuse, and stress.

1. **For purposes of screening, a brief approach during the general history taking** can provide the following information:
   - a. Whether there are **any major difficulties requiring further in-depth investigation** and **treatment** or **any minor problems that may develop into major dysfunctions and need correction.**
   - b. **If a dysfunction is discovered,** information to enable the clinician to decide whether the treatment can be handled by the physician or referred for more intensive therapy.
   - c. Correction of **misconceptions** and **education** of the patient.
   - d. **If a serious dysfunction is discovered,** it should be noted and deferred to another visit when an in-depth history can be taken. Even if a serious problem is found, the **rest of the screening history should be completed** since the discovery of major sexual problems is only one aspect of the screening history.
2. **Interviewing techniques.** How to conduct the sexual history depends on the preference of the physician and the circumstances of the patient's visit.
   - a. It is important to establish a **comfortable situation** in which the anxiety of both the physician and the patient is at its lowest.
   - b. The most important and helpful personal attributes for the clinician are a full recognition that gathering sexual data is as much a **professional obligation** as is gathering cardiovascular information, **a good preparation and training in human sexuality,** a **nonjudgmental and open-minded attitude** toward sexuality, an **awareness of one's own values and views about sex** while cognizant of other people's belief systems, and an **empathetic understanding** of others.
   - c. Sexual questions can be introduced anywhere in the history. However, in the course of the **urologic or gynecologic history, sexual topics seem to fit naturally.** The patient can be put at ease with opening comments from the physician that make an assumption of normality, such as "Many people experience . . ." or "When did you . . ." rather than "Did you ever . . ."
3. **Historic data.** At a minimum, the clinician should **ask the patient directly** whether a sexual dysfunction exists.

a. **The screening history for a sexual dysfunction should determine:**
   (1) **Date of onset.**
   (2) **Severity.**
   (3) **Whether there are multiple problems.**
   (4) **Whether the partner has a problem.**
   (5) **Severity of relationship discord.**
   (6) **Whether there has been any psychiatric treatment or counseling** for problems of sexual functioning, interpersonal relationships, or other related problems and, if so, the **outcome of the treatment.**
b. A suggested list of **problem areas,** citing the **least anxiety-provoking first,** includes:
   (1) **Frequency or timing of sexual relations.**
   (2) **Varieties of sexual activity.**
   (3) **Initiation and refusal of sexual advances.**
   (4) **Defining what is normal in sexual relations.**
   (5) **Myths about sex or lack of information.**
   (6) **Effects of medical conditions on sexuality.**
   (7) **Sexual outlets for persons living without sexual partners.**
   (8) **Children and sexuality—their own and that of adults.**
   (9) **Parents and adolescent sexuality.**
   (10) **Adolescents and adolescent sexuality.**
   (11) **Effects of aging on sexuality.**
   (12) **Anxiety and guilt about sexual activities.**
   (13) **Sexual dysfunctions.**
   (14) **Sexual deviations.**
c. A sexual history must **include** data pertaining to **diseases** and **drugs** that can interfere with sexual function.
   (1) **Chronic diseases** that can **influence sexual responses** include
      (a) **Diabetes.**
      (b) **Chronic renal failure.**
      (c) **Cardiac disease.**
      (d) **Respiratory diseases.**
      (e) **Arthritis.**
      (f) **Alcoholism.**
   (2) Many commonly used **drugs** can **interfere** with **sexual function,** especially those affecting the autonomic system and CNS and those that can elevate prolactin levels. These include:
      (a) **Antihypertensives.**
      (b) **Antidepressants.**
      (c) **Antipsychotics.**
      (d) **Sedatives.**
      (e) **Alcohol.**
      (f) **Narcotics.**
      (g) **Androgen antagonists.**
d. **If there are no previously identified problems such as the ones listed previously, then a more in-depth history should be taken to rule out organicity.** This allows a more informed decision as to whether referral or office treatment is appropriate, and the arrangement for a problem-oriented history should be made at the end of the screening history.

II. **Female sexual dysfunctions**
   A. **Anorgasmia** is the **inability to achieve orgasm.** Anatomic, circumstantial, and individual data have suggested that orgasm resulting from direct clitoral stimulation, such as masturbation and manual, oral, or mechanical stimulation of the clitoris, may be more intense than indirect stimulation by coitus. Thus, the determination of whether a pathologic condition such as anorgasmia actually exists depends on a **careful history of sexual prac-**

tices. The fact that a woman is anorgasmic during intercourse may not necessarily classify her as having a dysfunction until further exploration.

1. The classifications for anorgasmia may be categorized as follows (6):
    a. **Primary anorgasmia** is defined as the condition of a woman who has **never had an orgasmic experience under any circumstances.** It has been estimated that anywhere from 8% to 15% of women in the United States have never experienced orgasm.
    b. **Secondary anorgasmia** occurs when a woman has had at least one orgasmic experience, regardless of whether it was self-induced or partner-induced, induced by vaginal or rectal intercourse, or induced by oral-genital exchange. Secondary anorgasmia is situational, for which a woman can achieve **orgasm only under certain circumstances** such as by masturbation alone, by coitus alone, only at night, or while on vacation but not in the home.
2. **Etiologies.**
    a. **Organic factors** responsible for anorgasmia include any cause for dyspareunia, local genital or other pelvic pathologic processes, trauma, postsurgical conditions that produce discomfort, spinal cord injury, endocrinopathies, systemic diseases associated with pain, drugs affecting the CNS, infection, and pregnancy.
    b. **Psychological factors** include the historical antecedents that result in sexual inhibition such as poor parental role models, a negative self-concept, a restrictive home environment (e.g., sex was rarely mentioned or was associated with dirt, sin, anxiety, guilt, shame, and punishment; there was little nudity around the house), and a disturbed relationship or an absence of open affection between the parents.
    c. **Individual factors** that affect orgasm include fear of sexual intimacy or guilt, a poor relationship with the partner (e.g., indifference, poor communication, lack of trust, anger, or hostility), distractions, depression, and grief. Misinformation and ignorance of anatomy and physiology of orgasmic functioning are common.
3. **Management. Primary orgasmic dysfunction** often responds successfully to treatment. Two programs have been devised. Both have in common the technique of **desensitizing the woman in sexual situations to free her from anxiety and guilt while simultaneously developing and enhancing her sexual excitement and pleasure.** The specific focus is in learning what is pleasurable (sensate focus) and how to self-stimulate so that she is able to arrive at orgasm as well as communicate and share the experience with a partner after having learned it herself.

B. **Vaginismus** is an **involuntary reflex resulting in spastic contraction of the vaginal outlet** stimulated by imagined, anticipated, or real attempts at vaginal penetration. Vaginismus is a **psychophysiologic syndrome** affecting all components of the pelvic musculature of the perineum and outer third of the vagina. The diagnosis can be made only through physical examination and observation of the pelvic response, ruling out the presence of pelvic disorders. Patients **rarely complain of vaginismus directly.**

1. **Primary vaginismus** occurs if the reaction has **onset at the patient's first coital attempt.** She may have an unconsummated marriage or may present with the problem of infertility or other somatic complaint such as abdominal discomfort or respiratory or gastrointestinal difficulty.
2. **Secondary vaginismus** is vaginismus that has its **onset after a history of successful intercourse.** It may be a conditioned response to a negative stimulus such as local pathology and **can remain even after the pathologic process has been resolved.**
3. **Management of vaginismus includes assisting the woman in accepting the penetration of the introitus by introducing dilators with graduated diameters** until the vaginal vault can expand to accommodate an erect penis.

      a. This cannot be done effectively without a **clear understanding of the patient's fears** regarding sexual intercourse and her earlier negative conditioning, **which may include childhood abuse.**

      b. **Common fears associated with the vagina** are those of veneral disease, pregnancy, discomfort, and punishment. Ignorance, misinformation, and guilt reinforce the reflex and **must be resolved in addition to the physical exercise of dilation.**

C. **Dyspareunia** is painful intercourse. Conditions that result in painful coitus are multiple. The variety of subjective and objective factors that give rise to the psychophysiologic distress of pain before or after intercourse makes diagnosis difficult. Etiologies range from postcoital vaginal irritation to immobilizing abdominal pain.

    Unless a **careful history and pelvic and rectal examinations** are done, a diagnosis of dyspareunia cannot be made. There are positive pelvic and rectal findings that can and do objectively support the subjective complaint of coital discomfort.

    1. Etiology. The major sources of pelvic pathologic processes that contribute to dyspareunia are the following:

      a. **Disorders of the vaginal outlet** include postmenopausal atrophy and decreased lubrication, hymenal presence, episiotomy scars, infections, trauma, adhesions, and clitoral irritation.

      b. **Disorders of the vagina** include infection, decreased lubrication, pelvic relaxation resulting in rectocele, uterine prolapse, or cystocele, inflammatory or allergic response to foreign substances (e.g., douche products, suppositories, creams, perfumes), foreshortened vault resulting from surgery or radiation, and congenital malformations.

      c. **Disorders of the pelvic structures** include pelvic inflammatory disease, endometriosis, benign or malignant tumors of the uterus, ovarian pathology, pelvic adhesions secondary to abdominal surgery, disorders of the gastrointestinal and renal systems (e.g., inflammatory bowel disease, Crohn's disease, diverticulitis, or fistulas), and ureteral or bladder pathology.

    2. Management. The basic approach to dyspareunia is to **treat the discoverable disorder causing the complaint.** If a woman presents with a problem of painful intercourse, accept the complaint at face value and take the steps to identify the anatomic and physiologic source of the problem.

      a. **If the etiologic cause is treated, the discomfort is likely to be relieved.**

      b. However, with some problems, such as pelvic adhesions where **further treatment may not be feasible,** an **explanation of the cause of the pain** can be helpful. This reassures the patient and allays the fear and anxiety that something is seriously wrong. Furthermore, adaptation to the situation by **changes in sexual techniques may be helpful** and allow the patient access to sexual functioning with a lesser degree of discomfort.

      c. If the patient **continues to suffer sexual maladaptation** following a thorough workup to rule out treatable organic disease, a **referral for sexual** or **psychological** (or both) evaluation and treatment may be indicated.

      d. For a more thorough discussion on this problem, see Chapter 15.

D. **Disorders of desire** are defined as the **loss or absence of sexual desire or drive.**

    1. Definitions. Sexual desire (sex drive, libido) is defined as the **frequency or intensity with which one desires to participate in sexual activity** and is a function of both organic and psychological factors. The neural apparatus for sexual desire is separate from the other aspects of the sexual response. The **detection of a pathology occurs when there has been a substantial change** in either direction of the frequency of desire from an individual's baseline. Determination of a "normal" baseline is often difficult since individuals vary and statistics change with a given era, socioeconomic status, marital status, and educational, religious, geographic, and cultural factors.

The **frequency of intercourse does not reflect the frequency of desire** since intercourse itself does not represent the total picture of sexual outlets for the sexual response.

    a. **Primary desire phase dysfunction** is defined as the situation in which an individual **has always had either a very high or very low sex drive.**

    b. **Secondary desire phase dysfunction** occurs when there is a **significant and persistent decline** after a period of greater sexual interest. This condition is **not associated with the gradual decrease in interest found in aging or in chronic illness.** Interestingly, some women report increased sexual interest in the postmenopausal state rather than a decline.

2. **Evaluation.**
    a. **Subjective.** A diagnosis of a disorder of desire may be made on the basis of the following factors:
        (1) **What is the current sexual activity?**
        (2) **In how much sexual activity does the patient want to engage?** In how much does she wish to participate **relative to her partner's interest?**
        (3) Is the chief complaint truly a **loss of desire or is it another sexual dysfunction** (such as anorgasmia)?
        (4) Is there **confusion between desire and capability** such as with the woman who is monoorgasmic but feels that she should have multiple orgasms during every coitus?
        (5) Is the problem one of **inhibition or performance anxiety?**
        (6) Is the individual **simply not interested in the partner?**
        (7) Is the individual **withholding sex from the partner?**
    b. **Objective. A physical examination with laboratory studies to rule out endocrine or neurologic disorders** is indicated.
        (1) Some **organic factors to consider** are decreased testosterone levels; general weakness; malnutrition; chronic disease; CNS depressants, particularly alcohol, hallucinogens, opioids, and peripherally acting drugs (e.g., anticholinergics, antiadrenergics); neurologic diseases; diabetes; chronic renal failure; post-hysterectomy state; and pregnancy.
        (2) **Emotional factors** also affect sexual desire, such as loss of personal attractiveness; problems in marital intimacy; boring sexual routine; extramarital affairs; marital maladjustment; and situational disturbances such as a death, loss of a job, an illness, or a psychiatric condition.

3. **Management.** When the history, physical examination, and laboratory studies have **ruled out organicity, treatment plans can be made** (see section IV.).

III. **Conditions associated with sexual dysfunction**
  A. **Surgical effects on sexual function**
    1. **Any surgical intervention** that alters the anatomy of the sexual and reproductive structures will affect a woman's sexual functioning, both psychologically and physically. **Clarification of what specifically affects sexual function and what is myth is an integral aspect of the preparation of the patient for surgery.**
    2. **History.** The sexual history will provide data on her **sexual practices, her valuation of the specific organs** involved, and **what alterations in her sexual practices may be necessary** as a result of the surgical change.
      a. **A clitoridectomy or vulvar surgery** would require sexual adjustment, although **orgasmic potential is not always lost.**

      b. Hysterectomy is fraught with a mythologic **fear of loss of sexual responsiveness** because of uterine removal. The woman may need to be informed that the clitoris is the major organ of sexual function and that it remains intact.

      c. Mastectomy should have no anatomic basis for loss of sexuality. However, the **psychological loss can be sexually crippling** for some women, and preparation and counseling preoperatively and postoperatively are usually indicated.

  B. Hypoestrinism and menopause. The mythology and fear of instant aging and loss of femininity and desirability may affect the sexual functioning of some women who connect sexuality with only reproductivity. With the loss of ovarian function, some women emotionally discard sexual function. When women are made aware of the **distinction between the sexual and reproductive systems,** many become less depressed and feel restored to return to sexual activity. Some women have increased libido in menopause, either because of the relative increase in the testosterone-estrogen ratio or because of a disinhibition from no longer having a fear of pregnancy. **Estrogen replacement therapy is currently recommended** not only for preventing osteoporosis but also for improving vaginal lubrication and atrophic vaginal changes (see Chapter 25).

  C. Cancer. For those with malignant disease, the individual's sexual activity preferences should be incorporated into the treatment plan. Depending on the type of disease and the organ system affected, sexual concerns should be addressed. Even if the patient initially is more concerned with life and death issues, the reality of living with cancer with a good quality of life will surface eventually. **Management of sexual concerns will be intricately involved with such medical problems as organ loss, effects of radiation or chemotherapy, debilitation and malnutrition, depression, and side effects of drugs** other than cytotoxics all of which affect libido and sexual function. Its management will depend on the patient's life circumstances, such as whether she has a sexual partner or whether sexual release by masturbation has been important.

  D. Pregnancy. Research has been sparse and conflicting in the area of sexual desire and functioning in pregnancy. Some investigators are of the opinion that there is usually a decrease in coital frequency during the first trimester, then an increase in frequency and responsiveness occurs during the second trimester, possibly related to the increased pelvic congestion at that time. However, during the third trimester, because of physical discomfort and anticipation of childbirth, sexual interest tends to wane. Other studies suggest that women appear to have a progressively decreasing desire and frequency throughout pregnancy, being most pronounced in the third trimester. The decrease in sexuality is found mostly in primiparas, whereas multiparous women seem to have an increase in responsiveness and satisfaction. Women with a positive attitude toward pregnancy and who have good relationships with their partners appear to have increased sexual satisfaction. Generally, **although sexual interest may wax and wane during pregnancy, the desire for physical closeness, affection, and support is increased and is of utmost importance.**

IV. Treatment and referral. Although there is an increase in the availability of sexual therapy clinics, if there is no complicated relationship or psychiatric problem, **most complaints can be handled by the well-informed and trained primary clinician.** Patients often resist referral, feeling a rejection on the part of the primary care provider or are embarrassed to attend a specialized clinic as a public acknowledgment of a private issue. Women appear to be more willing to accept sex therapy than men.

  A. Indications for referral of a patient for sex therapy include the presence of psychopathology, poor doctor-patient rapport in discussing sexual matters, long history of marital partner discord, and multiple relationship problems. **Referral should also be made if the clinician has unresolved**

personal problems similar to the patient's, lacks resources or time to provide counseling or feels uncomfortable, or is untrained in the subject of human sexuality.

B. **Treatment of sexual problems by the primary care provider can be done in several dimensions.**

1. The **most basic approach** would include reassurance, dispelling myths, and giving accurate information on sexual function and permission to the patient to discuss sexual concerns.

2. **More intensive counseling** may include factors such as the need to assume mutual responsibility with the partner for the sexual problem, to obtain permission to engage in certain sexual acts, and to try techniques to remove performance anxiety and methods to improve couple communication.

V. **Prognosis.** Sexual dysfunction is frequently an important factor in relationship and family stress ending in separation or divorce. Prevention and avoidance of sexual problems is ideal and should begin with the provision of sex education starting in the elementary years. The education should include early intervention in dysfunctional or abusive family situations. A lack of controlled studies, standard definitions, uniform follow-up, and standard criteria for improvement pervades the literature. Information concerning the long-term outlook is guarded at best.

In general, orgasmic problems seem to respond to intervention with resolution occurring for the majority. Desire is the most difficult to treat with less than half reporting improvement. When the relationship is poor, behavioral approaches directed toward the sexual problem are rarely successful.

References

1. Goldfarb AF. Adolescent sexuality. *Acad Sci* 1997;816:395.
2. Risen CB. A guide to taking a sexual history. *Psychiatr Clin North Am* 1995;18:39.
3. Weisberg M. Physiology of female sexual function. *Clin Obstet Gynecol* 1984;27:697.
4. Watson JP, Davies T. ABC of mental health: psychosexual problems. *BMJ* 1997; 315:239.
5. Lewin J, King M. Sexual medicine. *BMJ* 1997;314:1432.
6. Steege JF, Ling FW. Dyspareunia: a special type of chronic pelvic pain. *Obstet Gynecol Clin North Am* 1993;20:779.
7. Meana M, et al. Dyspareunia: more than bad sex. *Pain* 1997;71;211.
8. Shen WW, Sata LS. Drugs that cause sexual dysfunction. *Med Lett Drugs Ther* 1987;29:65.
9. Lane RM. A critical review of selective serotonin reuptake inhibitor-related sexual dysfunction: incidence, possible aetiology, and implications for management. *J Psychopharmacol* 1997;11:72.
10. Schiavi RC, Segraves RT. The biology of sexual function. *Psychiatr Clin North Am* 1995;18:7.
11. Frank E, Anderson C, Rubinstein D. Frequency of sexual dysfunction in normal couples. *N Engl J Med* 1978;299:111.
12. Masters WH, Johnson VE. *Human sexual response,* 2nd ed. Boston: Little, Brown, 1970.
13. Mueller IW. Common questions about sex and sexuality in elders. *Am J Nurs* 1997; 97:61.
14. Rosen RC, Leiblum SR. Hypoactive sexual desire. *Psychiatr Clin North Am* 1995;18:107.
15. Hyde JS, et al. Sexuality during pregnancy and the year postpartum. *J Sex Res* 1996;33:143.
16. Kellett J. Functions of a sexual dysfunction clinic. *Int Rev Psychiatry* 1995;7:183.
17. Sarwer DB, Durlak JA. A field trial of the effectiveness of behavioral treatment for sexual dysfunctions. *J Sex Marital Ther* 1997;23:87.

28. DOMESTIC VIOLENCE

Patricia R. Salber

I. **Introduction.** Domestic violence (DV) is a term that is used to describe intimate partner violence and abuse (IPVA). In this chapter, the terminology used will be DV since this is the most common term used at this time.

DV is a common problem that impacts the health and safety of millions of women around the world. Extrapolating findings from 1998 National Violence Against Women Survey suggests that 1.5 million women annually are raped and/or physically assaulted by an intimate partner in the United States alone. Approximately 1,400 murders per year in the United States are attributable to intimates.

Domestic violence affects women from all economic, educational, social, racial, ethnic, and geographic groups. Young women, ages 16 to 24, experience the highest per capita rates of DV; however, it does occur in every age group. Dating violence has been reported in preteen and young teens and some cases of elder abuse are, in fact, DV. IPVA occurs in both heterosexual and lesbian relationships and in current or former dating, married, separated, or cohabiting relationships. Increasingly, it is recognized that DV has both short-term and long-term physical and emotional effects on children reared in violent homes even if they only witness the abuse.

Women with current or past histories of IPVA are seen frequently in outpatient clinical settings. Of 225 pregnant and 142 nonpregnant women presenting to an urban New England urgent care obstetrics and gynecology unit, 184 (46%) reported a history of physical or sexual abuse, and 38 (10%) reported recent abuse. Between 7% and 17% of pregnant women in this country are battered by their partners. Clinicians in outpatient settings, therefore, have a significant opportunity to identify and offer help to victims of domestic violence.

II. **Definition.** DV and abuse is a **pattern** of assaultive and coercive behaviors, including physical, sexual, psychological, and economic attacks and/or coercion that adults or adolescents use against their intimate partners. Perpetrators use a variety of tactics in frequent, sometimes daily, episodes to gain power and control over their partners. Examples of such tactics are as follows:
   - **Verbal abuse** "You're stupid. You're lucky I'm here to take care of you."
   - **Emotional abuse** Being forced to wait in the car while her partner visits his mistress.
   - **Using children** The partner takes the children away to force the victim to do what he wants.
   - **Isolation** The victims is cut off from family and friends.
   - **"Male privilege"** "It's the man's right to chose where and how we live."
   - **Economic abuse** The perpetrator controls all of the family money.
   - **Abuse of children, other dependents, or pets** "If you leave me I will kill the children, dog, your mother, and so forth."
   - **Threats** "I will kill you or I will commit suicide if you leave."
   - **Physical abuse** Pushing, punching, slapping, throwing, choking, stabbing, and shooting.

III. **Role of the clinician.** Clinicians and other members of the outpatient team play an important role in the lives of victims of IPVA through the following actions:
   - **Identify the violence and abuse.**
   - **Validate the victim's experience.**
   - **Assess immediate risk.**
   - **Document current and past abuse.**
   - **Refer victims to intimate partner violence experts, such as DV-trained social workers or community-based DV advocates.**

   Resources will vary from state to state and county to county. Often the Public Health Department or local Planned Parenthood Clinic will have a list of local resources.

IV. Presenting signs and symptoms
   A. Physical injuries. The most frequently recognized presentations of intimate partner violence are those of physical injuries. The most common sites of injury are the **head, face, neck,** and **areas** that are usually **covered by clothing** such as the chest, breast, and abdomen. In order to fully assess the woman, ask her to completely disrobe and to remove any hats, sunglasses, or other articles of clothing that could conceal an injury.

   Victims of DV often are reluctant to reveal the cause of their injuries due to fear, shame, and/or to protect their partner or children. It is important to note any **discrepancies** between the **nature of the injury and the reported cause.** For example, it is highly unlikely that an isolated periorbital ecchymosis would be caused by falling off a chair and landing on the floor.

   B. Sexual assault
      1. Sexual assault including marital rape, occurs commonly in the most violent relationships, whether heterosexual or homosexual. Battered women who have also been raped may present with acute or past injuries related to the rape (e.g., vaginal or anal tears) or they may report symptoms of **sexual dysfunction** such as **dyspareunia** or diminished libido.
      2. When sexual coercion occurs, the victim may be unable to use protection against unwanted pregnancy or sexually transmitted diseases (STDs). Therefore, she may present with a vaginal infection, pelvic inflammatory disease, chronic pelvic pain, or a urinary tract infection. Some HIV positive women may have contracted the virus from coerced sexual activity.
      3. The prevalence of violence during pregnancy is between 4% to 8%. Adverse consequences of violence during pregnancy include injuries to the mother and fetus; premature labor and delivery; and/or an increase in behaviors associated with poor pregnancy outcome such as smoking, alcohol and drug use, low maternal weight gain, and presenting late in pregnancy without prenatal care.

   C. Nontraumatic physical complaints. Victims of DV commonly have nontrauma presentations as well.
      1. Nontraumatic pain is a common presenting symptom and may manifest as a chronic pain syndrome such as chronic abdominal or pelvic pain. Such patients may have had a complete evaluation, including laparoscopy, without identification of the etiology of the pain.
      2. Battered women may also present with **physical symptoms** related to stress, anxiety, posttraumatic stress disorder, depression, sleep or appetite disturbances, decreased energy or fatigue, difficulty concentrating, palpitations, dizziness, paresthesias, dyspnea, and chest pain. Women who **attempt** or **commit suicide** often have a history of DV. Patients with **vague or diffuse complaints** can be particularly **difficult** and often frustrating to **assess;** however, these symptoms may also be manifestations of DV and **need to be taken seriously.**

   D. Substance abuse. The use of alcohol and drugs appears to increase after physical abuse begins. It is generally believed to be a consequence of the abuse, rather than a cause of the abuse. Clinicians may play an unwitting role in the overuse or abuse of psychoactive or sedating prescription medications by battered women in the attempt to treat the psychiatric and somatic manifestations of abuse.

   E. Chronic medical conditions. Battered women may have exacerbations or poor control of chronic medical conditions such as diabetes, hypertension, or heart disease. They may be prevented from obtaining or taking medication or even from seeking medical care. This is especially likely to be true for women with physical limitations.

V. History and routine screening for DV. The American College of Obstetricians and Gynecologists recommends that every woman and girl presenting to an obstetric and gynecologic provider be **screened** for **intimate partner violence.**

The rationale for universal screening is based on the prevalence of DV in women seen in obstetric and gynecologic settings, the high association of DV with an array of health problems, the lack of definitive markers to identify abuse, and the low level of suspicion and inquiry on the part of physicians. **This same recommendation should also be applied to any medical, family practice, urgent care, or emergency department clinician.**

Abused women may have a general unwillingness to volunteer information when not asked, but when directly asked about intimate partner abuse in their lives there is a high level of acceptance and response. **Screening** has been documented to **increase identification,** involves minimal to modest cost and little risk to the patient when implemented in a manner that ensures confidentiality and safety. Increased identification offers the opportunity to treat and refer appropriately. It also may decrease the chance for further abuse as well as decreasing children's exposure to violence thereby diminishing the chance for continuation of abusive behavior in future generations. There is anecdotal information that screening offers an opportunity to discuss the abuse, and to learn that health care providers care about DV and can serve as a resource.

National clinical guidelines on routine screening in outpatient obstetrics and gynecology as well as family planning settings have been published. These guidelines recommend that all females aged 14 years and older should be screened at every:
- Routine gynecologic visit.
- Family planning visit.
- STD clinic visit.
- Abortion clinic visit.
- New intimate relationship.
- Prenatal postpartum visit.

The screening should be part of a face-to-face encounter in a private setting without friends or relatives including children older than 2 years. Questioning should be **direct** and **nonjudgmental. Professional interpreters** should be used when translation is needed.

Examples of screening questions are the following:

Framing questions
- "Because violence is so common in many people's lives, I've begun to ask all my patients about it."
- "I'm concerned that your symptoms may have been caused by someone hurting you."
- "I don't know if this is a problem for you, but many women I see are dealing with abusive relationships. Some are too afraid or uncomfortable to bring it up, so I have started asking about it routinely."
- "Some of the lesbians I see here are hurt by their partners. Does your partner ever try to hurt you?"

Direct verbal questions
- "Are you in a relationship with a person who physically hurts or threatens you?"
- "Did someone cause these injuries? Was it your partner/husband?"
- "Has your partner or ex-partner ever hit you or physically hurt you? Has s/he ever threatened to hurt you or someone close to you?"
- "Do you feel controlled or isolated by your partner?"
- "Do you ever feel afraid of your partner? Do you feel you are in danger? Is it safe for you to go home?"
- "Has your partner ever forced you to have sex when you didn't want to?"
- "Has your partner ever refused to practice safe sex?"

A. **Validation of the patient's experience.** It is important that clinicians verbally acknowledge that hitting, punching, or other violent acts are a form of abuse and not part of a normal healthy relationship. Failure to do so may be interpreted by patients as **confirming the perpetrator's common assertions** that he will get away with it and that no one cares that there is abuse. **Validation involves telling the victim that violent behavior is**

wrong and **that nothing she has done or has failed to do makes the violence acceptable.**

Patients should be given a clear message that help is available. The patient should know that outpatient medical personnel can assist her in getting in touch with intimate partner violence experts (clinic-based or office-based trained social workers or community-based DV advocates). These IPV experts can help the person work through the logistics of leaving or assist with other safety strategies if the woman chooses to stay in the relationship.

Validation has been documented to serve as a turning point for women in abusive relationships. Knowing this may be helpful for clinicians who are frustrated by their inability to "fix" the problem of intimate partner violence at the time of the office visit. Leaving an abusive relationship is a process that generally requires advance planning to be accomplished safely and successfully.

B. Assess immediate risk. Safety assessment is a critical part of the evaluation. Clinicians must understand the correlates of lethality in intimate partner violence. An **escalating pattern** of violence can **signal** an increased risk of fatal outcome. Threats to kill the victim, the children, or self **must be taken seriously** since more than **one half of murder-suicides** take place in the setting of spousal or consortial relationships, often with a prior history of intimate partner violence:

Other risk factors for serious injury or death include:

- Substance abuse, especially drugs associated with an increase in violence, such as crack cocaine or amphetamines.
- Stalking or other behaviors suggestive of obsession with the victims.
- The presence of a firearm in the home.
- Evidence of violence behavior outside the home.

The **most dangerous period** for battered women is when they **attempt to leave** the relationship. Up to 75% of domestic assaults reported to law enforcement agencies are inflicted **after** separation of the couple. Women are most likely to be **murdered when attempting to report abuse or leave an abusive relationship.** During the early separation period, batterers often retaliate by abducting the children; more than one half of the 350,000 children kidnapped by parents each year occur in the context of intimate partner violence. In some instances, the heightened period of danger can last for several years.

C. Documentation

1. The medical record may be the only evidence that abuse has taken place.
    a. This documentation can provide pivotal information for criminal or civil legal remedies, such as divorce or child custody.
    b. Good documentation is also useful for physicians who are concerned about being unavailable for clinical practice secondary to court appearances.
    c. A legible, detailed, and accurate medical record may substitute for a personal appearance by a physician.
2. The medical record should include a description of the event in the patient's own words.
3. Abuse uncovered as a result of routine screening should also be documented.
4. Specify when and how the abuse was inflicted, as well as the name and relationship of the perpetrator. It is preferable to record "The patient states her husband, John Jones, punched her in the left eye yesterday evening about 11 PM" instead of "The patient alleges DV."
5. Prior episodes of abuse as well as abuse of children or other dependents should be described in detail regardless of whether that abuse required medical care.
6. Recent **changes** in the **pattern of abuse,** particularly **escalation** of the violence, coerced or forced sex, whether the perpetrator is abusing alcohol or other substances, and whether he has access to a firearm should be documented.

7. A prior history of abortions or treatment for STDs because of coerced unprotected sexual intercourse should also be noted.
8. The chart should include specific information on whether or not:
   - A social worker, DV advocate, or law enforcement officer was contacted.
   - The patient was seen by any of these individuals prior to leaving the office as well as the results of these contacts.
   - If the patient was not seen by a DV specialist or law enforcement prior to discharge, the chart should include the details of the assessment of the patient's immediate risk of injury (see previous discussion).
9. If the patient is not at risk for immediate harm and if she prefers, up-to-date information about community DV agencies should be given so that the patient can arrange follow-up on her own. This should also be recorded in the chart.

VI. **Physical examination.** A complete physical examination should be performed, paying close attention to areas of the body in which physical signs of abuse can be hidden, such as the scalp and areas generally concealed by clothing. Areas of tenderness and injuries that are not visible should be noted on a preprinted or hand-drawn outline of a human body. This includes injuries to the scalp concealed by hair as well as soft tissue injuries that are not yet discolored.

If sexual abuse is suspected, a sexual assault examination should be performed. Many counties have agreements with specific agencies or emergency rooms to perform all evidentiary examinations for their service area. If the clinician is not equipped or versed in the specifics of this type of examination, then referral to the designated agency is appropriate.

In the event that the clinician's office is willing to do an evidentiary examination, all visible injuries should be photographed, after obtaining the patient's consent. It is usually easiest to use a Polaroid camera so that the adequacy of the photographs can be assessed before the patient leaves the office.

VII. **Referral.** Every effort should be made to ensure high-risk individuals see or speak with an intimate partner violence specialist prior to leaving the office. Specialists trained in DV, such as trained social workers or community-based DV advocates, can help the victim assess the situation, discuss options, develop a detailed safety plan, and arrange a safe haven including shelter. If the patient is willing, arrangements should be made for those not in immediate danger to speak with an DV specialist prior to discharge. All patients should be advised of the option of calling law enforcement.

Although clinicians are often tempted to make disposition decisions for a battered woman, the patient is in the best position to ultimately determine where the safest location is for her. She knows the batterer; she may be afraid for the safety of her loved ones, such as her children, parents, or siblings; and she may know, from prior attempts to leave, that the criminal justice system cannot ensure her safety. The decision to go or not to go home must ultimately be made by the patient and respected by the clinician.

VIII. **Follow-up.** Leaving a violent relationship is a process that can take months to years to accomplish. It is important that clinicians continue to inquire about the violence and offer validation and support in subsequent visits. When possible, telephone follow-up in 1 to 2 weeks after the index visit can be safely accomplished if prior arrangements are made with her to ensure safe times and safe telephone numbers to use. Never leave information on a home answering machine or send written correspondence including bills that indicate DV to the woman's home. These can suggest to the perpetrator that she has disclosed information regarding the abuse.

IX. **Legal considerations.** Many states have laws that require health care providers to report known or suspected cases of abuse to the police. The indications for initiating a report vary from state to state. Victims of DV must be apprised of the duty to report and its potential ramifications. Unfortunately, in some jurisdictions the criminal justice response to victims of DV may place the victim at increased risk for harm. For example, a report that triggers a police home visit and not arrest, or an arrest with only a few hours in jail may enrage the perpetrator and lead to retaliation and more serious injury or death. Clinicians also have a duty to report a patient's intent to harm a third party.

Victims of IPVA often need legal help as they seek to protect themselves and their children. Civil protection orders are available to battered women in every U.S. state and the District of Columbia. Protection orders, as well as information on other legal services for victims of partner violence, can often be obtained through the assistance of community DV shelters or agencies.

X. Promoting office awareness of DV. Every outpatient office should have a plan for continuing education of all staff about the dynamics, identification, and appropriate interventions for intimate partner violence. Evidence suggests that traditional continuing education programs are more effective if combined with enablers, such as chart stamps that remind clinicians to ask about IPV, exam room posters, or lapel buttons that send a message to patients that it is safe to discuss IPV in this setting.

Educational materials and background information on intimate partner violence can be obtained by calling or emailing one of the following organizations:

* Physician for a Violence-free Society (415-621-3582; pvs@pvs.org).
* The Family Violence Prevention Fund's Health Resource Center (1-800-313-1310).
* National Domestic Violence Hotline (1-800-799-SAFE). Identify yourself as a provider and state your question.

Suggested Reading

Campbell J, ed. Assessing dangerousness: potential for further violence of sexual offenders, batterers, and child abusers. Newbury Park, CA: Sage, 1995.

Cokkinides VE, Coker AL, Sanderson M, et al. Physical violence during pregnancy: maternal complications and birth outcomes. *Obstet Gynecol* 1999;93(5).

El-Bassel N, Gilbert L, Rajah V, et al. Fear and violence: raising the HIV stakes. *AIDS Education and Prevention* 2000;12(1):154–170.

Felitti VJ, Anda RF, Nordenberg D, et al. Relationship of childhood abuse and household dysfunction to many of the leading causes of death in adults: the adverse childhood experience (ACE) study. *Am J Prev Med* 1998;14:245–258.

Gazmararian JA, Petersen R, Spitz AM, et al. Violence and reproductive health: current knowledge and future research directions. *Matern Child Health J* 2000;4(2).

Gerbert B, Abercrombie P, Caspers N, et al. How health care providers help battered women: the survivor's perspective. *Women and Health* 1999;29(3):115–135.

Gerbert B, Caspers N, Bronstone A, et al. A qualitative analysis of how physicians with expertise in domestic violence approach the identification of victims. *Ann Intern Med* 1999;131:578–584.

Hamberger LK, Ambuel B. Dating violence. *Ped Clinic North Am* 1998;45:381–390.

Lee D, James L, Sawires P. *Preventing domestic violence: clinical guidelines on routine screening.* San Francisco: The Family Violence Prevention Fund, October 1999.

Renzetti C. Violent betrayal: partner abuse in lesbian relationships. Newbury Park, CA: Sage, 1992.

Roberts GL, Williams GM, Lawrence JM, et al. How does domestic violence affect women's mental health? *Aust Womens Health* 1998;117–129.

Salber P, Taliaferro E. *The physician's guide to domestic violence: how to ask the right questions and recognize abuse.* Volcano, CA: Volcano, 1995.

Tjaden P, Thoennes N. Prevalence, incidence, and consequences of violence against women: findings from the national violence against women survey. NIJCDC, NCJ-172837, 1–14, Nov 1998.

Thompson RS, Rivara FP, Thompson DC, et al. Identification and management of domestic violence: a randomized trial. *Am J Prev Med* 2000;19(4).

29. SEXUAL HARASSMENT, SEXUAL EXPLOITATION OF PATIENTS AND CHILD MOLESTATION

Ty Yarnel

Public and professional awareness of sexual harassment, sexual exploitation of patients by health care workers, and sexual abuse of children has greatly increased in the past decade. This is the result of multiple factors: greater media coverage, legislative mandates affecting how professionals report suspected abuse, increased litigation surrounding such cases, and the development of professional training programs designed to aid in identification and prevention of abuse. The clinician's responsibility for dealing with sexual abuse starts with a willingness to **acknowledge** that such **abuses do occur, sensitivity** to the special **needs** of **victims,** and an **objective approach** to examination and assessment. It is also important for practitioners to keep updated on the periodic amendments in the law relative to mandated reporting as these laws change from state to state and from year to year. There are also both legal and ethical obligations to inform patients of the options that are available to them that many laws address. The increasing frequencies of accusations of sexual abuse in divorce and/or custody cases and litigation surrounding recovered memories of abuse (19,15) also calls for a cautious and objective approach by the provider.

I. **Sexual harassment** is a widespread and serious form of sexual discrimination that was prohibited by Title VI of the Civil Rights Act of 1964 (23). Expanded provisions for victims were offered under the 1991 Civil Rights Act, and additional guidelines from the U.S. Department of Education Office for Civil Rights were released in January 1999. Yet complaints have continued to be met with invalidation and disbelief, resulting in a reluctance to report this trauma (6,9,24). When complaints are made, they are frequently ignored, discredited, and blamed on the victim, who often loses job and career in the course of seeking redress. Although both men and women can be victims, the majority of reported sexual harassment cases affect women (6,15,22).

   A. **Description and definition. Sexual harassment** is defined as **unwelcome sexual advances or visual, verbal, or actual conduct of a sexual nature.** This misconduct may include unwanted requests for sexual favors; sexual gestures; computer communication; and displaying posters, pictures, cartoons, or similar objects that are sexually suggestive. It also includes making derogatory comments, physical or verbal abuse inflicted in a sexual manner, comments about a person's anatomy, or using sexually degrading words. The offensive conduct is usually made by a person in a position of power to one of lesser status and, therefore, is **not generally a sexually motivated act but rather an act of power** expressed sexually. Sexual harassment can range from subtle but inappropriate sexual innuendoes to violent and forced sexual acts (rape). Harassment may take the form of emotional, psychological, and/or physical trauma. It is important to recognize that men and women are likely to differ in their assessments of what constitutes sexually offensive behavior. Many courts refer to this as the "reasonable woman" standard in evaluating harassment cases (6).

      1. **Legal definition.** Two types of sexual harassment are specifically defined and prohibited by Title VI of the Civil Rights Act as *Quid Pro Quo* and *Hostile Work Environment* (23).

         a. **Quid pro quo harassment** involves explicitly or implicitly offering, granting, or denying a work-related benefit in exchange for sexual favors. In an educational environment **Quid Pro Quo** harassment occurs when a school employee causes a student to believe s/he must

This chapter is a revision from the third edition by Phyllis A. Kaufman and Mary Lou Hyde.

submit to unwelcome sexual conduct to participate in or benefit from a school program or activity or to receive desired grades (16).

b. **Hostile work environment** involves unreasonable interference with an individual's work performance or workplace making it intimidating, hostile, or offensive and interfering with the right to work in an environment that is free from discriminatory intimidation, ridicule, and insult. In an educational environment a **hostile environment** occurs when unwelcome conduct of a sexual nature is so severe, persistent, or pervasive that it affects a student's ability to participate in or benefit from an education program or activity or creates an intimidating, threatening, or abusive educational environment (16).

B. **Incidence.** The latest surveys (25,14,24) show that over the past 15 years there has been no change—40% to 50% of working women and up to 15% of working men experience sexual harassment and 85% of girls and 76% of boys reported experiencing some form of sexual harassment in school. It is reported that 90% of all harassers are men. Among women who have been sexually harassed, 64% said they did not report the harassment, and over half of those who did said the problem was not resolved to their satisfaction. At least 75% of women who have been harassed said they have felt one or more symptoms of emotional or physical distress because of the harassment. Surveys documenting sexual harassment of students usually focus on female students and indicate that graduate students are more likely to be harassed by professors than are undergraduate students and that this harassment is widespread.

C. **Symptoms.** Victims of sexual harassment often present with symptoms that are frequently associated with **stress-related illness.** Such complaints may include headaches, backaches, neck pain, gastrointestinal complaints, sleep disturbance, fatigue, change in appetite, and excessive use of sick leave. Victims often meet the *Diagnostic and Statistical Manual of Mental Disorders, fourth edition (DSM-IV)* criteria for **major depression and post-traumatic stress disorder** (PTSD) (1). The following cluster of symptoms typically follows incidents of sexual harassment when the victim has felt powerless and trapped.

1. **Reexperiencing the harassment** in one (or more) of the following ways:
   a. **Recurrent and intrusive recollections of the harassment.**
   b. **Recurrent and distressing dreams of the events.**
   c. **Acting or feeling as if the abusive events were recurring or being relived** (includes illusions, hallucinations, dissociative flashbacks, and such).
   d. **Intense psychological distress** when exposed to **internal** or **external** stimuli that symbolizes or resembles an aspect of the trauma. Emotional or psychological symptoms may include:
      (1) Guilt and self-blame.
      (2) Anger, rage, and obsessions with vengeance.
      (3) Shame and embarrassment.
      (4) **Feelings** of **vulnerability** and/or **fears of retaliation** by the harasser.
      (5) **Physical and/or psychological discomfort with physical intimacy.**
   e. **Physiologic reactivity** on exposure to internal or external cues that symbolize or resemble an aspect of the trauma. Complaints may include:
      (1) Headaches, backaches, and neck pain.
      (2) Skin rashes.
      (3) Gastrointestinal complaints, including nausea, constipation, diarrhea, and appetite disturbances.
      (4) Sleep disturbance and fatigue.
      (5) Menstrual problems.

2. **Persistent avoidance of stimuli associated** with the **trauma** and a **numbing of responsiveness** (not present before the sexual harassment) as evidenced by **at least three** of the following:
   a. Efforts to **avoid thoughts, feelings,** or **conversations** about the traumatic events.
   b. Efforts to **avoid activities, places, or people** who arouse recollections of the traumatic events.
   c. **Inability to recall important aspects of the trauma.**
   d. Markedly **diminished interest or participation in significant activities.**
   e. **Feeling of detachment or estrangement from others.**
   f. **Restricted range of affect.**
   g. **Sense of a foreshortened future** (e.g., career, marriage, children, or normal life span).
3. **Persistent symptoms of increased arousal, not present before the trauma** as indicated by **two** or more of the following:
   a. **Difficulty falling or staying asleep.**
   b. **Irritability or outbursts of anger.**
   c. **Difficulty concentrating.**
   d. **Hypervigilance.**
   e. **Exaggerated startle response.**
D. Some victims progress through **predictable stages** that may overlap and include **self-blame, confusion, fear and anxiety, depression, anger,** and **disillusionment.** There is also a **profound and prolonged sense of powerlessness.** If the victim is involved in litigation (workers compensation or a personal injury suit), all symptoms may be exacerbated or prolonged by what is sometimes referred to as "the second wound."
E. **History**
   1. A thorough history of complaints, including any physical injuries, must be accurately documented.
   2. It is important to **relate the symptom onset,** if possible, to **environmental events that indicate harassment.** For example, ask about the relationships with employers, landlords, teachers, and health care providers.
   3. The clinician should listen carefully and empathically and **withhold all moral and legal judgments.** Attitudes that blame the victim or express disbelief are invalidating and only compound the trauma and reinforce self-blame.
F. **Physical examination techniques**
   1. The **coercion in sexual harassment is often subtle and not necessarily accompanied by physical violence** or **assault. Consequently, a physical examination may not be indicated** except in cases for whom there is reason to believe that there will be evidence of assault or physical injury.
   2. If a physical or gynecologic examination is indicated, a **female health care professional should attend the physician, whether male or female.** The patient may perceive sexual harassment during the physical examination if left alone with the provider. When a sexual assault examination is necessary refer to that discussion in Chapter 30.
   3. **Bruises, abrasions, and scratches** should be accurately measured, recorded, and treated as indicated. When possible, photographs of the injuries may be useful to accurately reflect the nature of the assault.
   4. A **psychiatric examination** and referral for **psychological testing may be useful** in assessing the degree of mental trauma.
G. **Management.** A referral for supportive **psychotherapy or counseling** with medical management of **antidepressants** is often indicated. Muscle relaxants, minor tranquilizers, and sedatives provide only short-term symptom relief and should be used sparingly and cautiously.

H. Sequelae. Sexual harassment has an **emotional effect** on those who experience its trauma. Victims of harassment report feeling angry, upset, frightened, and guilty. Other specific effects reported include becoming more self-conscious about appearance, feeling trapped or powerless, feelings of defeat, diminished ambition, decreased job satisfaction, impaired job performance, and difficulties in trusting certain authority figures who might represent the harasser.

II. Sexual exploitation of patients by health care professionals. Prohibition against engaging in sexual intimacies with a patient is one of the oldest ethical mandates in the health care professions and predates the 2,500-year-old Hippocratic Oath by appearing in the even more ancient code of the Nigerian healing arts (4). The destructive effects of such exploitation have been documented by systematic research and case studies over the past decade (9,20).

    A. Description and definition. Clinician-patient sexual involvement is characterized by the physician, therapist, or other health care professional **using his or her power and status to exert sexual dominance over the patient.** The trust and vulnerability of the patient enhances this power of the health care professional. There is a clear **prohibition against any sexual intimacies with patients; and no cause, situation, or condition could ever legitimize such intimacies.** The prohibition stands as a fundamental ethical mandate no matter what the rationalization (11,20).

    B. Incidence. The actual incidence **is unknown** because patients are reluctant to report, and estimates are generally based upon anonymous surveys. Less than candid reporting is suspected owing to the growing number of states in which therapist-patient sexual intimacy has become criminalized and to the increase in awareness among patients in how to file complaints. The surveys do reveal some consistent trends:

        1. There are no significant differences in exploitation of patients among the various health care professions.

        2. Male physicians and therapists engage in sex with their patients at much higher rates than do female health care professionals (20).

        3. Studies of risk factors reveal no personal histories or characteristics of clients that can predict risk.

        4. The most effective **predictor of risk is whether the therapist or physician has engaged in sex with another patient.** Data from surveys and actuarial data reveal that 80% of exploiting health care professionals have exploited other patients (7,20).

        5. Sexual exploitation is not limited to adult patients. A national survey found a significant number of cases involving minor children (4,20). The average age of the boys was 12 years with a range from 7 to 16 years of age. The average age of the girls was 14 years with a range of 3 to 17 years old.

    C. Symptoms. Victims of sexual exploitation by health care professionals (like victims of sexual harassment) may present with symptoms that are frequently associated with **stress-related illness.** They often meet the *DSM-IV* criteria for **PTSD and major depression** (see section I.C.) (3).

        1. Patients may be **secretive** about the abuses and will have difficulty trusting those who subsequently treat them.

        2. Victims may remain ambivalent about the former abusing provider and therefore, reluctant to report the abuse. They may even **blame themselves** for the abuse and **feel guilty** or **ashamed.**

        3. Patients may not know that such abuses are considered unethical or illegal and may anticipate that subsequent health care professionals will similarly exploit them. This may **result in avoidance of physical examinations** or therapy for many years.

    D. History. A thorough and detailed history of the complaints and any physical injuries must be accurately documented.

        1. It is essential to **obtain a detailed medical history** as well as a **full personal history** including **any** prior sexual victimization, current or prior substance abuse, and prior claims of physician or therapist exploitation.

2. It is important to **relate the symptom onset, if possible, to environmental events** that indicate exploitation. For example, ask about the relationship with the health care provider inside and outside the actual treatment setting.

3. The clinician should **listen carefully and empathically.** Attitudes that blame the victim or express disbelief are invalidating and only **compound** the **trauma** and **reinforce self-blame.**

E. **Examination techniques.** A physical examination may not be indicated since sexual exploitation is often subtle, lengthy, and usually not accompanied by physical violence. An examination may increase the patient's anxiety and resistance.

1. If a physical or gynecologic examination is indicated, a **female health care professional should attend the provider.**

2. A **psychiatric examination** and referral for **psychological testing may be useful** in assessing the degree of mental trauma. Such a referral should be made to a mental health specialist with expertise in this area.

F. **Sequelae.** The consequences of sexual exploitation for clients seem to cluster into ten very general categories (18).

1. **Ambivalence** about the abuser.

2. **Guilt** and **self-blame** over the sexual involvement as well as for the abuse reporting.

3. **Emptiness and isolation** as a result of loss of connection to the abusing professional.

4. **Sexual confusion** may be intensified by the abuse.

5. **Impaired ability to trust** which often prevents the patient from obtaining future treatment.

6. **Confused roles and boundaries** causing the patient to take the role of counselor with the abusing professional.

7. **Emotional lability** often resulting in extreme disequilibrium, mood swings, and profound depression.

8. **Suppressed rage** owing to ambivalence, guilt, and confusion. Rage is a **natural reaction** to betrayal and exploitation.

9. **Increased suicidal risk.**

10. **Cognitive dysfunction,** often occurring in the areas of concentration and memory and often involving flashbacks, intrusive thoughts, and nightmares.

G. **Management. Damage is usually extensive and profound;** and long-term management that involves supportive, educative, and cognitive **psychotherapy is usually indicated.**

1. Referral to a psychotherapist with expertise in the area of sexual exploitation of patients is indicated. The treatment of choice may combine both **individual and group treatment** with other victims who have been similarly exploited.

2. The patient should be informed that **sexual exploitation is unethical, illegal, and harmful.** All options for remedy should be discussed with the patient:

   a. Formal complaint to the **state licensing board.**

   b. Complaint to the **professional ethics committee.**

   c. **Criminal charges** may be filed with law enforcement officials in some states.

   d. The patient may be able to sue the abusing professional in **civil court for personal injury** and damages.

3. Every treating clinician should be familiar with their own **state laws** that may **mandate a special response** in such cases. For example, in 1990 the California Department of Consumer Affairs (7) published a document that is sent to all licensed therapists and counselors in California

and that must, according to California law, be **provided** to any **patient who reports** having been **sexually involved** with a **prior therapist.**

III. **Child molestation: sexual abuse of children and adolescents:**
   A. **Description and definition.** Child molestation refers to sexual abuse or sexual exploitation of a child by an adult or older person exerting power and authority over the child. The child is incapable of comprehending the nature of activities and is developmentally unprepared to give consent (2).
      1. Its **three major forms** include:
         a. **Exploitation within the home** by parent, parenting figures, or older children (incest).
         b. **Assault or exploitation by a nonrelated adult** (usually a pedophile).
         c. **Habitual exploitation for money** (child pornography, child prostitution).
      2. The molestation may be **assaultive and violent, resulting in both physical injury and emotional trauma, or nonassaultive and subtle, resulting in emotional trauma.**
      3. **Sexual abuse includes:**
         a. Finger manipulation.
         b. Intercourse.
         c. Oral-genital contact.
         d. Genital contact.
         e. Anal intercourse.
         f. Fondling.
         g. Exposure to verbal or visually explicit sexual material.
      4. **Sexual play** between children the same age, without coercion, is considered normal. Children who are coercive or threatening or who engage in developmentally inappropriate play (e.g., oral-genital contact) may be reacting to their own abuse. These incidents should be reported for evaluation to local law enforcement or child welfare agencies.
   B. **Incidence.** Incestuous assault within families bears **no relation to class, race, economic status, or social background.** Recent statistics indicate that the rate of sexual victimization is between 12% to 25% for girls and 8% to 10% for boys (2). Statistics inadequately reflect middle-class and upper-class reporting of abuse; however, they do reflect a dramatic increase in allegations in the past 15 to 20 years. **It is unclear whether there is an increase in actual abuse, an increase in the reporting of abuse, or better investigative and reporting techniques.** Generalizations that can be made are:
      1. **The perpetrator** is likely to be male and known to the child.
      2. **Adolescents** are perpetrators in at least 20% of reported cases.
      3. **Incest is the most common form of molestation** reported with more than 75% of the cases involving a relative or friend.
      4. **The most common perpetrator is the father, followed by the stepfather and uncle.** Mother-son incest is rarely reported.
      5. **Women** may be perpetrators but they represent a small minority of sexual abuse allegations.
      6. **False accusations do occur** and may be seen when divorce or custody dispute issues are involved (2,12).
      7. **Recent research** also informs that suggestion and misleading or repeated questioning of **children may result in false accusations** (1,5,8,15).
   C. **Symptoms.** The initial symptoms and long-term physical and emotional sequelae of sexual abuse vary depending on the trauma, age, and sex of the child (21).
      1. **Physical symptoms and evidence of abuse.**
         a. Infants and toddlers may have **general irritability** secondary to oral or rectal abrasions that cannot be visualized by the parent or clinician.

      b. Dysuria from genital trauma may suggest a urinary tract infection.

      c. Abdominal pain.

      d. Laceration to the anus, vestibule, or hymen may be associated with bleeding.

          (1) An anal fissure from penetration may be misdiagnosed and attributed to passing large stools or falling on an object.

          (2) Rarely does any object accidentally penetrate the rectum or vagina.

          (3) Anal fissures from large stools may be differentiated from trauma by using a colposcope during examination (1).

      e. Any trauma to the genitalia of preverbal children should be reported as probable sexual abuse unless the incident was witnessed.

      f. Any sexually transmitted disease in a child is to be reported as sexual abuse.

  2. Behavioral symptoms of sexual abuse vary with age and sex of the child and the abuse experience.

      a. Symptoms may be overt (e.g., fear and avoidance of the perpetrator).

      b. General and nonspecific symptoms may include (but not be limited to):

          (1) Sleep disorders.

          (2) Developmental delay.

          (3) Regression (particularly related to toilet training).

          (4) Sexual acting out (developmentally unusual).

          (5) Generalized anxiety.

          (6) Phobias.

          (7) Behavioral problems.

          (8) Enuresis and encopresis.

          (9) Fear of dying.

          (10) Running away.

          (11) Prostitution.

          (12) Low self-esteem.

          (13) Attempted suicide.

          (14) Fatigue.

          (15) Eating disorders.

          (16) Identity confusion.

          (17) Psychosomatic complaints including gastrointestinal disorders, headaches, and exaggerated gag response.

          (18) School failure or a sudden drop in academic achievement.

          (19) Overly compliant behavior in an exaggerated attempt to please adults and to be perfect.

          (20) Lying or exaggerating.

          (21) Isolation from one's peer group and friendships.

      c. Many children will not disclose abuse unless asked directly in a nonaccusing or judgmental manner.

      d. An older child may be able to tell about the abuse, but be reluctant to do so for fear of **reprisals, guilt associated** with the **act, or acceptance of bribes,** or for **fear** of **dissolution** of the **family.**

      e. Disbelief or denial as well as anticipation of the trauma engendered by the legal system (court testimony facing the accused) may cause the child to recant (11).

D. Techniques for examination and history taking. The doctor-patient relationship is important **not only for competent medical care but also for support** in helping to allay the intense anxiety, to redefine the event as a treatable physical injury rather than a moral lapse or sexual perversion, to treat sequelae in the victim, and to provide continuity of relationship (especially important if the child has been removed to a strange, new environment).

    Investigative interviews should be conducted by law enforcement or designated members of the community to minimize the repetitive questioning of the child and thus reducing the potential for **secondary trauma.** However, this does not preclude the medical professional from obtaining a detailed medical history and review of symptoms (1).

1. A thorough, methodical, and sensitive **interview** includes a **history from both** the child and the parent **(separately if possible), a physical examination,** and **direct observation** of the interaction between the child and parents. Care should be taken to avoid closed-ended or leading questions the prevent the possibility of directing the child's rendition of events.

2. **Guidelines** for interviewing physically or sexually abused children have been published by the American Academy of Child and Adolescent Psychiatry (1,8). Children have often made spontaneous statements during the history and physical examination.

   a. Interview the child and caregiver **separately** when possible.

   b. **Avoid judgment** and expression of **strong emotion.**

   c. **Reassure** the child that she or he lacks any responsibility for the abuse.

   d. Be prepared for **spontaneous statements** obtained while taking a routine medical history.

   e. Use **open-ended questions** to facilitate increased opportunity for spontaneous statements.

3. A physical examination by a clinician who is present during the interview **decreases** the child's anxiety and resistance for this necessary procedure.

   a. **Any abuse or acute injury** suspected to have occurred in the previous 72 hours should be examined **immediately.** If there is no acute injury or the reported abuse is more than 72-hours old, an evaluation should be **rescheduled** if there is an appropriate investigations team available (1).

   b. The genital examination should be a matter-of-fact part of the head-to-toe physical examination. It is important to **explain what will be done and why and to ask if the child has questions.** The child should have as much control over the examination as possible. Ask that the child remove his or her own clothing and participate by holding swabs for you. **Abused children appreciate** any **comments** that **reassure** them that **they are intact, normally developed, and without defect.**

   c. Often there are **no physical findings** on examination. Many types of abuse leave no evidence and injuries to the genitalia heal quickly.

   d. Internal genital examinations should be performed **only** in instances of internal genital bleeding.

   e. **Physical findings** may be present **without** specific **abuse history.** Further investigation is necessary by law enforcement or child welfare agencies.

4. **Investigative procedures.**

   a. The colposcope, when available, can be used externally to improve lighting and to provide magnification and photographic documentation of the examination. There may be a special medical team in your area to complete these examinations as follow-up.

   b. **Blood specimens** should be drawn for syphilis serology, and a complete blood cell count should be obtained to determine anemia on the basis of nutritional neglect or bleeding secondary to trauma.

   c. **A urine specimen** should be taken for urinalysis and, if indicated, for **determination of the presence of spermatozoa.**

   d. **Pregnancy test** (blood or urine) in the pubertal or older girl should be done.

   e. Samples for *Chlamydia* and *Neisseria gonorrhoeae* cultures are obtained from **pharynx** and **rectum** in **both sexes** and from the

vagina in girls. Generally, the **throat culture** is reported to be the **most traumatic** part of the examination by the child.

  f. **Herpes virus** testing should be done when suspicious lesions are present.

  g. Human immunodeficiency virus **(HIV)** and **hepatitis B** testing should be done when indicated by history.

  h. Aspirates from the vaginal vault should be collected and examined for sperm, acid phosphatase, and pathogenic organisms, when indicated by history.

  i. **Evidence of sperm and acid phosphatase may be detected in swabs from between the molars** up to 1 week after the last incident in cases of fellatio.

  j. The child's **head hair may be combed for evidence of pubic hairs** when indicated by history.

  k. **Stools** should be guaiac-tested for the **presence of occult blood** if sodomy has been part of the abuse.

  l. Swabs from the perianal area can be tested for sperm and acid phosphatase and cultured for gonorrhea.

  m. The results of the assessment should be recorded on a standardized form to ensure that all information has been gathered and documented and subsequently submitted to the investigative team.

E. **Management**

  1. In most states there is a **reporting law that mandates that health practitioners and other professionals who work with children report** suspected abuse **to child protective agencies** (law enforcement agencies such as police and sheriff departments, probation departments, departments of justice, and county welfare agencies). Each state has different laws and regulations. It is crucial and mandatory that the clinician know and **report appropriately.** Usually, there is a standardized form that must be completed following an immediate telephone report. [Figure 29.1 is an example of the Suspected Child Abuse Report used in California (Rev. 1/93). Copies of this completed report are sent to the agency contacted within 36 hours of the immediate telephone report. Copies are distributed to police or sheriff, county welfare or probation, and the district attorney.]

  2. Administer **treatment** as **appropriate** for any physical injuries (e.g., trauma, abrasions).

  3. Schedule **follow-up appointments** for reevaluation or treatment of gonorrhea (1 week), syphilis (4–6 weeks), pregnancy (at the latest, 6 weeks), HIV (6 weeks, 3 and 6 months), and HBsAg positive (4–6 weeks).

  4. If the child is in **danger of continued abuse or retaliation** for having reported the abuse, protection can be afforded by either **hospitalization or release to the community children's protective services.** It is the practitioner's responsibility to **report suspected sexual abuse of children and to be familiar with local reporting requirements.**

  5. Because the child's suffering goes far beyond any visible physical evidence of abuse, **a referral for counseling should be made immediately and should include the child and all family members involved in that child's care.**

F. **Sequelae.** The experiences of early and continuing sexual assault are carried into adulthood. **Counseling is indicated** for the victim's comfort as well as for interrupting the abuse cycle. The following sequelae often appear in some combination in both male and female victims of abuse.

  1. **Physical trauma residuals from untreated sexually transmitted disease or bodily injury.**

  2. **Psychosomatic complaints.**

  3. **Distorted self-image,** which may present with **hypersexuality, eroticized behavior, denial of sexual feelings or desirability,**

SUSPECTED CHILD ABUSE REPORT
To Be Completed by Reporting Party
Pursuant to Penal Code Section 11166

A. CASE IDENTIFICATION

TO BE COMPLETED BY INVESTIGATING CPA

VICTIM NAME:

REPORT NO./CASE NAME:

DATE OF REPORT:

B. REPORTING PARTY

NAME/TITLE

ADDRESS

PHONE ( )

DATE OF REPORT

SIGNATURE

C. REPORT SENT TO

☐ POLICE DEPARTMENT   ☐ SHERIFF'S OFFICE   ☐ COUNTY WELFARE   ☐ COUNTY PROBATION

AGENCY

ADDRESS

OFFICIAL CONTACTED

PHONE ( )

DATE/TIME

D. INVOLVED PARTIES

VICTIM

NAME (LAST, FIRST, MIDDLE)

ADDRESS

BIRTHDATE   SEX   RACE

PRESENT LOCATION OF CHILD

PHONE ( )

SIBLINGS

	NAME	BIRTHDATE	SEX	RACE		NAME	BIRTHDATE	SEX	RACE
1.					4.				
2.					5.				
3.					6.				

PARENTS

NAME (LAST, FIRST, MIDDLE)

BIRTHDATE   SEX   RACE

NAME (LAST, FIRST, MIDDLE)

BIRTHDATE   SEX   RACE

ADDRESS

ADDRESS

HOME PHONE ( )

BUSINESS PHONE ( )

HOME PHONE ( )

BUSINESS PHONE ( )

E. INCIDENT INFORMATION

IF NECESSARY, ATTACH EXTRA SHEET OR OTHER FORM AND CHECK THIS BOX. ☐

1. DATE/TIME OF INCIDENT

PLACE OF INCIDENT *(CHECK ONE)* ☐ OCCURRED ☐ OBSERVED

IF CHILD WAS IN OUT-OF-HOME CARE AT TIME OF INCIDENT, CHECK TYPE OF CARE:

☐ FAMILY DAY CARE ☐ CHILD CARE CENTER ☐ FOSTER FAMILY HOME ☐ SMALL FAMILY HOME ☐ GROUP HOME OR INSTITUTION

2. TYPE OF ABUSE: *(CHECK ONE OR MORE)* ☐ PHYSICAL ☐ MENTAL ☐ SEXUAL ASSAULT ☐ NEGLECT ☐ OTHER

3. NARRATIVE DESCRIPTION:

4. SUMMARIZE WHAT THE ABUSED CHILD OR PERSON ACCOMPANYING THE CHILD SAID HAPPENED:

5. EXPLAIN KNOWN HISTORY OF SIMILAR INCIDENT(S) FOR THIS CHILD:

SS 8572 (Rev. 1/93)

INSTRUCTIONS AND DISTRIBUTION ON REVERSE

DO NOT submit a copy of this form to the Department of Justice (DOJ). A CPA is required under Penal Code Section 11169 to submit to DOJ a Child Abuse Investigation Report Form SS-8583 if (1) an active investigation has been conducted and (2) the incident is **not** unfounded.

Police or Sheriff-WHITE Copy; County Welfare or Probation-BLUE Copy; District Attorney-GREEN Copy; Reporting Party-YELLOW Copy

FIG. 29.1. Sample reporting form.

anorexia or obesity, **or a facade that masks complaints** of emptiness inside and a belief that "I am not what I appear to others."
4. **Inability to verbalize sexual, erotic, or intimate feelings.**
5. **Feelings of being different from others and being alone** with the "secret."
6. **Low self-esteem, self-blame, and guilt.**
7. **Isolation and loneliness.**
8. **Amnesia,** especially for events surrounding the molestation.
9. **Suppression of affect or feeling.**
10. **Chronic PTSD** as described in *DSM-IV* (see summary of those symptoms, section I.C.). When PTSD becomes chronic, it is sometimes confused with borderline personality disorder as described in *DSM-IV*.
11. **Those who have histories of physical or sexual abuse are at risk for repeating this behavior.** They are often vulnerable to repeated victimization and are at risk for either sexually abusing others or choosing partners who will. The treatment goal is to relieve symptoms to promote more adaptive functioning. It also includes breaking the cycle to prevent victimization of the next generation of children.

References

1. American Academy of Child & Adolescent Psychiatry. Practice parameters for the forensic evaluation of children and adolescents who may have been physically or sexually abused. *J Am Acad Child Adolesc Psychiatry* 1997;36:423–442.
2. American Academy of Pediatrics. Policy statement; guidelines for the evaluation of sexual abuse of children: subject review (RE9819). *Pediatrics* 1999;103(1):186–191.
3. American Psychiatric Association (APA). *Diagnostic and Statistical Manual, 4th ed* (DSM-IV). Washington, DC: APA, 1994.
4. Bajt T, Pope K. Therapist–patient sexual intimacy involving children and adolescents. *Am Psychol* 1989;44:455.
5. Batterman-Faunce JM, Goodman GS. Effects of context on the accuracy and suggestibility of child witnesses. In: Goodman GG, Bottoms BL, eds. *Child victims, child witnesses.* New York: Guilford, 1993.
6. Blumenthal JA. The reasonable woman standard: a meta-analytic review of gender differences in perceptions of sexual harassment. *Law & Behav* 1998;22(1):33–57.
7. California Department of Consumer Affairs. *Professional therapy never includes sex,* 1990. (Available from Board of Psychology, 1430 Howe Avenue, Sacramento, CA 95825.)
8. Ceci SJ, Bruck M. Suggestibility of the child witness: a historical review and synthesis. *Psychol Bull* 1993;113:403.
9. Charney D, Russell R. An overview of sexual harassment. *Am J Psychiatry* 1994; 151:10.
10. Finkelhor D, et al. *A sourcebook on child sexual abuse.* Beverly Hills, CA: Sage, 1986.
11. Fitzgerald L. Sexual harassment: violence against women in the workplace. *Am Psychol* 1993;48:1070.
12. Gardner R. *True and false accusations of child abuse.* Cresskill, NJ: Creative Therapeutics, 1992.
13. Groth N. The incest offender. In: Sgroi S, ed. *Handbook of clinical intervention in child sexual abuse,* 2nd ed. New York: Lexington, 1993.
14. Kopels S, Dupper DR. School based peer harassment. *Child Welfare* 1999;78: 435–460.
15. Loftus E. The reality of repressed memories. *Am Psychol* 1993;48:518.
16. Office for Civil Rights (OCR). *Sexual harassment guidance: harassment of students by school employees, other students, or third parties.* (1997 guidance).
17. McDonald M. The myth of epidemic false allegations of sexual abuse in divorce cases. *Court Review* Spring 1998.
18. Pope K. How clients are harmed by sexual contact with mental health professionals: the syndrome and its prevalence. *J Counsel Dev* 1988;67:222.
19. Pope KS, Brown LS. Memory, abuse, and science: questioning claims about the false memory syndrome epidemic. *Am Psychol* 1996;51:957–974.

20. Schoener GE, Stewart DE. A curriculum of physician-patient sexual misconduct and teacher-learner mistreatment. *Can Med Assoc J* 1996;154:643–649.
21. Sgroi SM, ed. *Handbook of clinical intervention in child sexual abuse,* 2nd ed. New York: Lexington, 1993.
22. U.S. Department of Education Office for Civil Rights. Protecting students from harassment and hate crime—a guide for schools. January 1999.
23. U.S. Equal Employment Opportunity Commission. Discrimination because of sex under Title VI of the 1964 Civil Rights Act as amended: adoption of interim guidelines—sexual harassment. *Fed Regist* 1980;45:25024–25025.
24. U.S. Merit Systems Protection Board. Sexual harassment in the federal workplace trends, progress, and continuing challenges: a report to the President and the Congress of the United States by the. 1994:14.
25. Webb S. *Step forward: sexual harassment in the workplace.* New York: Master-Media, 1991.

30. RAPE

William M. Green

I. **Definition.** The traditional definition of *rape* (**"the unlawful carnal knowledge of a woman by force and against her will"**) has persisted since the sixteenth century. It has been only in the last 25 years that many states have revised and expanded their sexual assault statutes to be **gender-neutral** and to specify that **any sexual penetration (by any bodily part or foreign body)** completes the crime. Lack of consent to sexual activity is a key facet of the crime. Physical force, fraud, and threats to harm the victim or third parties are all sufficiently coercive to invalidate consent.

II. **Incidence.** More than 89,000 rapes were reported to the Federal Bureau of Investigations in 1999 compared with about 82,000 in 1980 and 37,000 in 1970. Rape is the **most underreported violent crime.** Some experts estimate that 70% of rapes are not reported; others believe that as many as 90% of sexual assaults never reach the attention of authorities. Fear of reprisal, shame, guilt, distrust of the criminal justice system, and recognition of the many negative stereotypes associated with sexual assault deter the majority of victims from contacting the police.

III. **Psychological impact.** Rape is a violent assault on both the body and the psyche whereby the assailant uses sex as a weapon to dominate, subjugate, degrade, or punish the victim. Rape is a pseudosexual crime with sexual behavior in service of nonsexual needs. Rape is not the result of uncontrolled sexual passion.

   The rape survivor has been through an unforgettable life crisis that disrupts her psychological equilibrium. **Victims almost uniformly report fear of death as the predominant emotion during the attack.** The violence, intimidation, and loss of control associated with the assault are much more potent stressors than the sexual aspects.

IV. **Approach to the victim.** A sympathetic and well-informed examiner who provides the necessary support, information, and guidance can be pivotal in helping the victim cope with, and recover from, her ordeal. A few simple techniques used at the initial encounter can facilitate the restoration of emotional equilibrium.

   A. Sexual assault is a crisis and should be viewed as a **medicolegal emergency.** The victim should be evaluated promptly and in an environment that is calm, supportive, and organized. Subjecting the victim to delays and the chaos of the emergency room heightens the victim's anxiety and apprehension and allows valuable forensic evidence to be lost.

   B. **Offer privacy.** A separate examination room is mandatory so that the victim may feel less vulnerable and the circumstances of the rape may be described in private. If a man conducts the examination, a female assistant **must** be present.

   C. **Establish rapport and initiate a supportive relationship.** Project a calm, professional, and nonjudgmental demeanor. Acknowledge the victim's feelings.

   D. **Help the victim regain a sense of control.**
      1. Encourage (but do not force) the victim to verbalize about the assault.
      2. Allow the victim to set the interview pace.
      3. Describe the sexual assault evaluation procedure.
      4. Ask permission before beginning examination or evidence collection procedures.

   E. **Acknowledge fear as the predominant emotion during rape.**
      1. Reassure the victim that she is now safe.
      2. Do not leave the victim alone; a nurse, family member, or rape crisis center advocate should stay with the victim.

F. Reassure the victim about her physical condition.
G. Acknowledge guilt as a universal feeling after sexual assault.
   1. Avoid phrases or innuendo that may seem judgmental.
   2. Use reflections or clarification to convey understanding.
H. Bolster self-esteem and support coping skills. Assure the victim that her **options during** the **assault** were **extremely limited** and that her **survival is testament** to her **strength** and **successful coping abilities.**
I. Reduce shame and embarrassment.
   1. Start with general questions before moving to specific sexual questions.
   2. Acknowledge the difficulty of discussing sexually explicit material.
   3. Explain that a complete and candid description of all sexual acts is necessary to search for injury or other findings. Also explain that each illegal act incurs a separate penalty.
V. History. Most states have forensic protocol that specifies the details required for the history, examination, and evidence collection. Medical information not specifically required by the protocol should be entered in a separate medical record. The history must also include basic demographic and past medical data plus the specific details of the assault.
   A. General medical history
      1. Demographic: victim's age and ethnicity, use of interpreter (if appropriate).
      2. Medical history.
         a. Medications.
         b. Allergies.
         c. Tetanus immunizations status.
         d. Preexisting injuries.
         e. Current illnesses (acute or chronic).
      3. Gynecologic history.
         a. Last menstrual period.
         b. Recent gynecologic injury, procedure, infection, or treatment that may influence the interpretation of current examination findings.
         c. Document the date and time of any consensual sexual activity that occurred within 5 days prior to the rape. This is essential to avoid confusion in the forensic analysis of semen evidence.
         d. Any additional gynecologic history that directly or indirectly implies prior sexual activity should be omitted, unless there is absolute medical relevance. At trial this information can be misused to humiliate the victim and to cause the jury to focus on her behavior rather than that of the assailant.
   B. Assault history
      1. Date and time of assault.
      2. Description of the assault surroundings with which the victim may have had direct contact (trace evidence) including location.
      3. The assailant(s).
         a. Name (if known) or brief description.
         b. Number.
         c. Ethnicity.
         d. Who did what.
      4. Method(s) of coercion.
         a. Weapon (threatened or used).
         b. Restraints.
         c. Threats (to the victim or others).
         d. Description of physical contact or struggle.
         e. Drug and/or alcohol use.
      5. Sexual acts.
         a. Penetration (attempted or accomplished) of vagina, rectum, or both.
         b. Oral acts.
         c. Foreign bodies.
         d. Prohibited touching.

      e. Use of lubricant.

      f. Use of condom.

      g. Ejaculation (site).

    6. Postassault cleanup (forensic implications).

      a. Genital wipe.

      b. Bathing.

      c. Douching.

      d. Clothing change.

      e. Gargling, eating, drinking, brushing teeth.

VI. Physical examination and evidence collection. Every jurisdiction has specific and detailed protocols for conducting the evidentiary examination and collecting forensic evidence. It is mandatory that the local protocol be followed exactly. Even the slightest deviation jeopardizes the integrity of the case. **A complete and legible record facilitates justice and decreases the probability of a court appearance; photographs of injuries and findings are particularly helpful.**

    A. Physical examination should include:

      1. Date and time of the examination and evidence collection.

      2. Assessment of demeanor and mental status.

      3. General physical examination with special attention to areas of complaint or injury.

      4. Complete dermal examination to document injury, foreign material, or stains.

      5. Pelvic examination to document trauma, stains, and foreign material and to collect samples for forensic sampling and evaluation.

      6. Rectal examination and anoscopy (if indicated) for evidence of trauma, stains, and foreign material and for forensic sampling and evaluation.

      7. Oral examination (if indicated) for evidence of trauma, foreign material, and forensic sampling.

      8. Alternative light source scanning to highlight stains and secretions.

      9. Many jurisdictions recommend a colposcopic examination of the vulva and vagina to document the presence of microtrauma.

    B. Investigative procedures and evidence collection usually include:

      1. Assault clothing.

      2. Reference hair samples (head and pubic).

      3. Pubic hair combings.

      4. Fingernail scrapings.

      5. Vaginal pool sampling for immediate motile sperm evaluation and swabs for forensic analysis to establish the presence of semen and detect genetic markers that will help include or exclude potential suspects. Additional swabs for possible DNA analysis may be needed, depending on the specific protocol. Cervical swabs may be requested in an attempt to recover sperm if the assault occurred more than 48 hours prior to the examination (see section VIII C.).

      6. A saliva sample (obtained from a chewed 2 × 2 gauze pad) and a blood sample are collected to help the crime laboratory identify and interpret and foreign antigens (which may have been left by the assailant) that are found in any of the evidence material.

      7. Sensitive urine or serum pregnancy test.

      8. Blood alcohol or toxicology screen (if indicated by the local protocol). Documented intoxication may invalidate the victim's ability to grant lawful consent to sexual activity. Toxicology sampling may also be helpful if drug-facilitated rape is suspected.

VII. Management. The treatment of the sexual assault victim is multifaceted. Both curative and preservative issues must be addressed. Acute injuries or complaints **must be evaluated and treated in the same expeditious way as for any emergency department patient.**

    A. Crisis intervention will be necessary to some degree for all victims. The use of consultation, medication, referral, and follow-up should be individualized to each victim. Medication should be used sparingly because chemical suppression of the responses to the event may prolong symptomatology and sequelae. Rape crisis advocacy is particularly helpful to facilitate both immediate crisis intervention and ongoing counseling.

B. Pregnancy prevention should be discussed with every victim of reproductive age. The risk of pregnancy varies with many factors. The probability of conception from a single act of coitus at midcycle is up to 30%. The overall average for pregnancy from a single, random intercourse is 2% to 4%. The alternatives for dealing with the potential pregnancy issues include:

1. **Repeat pregnancy test** in 2 weeks. A positive test will require a decision about continuing or terminating the pregnancy.
2. **Menstrual extraction** if the subsequent menses is delayed.
3. **Insertion of a copper-containing intrauterine device (IUD).** The insertion must be done within 5 days of the exposure, and the victim must accept the standard risks of IUD use (perforation, hemorrhage, infection, and infertility). This method also provides ongoing contraception.
4. **Postcoital hormonal treatment.** The best-tolerated method that is effective uses 100 mg ethinyl estradiol plus 1 mg norgestrel (equivalent to two Ovral tablets) at the time of the examination and again 12 hours later. Other combination oral contraceptive pills or progestin-only oral contraceptives also may be used.
   a. Treatment **must** be initiated within 72 hours of exposure.
   b. Side effects are usually mild (nausea, vomiting, irregular menstrual bleeding).
   c. The failure rate is less than 2%.
   d. The victim must be reevaluated if she has not had a menstrual period within 3 weeks of the treatment.

C. Sexually transmitted disease (STD) prophylaxis. The main preventable STD risks to the rape victim are gonorrhea, chlamydia infection, and syphilis. **Every victim should be strongly encouraged to take prophylaxis.** If the victim takes prophylaxis at the time of the examination, STD cultures are optional. If the patient declines prophylaxis, cultures are prudent and follow-up evaluation is required. The **minimum antibiotic regimen must include medication effective against** *Neisseria gonorrhoeae* and *Chlamydia trachomatis*. Although clinical data on incubating syphilis treatment is lacking, ceftriaxone, cefixime, erythromycin, doxycycline, and azithromycin have activity against *Treponema pallidum*. Age, allergy history, and potential pregnancy must be considered when selecting medications.

1. **Gonorrhea.**
   a. Ceftriaxone, 125 mg IM **or**
   b. Cefixime, 400 mg PO **or**
   c. Ciprofloxacin, 500 mg PO **or**
   d. Ofloxacin, 400 mg PO plus Azithromycin 1 g PO **or**
   e. Spectinomycin, 2 g IM, **or**
   f. Cefotetan, 1 g IM.
2. **Chlamydia.**
   a. Azithromycin 1 g PO **or**
   b. Doxycycline, 100 mg PO bid for 7 days **or**
   c. Erythromycin base, 500 mg PO qid for 7 days **or**
   d. Erythromycin ethylsuccinate, 800 mg PO qid for 7 days **or**
   e. Ofloxacin, 300 mg PO bid for 7 days.
3. The risk of contracting **aquired immunodeficiency syndrome** from sexual assault is of obvious concern to the rape victim. Unfortunately, there are no current data to define the degree of risk and no consensus regarding prophylaxis. Victims should be educated about HIV testing and given information about local resources. Ideally, blood for HIV testing should be drawn at the time of the postassault examination and repeated at 6, 12, and 24 weeks.
4. **Herpes virus** and **human papillomavirus infections** are also STD risks, but prophylaxis is not currently available.

5. The risk of acquiring **hepatitis B** after rape is unknown. Nonimmune victims should be offered postexposure vaccination (with follow-up immunization at 1 to 2 months and 4 to 6 months).

6. Vaginitis secondary to **trichomonal infection** or **bacterial vaginosis** has been reported after sexual assault. Although these infections are without significant morbidity and commonly diagnosed in sexually active women, **prophylaxis** with **metronidazole, 2 g PO should be offered** to the victim.

D. Arrangements should be made to ensure that the victim has a safe place to return to and that transportation is available.

E. Follow-up. Two follow-up visits are recommended after the initial examination.

   1. One to 2 weeks.

     a. Repeat cultures are obtained, if indicated.

     b. Pregnancy testing can be repeated, if indicated.

     c. A general assessment of the victim's emotional status is appropriate.

     d. A counseling referral should be made, if not already initiated.

     e. Forensic follow-up to document and photograph developing or healing injuries.

   2. Six to 12 weeks.

     a. Repeat Venereal Disease Research Laboratory (VDRL) test sample is drawn and laboratory work is reviewed.

     b. Treatment decisions, medical and psychological, should be tailored to the needs of the individual victim.

     c. HIV testing should be repeated at 6, 12, and 24 weeks.

F. Counseling

   1. Every rape victim can benefit from counseling and should be encouraged to take advantage of local resources. Most communities have some form of rape crisis center or hotline that offers an excellent starting place for support.

   2. Victims who were emotionally or psychiatrically disturbed before the assault may experience a **compound reaction,** with severe disorientation and symptomatology. For these victims, urgent psychiatric evaluation is mandatory.

VIII. Sequelae. The exact nature of the attack; the victim's age; and her coping style, support system, and preexisting mental health all influence the response to, and recovery from, sexual assault. Most victims, however, experience a **basic sequence of psychological events in the aftermath of rape.**

A. The **acute phase** may last from days to months.

   1. Shock and disbelief are very common initial reactions. The victim may appear calm and collected, her affect may be blunted, or she may seem somewhat withdrawn. Denial may effectively suppress her fear and anxiety. The outward appearance is a poor indicator of the inner turmoil she experiences.

   2. Shame and **guilt** may be very potent. Most victims believe they could, or should, have handled the situation differently for a better outcome. "If only" and "I should have" statements are frequent.

   3. Somatic complaints are common. She may have problems related to the specific physical trauma of the assault or she may experience generalized, nonspecific symptoms such as fatigue, headaches, diffuse soreness, and so forth.

B. The **recovery phase** is often preceded by a period of pseudoadjustment in which denial masks the patient's true emotions, and she appears to be "back to normal."

   1. As denial fades and defenses weaken, **depression** commonly develops. Sleep disturbance, nightmares, phobias, and the emergence of previously unresolved issues become problematic and cause many victims to initiate, or renew, counseling.

2. **Increased motor activity** affects many victims. Changing residence, changing phone numbers, taking trips (especially to see family members), or beginning new social networks are common.
3. **Anger** is uncommon before the recovery phase is well established. Mastery dreams, in which the victim kills or maims the rapist, are common and a healthy expression of anger.
4. **Integration and resolution** occur after the victim comes to terms with her feelings about the assault, the assailant, and her own sense of self-esteem and self-reliance.

References

1. Galsier A. Emergency postcoital contraception. *N Engl J Med* 1997;337:1058–1064.
2. Bienen L. Rape III: national development in rape reform legislation. 6 *Womens Rights L Rep* 1980;170(Spring).
3. Braen GR. *The rape examination.* North Chicago, IL: Abbott Laboratories, 1976.
4. Burgess A, Holmstrom L. Rape trauma syndrome. *Am J Psychiatry* 1974;131:981.
5. Centers for Disease Control. 1998 Sexually transmitted disease treatment guidelines. *MMWR* 47(RR-1), 1998.
6. Glaser J, Hammerschlag MR, McCormack MW. Epidemiology of sexually transmitted diseases in rape victims. *Rev Infect Dis* 1981;2:246.
7. Green WM. *Rape: the evidential examination and management of the adult female victim.* Lexington, MA: DC Health, 1988.
8. Hicks DJ. Rape: sexual assault. *Obstet Gynecol Ann* 1978;7:447.
9. Lippes J, et al. Postcoital copper IUDs. *J Assoc Planned Parenthood Phys* 1979; 14(3):87.
10. Notman MT, Nadelson CC. Psychodynamic and life-stage considerations. In: McCombie SL, ed. *The rape crisis intervention handbook.* New York: Plenum, 1980.
11. Office of Criminal Justice Planning. *State of California medical protocol for examination of sexual assault and child sexual abuse victims.* CA: Office of Criminal Justice Planning, 2001.
12. Sensabaugh GF, Bashinski J, Blake ET. The laboratory's role in investigating rape. *Diagn Med* 1985;March:46.
13. Shiff AF. Rape in the United States. *J Forensic Sci* 1978;23:850.
14. Sutherland S, Scherl D. Patterns of response among victims of rape. *Am J Orthopsychiatry* 1970;40:503.
15. Tietze C. Probability of pregnancy resulting from a single unprotected coitus. *Fertil Steril* 1960;11:485.
16. Vollman RF. Assessment of the fertile and sterile phases of the menstrual cycle. *Int Rev Nat Fam Plann* 1977;1:40.
17. Wooding BA, Evans JR, Bradbury MD. Sexual assault: rape and molestation. *Clin Obstet Gynecol* 1977;20:509.
18. Federal Bureau of Investigation, U.S. Department of Justice, Crime in the United States 1999. *Uniform crime reports.* 1999.

31. LESBIAN HEALTH ISSUES

Patricia A. Robertson

Only recently has attention been focused on health care issues for lesbians. A significant proportion (5%–10%) of female patients are lesbian. However, many lesbians do not disclose their sexual identity to practitioners because of previous negative experiences. It is important that the office environment be comfortable for all women, including lesbians. Sensitive support staff, patient educational materials that acknowledge and are inclusive of lesbian lifestyles, a diversity of magazines in the waiting room, and office forms that include a category for domestic partner (as well as for married or single) all help to accomplish a comfortable environment for lesbians.

A 1992 study revealed that 70% of self-identified lesbians are exclusively lesbian (engaging in sexual behavior with women only), 22% are primarily sexually active with women, and 6% are bisexual (10). The social support network for lesbians differs from that of heterosexual patients and includes friends, partners, family of origin, and co-workers. Acknowledgment of these social supports is fostered by not restricting visits in the intensive care unit to family of origin, but rather to the family of choice for the lesbian patient. According to national studies, 60% to 65% of lesbians are partnered in committed relationships.

I. **Approach to the lesbian patient**
   A. **Technique.** Lesbians are as varied as heterosexual women in their body physiques, personalities, education, and income. Most lesbians will not spontaneously inform their practitioner of their sexual orientation, although the majority would like their practitioners to know that they are lesbian (2).
      1. In the approach to history taking of any patient, **open-ended questions should be used** (e.g., "Are you sexually active, and if so, are you active with men, women, or both?").
      2. **Sensitivity and reassurance that all information will be confidential should be emphasized.** Before documenting the patient's lesbian lifestyle into the medical record, obtain permission to do so since employers might review their employee's medical records if the company is self-insured. Lesbian patients may be at risk for losing their jobs if employers discover their lifestyle (the majority of states do not have statutes protecting lesbians from discrimination based on sexual orientation). The lesbian patient may prefer that her lifestyle not be disclosed in the medical records for this or other reasons. However, other women may prefer that their lifestyle be documented in the medical record so that during future visits, the practitioner will not assume that they are heterosexual.
      3. The most frequent complaint by lesbians about their health care is that they are **automatically assumed to be heterosexual and are often inappropriately tested** [e.g., for sexually transmitted diseases (STDs)] **and counseled** (e.g., for birth control).
   B. **History.** A complete history should be taken, including a focus on the presenting problem with attention to:
      1. **Substance use:** tobacco, alcohol, injectable drugs.
      2. **Depression symptoms.**
      3. **Pregnancy plans,** if in reproductive age.
      4. **Number and gender of current partners** with assessment of patient knowledge base about STDs and contraception.
   C. **Physical examination** should be as comfortable as possible. Factors that influence this include the **partner's presence if requested** by the patient, the use of small **warmed speculums,** and an ongoing **explanation of each part of the examination.**

D. Investigative procedures
  1. **Mammography** and its importance in diagnosing early breast cancers need to be discussed, with initiation of regular mammography based on risk factors.
  2. A **Papanicolaou** (Pap) **smear** should be done according to risk factors and even if the lesbian patient has never been sexually active with men since the human papillomavirus can be transmitted between women (7).
  3. **Cultures** for gonorrhea and chlamydial infections are probably **not** indicated in lesbian patients **unless** a history of **heterosexual activity** or symptoms are present.
  4. **Guaiac** (Hemoccult) testing on stool and screening sigmoidoscopy should be done according to current guidelines (see Chapter 32).
  5. **HIV** testing should be offered to lesbians who are at risk. A recent study by the San Francisco Department of Public Health revealed the prevalence of HIV in lesbian and bisexual women to be 1.2%. This is more than three times higher than that estimated for all adult and adolescent women in San Francisco (0.35%) (9). For HIV-discordant lesbian couples, latex gloves or cut-up latex condoms may be useful in preventing transmission of HIV to the uninfected partner.
E. Referrals. It is important that the lesbian patient not be referred to homophobic practitioners or subspecialists. Past negative experience with homophobia in the health care system is probably the primary reason that lesbians have underutilized medical care. It is important to know which colleagues are sensitive to lesbian patients and to refer lesbians **only** to them. Several institutions have generated lists of lesbian-sensitive providers within the institution. The Gay and Lesbian Medical Association also maintains a list that covers a large geographical area (1-415-255-4547).

II. Specific medical issues
  A. STDs. For any woman who has been sexually active with men, including lesbians, baseline cervical cultures for chlamydia and gonorrhea should be obtained and blood tests ordered based on individual risk for syphilis, hepatitis C, and HIV. Hepatitis B immunization should be administered unless there is evidence of hepatitis B antibodies or a history of previous immunization. If the lesbian patient remains monogamous and her initial cervical cultures are negative, there is probably no need to do annual cervical cultures.
  B. Vaginitis does occur in lesbians. In one study of lesbians presenting to a lesbian clinic, 11% were diagnosed with bacterial vaginosis, 5% with monilial vaginitis, and 1% with trichomonal vaginitis (8). All women who had vaginitis responded to conventional therapy. Although there is no study on the transmission of vaginitis between female partners, there has been a high concordance (up to 80%) of bacterial vaginosis of partnered lesbians. **If the vaginitis recurs** after one treatment, **then** the lesbian **partner should be examined and treated** appropriately.
  C. Breast cancer. The incidence of breast cancer in women is 1:10 and is more common in those who have not had children at a relatively early age. Since 70% of lesbians have not had children, they may be **at increased risk for the development of breast cancer** compared with heterosexual women. **Routine breast screening with the breast self-examination should be encouraged,** as well as compliance with established mammography guidelines (see Chapter 9).
  D. Endometriosis may occur more often in lesbians than in heterosexual women because most lesbians have not had their menstrual cycles interrupted by pregnancy or prolonged exposure to oral contraceptives. **Dysmenorrhea, irregular intermenstrual spotting, and any clinical evidence of endometriosis** (e.g., adnexal mass, uterosacral nodularity) **should be thoroughly evaluated** to rule out endometriosis. The only accurate diagnosis for endometriosis is by **laparoscopy** (see Chapter 16).

III. Motherhood in lesbians. Currently, about 50% of lesbians seriously consider the option of motherhood (7) by **adoption, donor insemination, or intercourse.**

   A. **Studies** have been done **comparing children raised in lesbian households with those raised by single heterosexual mothers and no differences were noted** (1). Studies of the sexual identity of children raised in lesbian parented households show that the children are **not** more likely to be homosexual in orientation than those children raised by heterosexual parents.

   B. **In discussing parenting options with a lesbian patient,** a practitioner should be supportive of her decision and should provide the information she may need, such as medical issues and referrals for legal counseling. (The National Center for Lesbian Rights has a packet for prospective lesbian parents: 1-415-392-6257.) For lesbians who opt for pregnancy by **donor insemination,** frozen semen (not fresh) is recommended to allow a time lapse for HIV testing from the donor. If the semen is obtained through a sperm bank, then usually extensive donor testing has already been done. A known donor must be screened for HIV, hepatitis B surface antigen (HBsAg), rapid plasma reagin (RPR), and so forth by his primary care practitioner prior to insemination. If the lesbian couple plans to have a pregnancy by co-maternity (an egg is aspirated from one member of the couple and fertilized with sperm, and the embryo is placed in the uterus of the other member of the couple), then access to an *in vitro* fertilization program is needed.

      1. For the lesbian patient **planning a pregnancy, a complete medical examination should be done,** which should **include** a **history, physical examination,** and **laboratory testing** (Pap smear, urinalysis, complete blood cell count, rubella titer, blood type, Rh factor, HIV screening, RPR, HBsAg, and purified protein derivative).
      2. **Gonorrhea and chlamydial cultures** should be done if the woman has had **a history of sexual activity with men.**
      3. **Other screening should be done as appropriate** (e.g., Tay-Sachs, sickle cell).
      4. Three months prior to the insemination, the patient should begin taking either multivitamins, containing 0.4 mg of folic acid every day or prenatal vitamins (usually containing 1 mg of folic acid) to decrease the risk of birth defects in the fetus.
      5. Counseling should be done discussing the importance of abstaining from alcohol completely during the insemination period as well as avoiding exposure to environmental toxins during time of embryo development.

IV. Medicosocial issues

   A. **Rape.** Of the 148 lesbians in the San Francisco study (8), 40 reported having been **victims of rape** at some time in their lives. This is **similar to a comparable female heterosexual population.** Thirty percent of these women reported current sexual problems that they attributed directly to this traumatic event in their lives. None of the lesbians who had been raped had received counseling afterward. Lesbians and their partners should have **access to rape counseling programs that have staff trained in working with lesbians.** For further information, see Chapter 30.

   B. **Alcoholism.** There is increased use of alcohol in lesbians ages 20 to 40 compared with heterosexual women (4). Lesbian Alcoholics Anonymous (AA) groups are more effective in the treatment of lesbian alcoholics than are heterosexual AA groups (5). The provider should refer the patient to whatever appropriate resources are available in the community.

   C. **Suicide.** The incidence of suicide attempts and completed suicide in lesbian youths are increased compared with heterosexual female youths, possibly at a three times higher frequency rate (2). Thus, **increased sensitivity to adolescent females** struggling with sexual identity is important. Prompt appropriate psychotherapy referrals for youths with symptoms of depression are strongly recommended.

   D. **Hate crimes.** A number of lesbians have been victims of hate crimes (verbal abuse, threats of violence, property damage, physical violence, and murder).

One study in Philadelphia reported an incidence of 25% of lesbians being the victims of hate crime by a family member (6). It is important to **diagnose depression** and **stress-related illnesses** caused by societal homophobia and refer appropriately for supportive psychotherapy.

E. **Domestic violence.** Domestic violence does occur in lesbian relationships at approximately the same rate as in heterosexual relationships (11%), with some violence being in the context of alcohol abuse. Detection of battering in lesbians needs the same diligence as in heterosexual women. If there are no local resources in your area for lesbians who are in relationships with domestic violence, there is a hotline number that may be useful to them (1-800-799-SAFE). The counselors have received training in lesbian domestic violence. All victims of domestic violence should be encouraged to contact the local domestic violence center for counseling, if available (see Chapter 28).

References
1. Chan R, Raboy B, Patterson C. Psychosocial adjustment among children conceived via donor insemination by lesbian and heterosexual mothers. *Child Development* 1998;69:443–457.
2. Dardick L, Grady KE. Openness between gay persons and health professionals. *Ann Intern Med* 1980;93:115.
3. Feinlieb MR. *Report of the secretary's task force on youth suicide.* Rockville, MD: U.S. Department of Health and Human Services, 1989.
4. Gruskin E, et al. Patterns of cigarette smoking and alcohol use among lesbian and bisexual women enrolled in a large health maintenance organization. *Am J Pub Health* 2001;91:19.
5. Hall J. Alcoholism in lesbians: developmental, symbolic, interactionist, and critical perspectives. *Health Care Wom Int* 1990;11:89.
6. Herek GH. Hate crimes against lesbians and gay men: issues for research and policy. *Am Psychol* 1989;44:948.
7. Johnson S, Guenther S, Laube D, et al. Factors influencing lesbian gynecologic care: a preliminary study. *Am J Obstet Gynecol* 1981;140:20.
8. Marrazo JM, et al. Genital human papillomavirus infection in women who have sex with women. *J Infect Dis* 1998;178(6):1604–1609.
9. Robertson P, Schacter J. Failure to identify venereal disease in a lesbian population. *Sex Transm Dis* 1981;8:75.
10. Surveillance Branch, AIDS Office, San Francisco Department of Public Health. *HIV seroprevalence and risk behaviors among lesbians and bisexual women. The 1993 San Francisco/Berkeley women's survey,* October 19, 1993.
11. Warshafsky L. *Lesbian health needs assessment.* Los Angeles Gay and Lesbian Community Services, Los Angeles, 1992.

Additional Reading
Carroll NM. Optimal gynecological and obstetric care for lesbians. *Obstet Gynecol* 1999;93:611–613.
Koh A. Use of preventive health behaviors by lesbian, bisexual, and heterosexual women: questionnaire survey. *West J Med* 2000;172:379–384.
The National Institutes of Health. Solarz A, ed. *Lesbian health: current assessment and direction for the future.* Washington, DC: National Academy Press, 1999.
White J, Levinson W. Primary care of lesbian patients. *J Gen Intern Med* 1993;8:41.

Resources and Patient Education Materials
American College of Obstetricians and Gynecologists. *Lesbian health* Patient Pamphlet. 1-800-762-2264, ext. 183 or sales.acog.com
Domestic Violence Prevention Fund: Pink triangle wallet-sized card (wall dispenser available: ideal for bathroom in office) with domestic violence hotline number on it, as well as safety plan tips: www.fvps.org
Hotline number for lesbians in domestic violence relationships: 1-800-799-SAFE.
National Center for Lesbian Rights: 1-415-392-6257.
Office on Women's Health. *Lesbian Health Fact Sheet.* 200 Independence Avenue SW, Room 712E, Washington, DC 20201, 1-202-690-7650, www.4woman.gov, 1-800-994-WOMAN.

32. HEALTH CARE MAINTENANCE

Nancy D. Sullivan and Caryn Rybczynski

General health care maintenance, which includes screening procedures, education, and counseling as well as a good history and physical examination, is the responsibility of the primary health care provider. Since the specialties of medicine, family practice, obstetrics and gynecology, and pediatrics all may provide primary care, age-specific charts for periodic health examinations are included. These charts are from the U.S. Preventive Services Task Force and are the result of years of intensive research. Since many female patients inquire about health care issues for their male partners and children, these tables are all-inclusive (see Appendix).

I. **History**
   A. **General medical history**
      1. **A general medical history** should be obtained, including the patient's identification; medical history; surgeries and sequelae; history of trauma, allergies (agent and type of reaction), or transfusions (number, reasons, reactions); medications (prescription and over-the-counter, including any herbal remedies); breast self-examination (BSE); diethylstilbestrol (DES) exposure; occupational exposures and habits (quantitative use of alcohol, tobacco, caffeine, street drugs); and exercise patterns. Providers should also inquire into any history of and/or current abusive relationships including domestic violence and emotional and/or sexual abuse (see Chapters 28 and 29).
      2. **A family history** should include the age and health of parents, siblings, and children as well as any history of hypertension, heart disease, diabetes, cancer, kidney disease, anemia, muscular disorders, neurologic diseases, or birth defects.
   B. **Obstetric and gynecologic history**
      1. **The menstrual history** includes age of onset (menarche), length and duration of cycles, heavy or painful periods, last menstrual period, abnormal bleeding including intermenstrual bleeding, and menopause.
      2. **An infection history** includes herpes, gonorrhea, syphilis, chlamydia, human papillomavirus (HPV), HIV, hepatitis B, pelvic inflammatory disease, and vaginitis.
      3. **A neoplastic history** includes last Papanicolaou (Pap) smear; a history of an abnormal Pap smear or biopsies; and a history of ovarian, tubal, endometrial, cervical, vaginal, and vulvar cancer. Any cancer history must be documented regardless of type or organ involvement.
      4. **A history of DES exposure** must be obtained.
      5. The patient should be asked if there is any **history of unusual vaginal discharge or pelvic pain.**
      6. **A history of any gynecologic surgery** and the dates, indication for the surgery, and sequelae should be obtained.
      7. **An obstetric history** should include difficulty in conceiving; date of each pregnancy and outcome; therapeutic and/or spontaneous abortion; duration of pregnancy; sex and weight at birth of children; type of delivery; and problems during pregnancy, delivery, or the postpartum period.
   C. **Sexual history is essential.** It is best obtained in a nonjudgmental way without assumptions (i.e., that the patient is sexually active, monogamous, or heterosexual).
      1. **Possible ways to open the discussion** include "Are you satisfied with the sexual aspects of your life?" or "Do you have any questions or

This is a revision from the third edition chapter by Nancy D. Sullivan and Patti Tilton.

sexual difficulties that you would like to discuss?" or "Do you have a desire or need for contraception?" For lesbian patients or others who do not need contraception, it is still important to educate them about the noncontraceptive benefits of the birth control pill, especially if they are at high risk for ovarian or endometrial cancer.

2. **If a problem is identified,** assessment should include clarification of the problem including the duration of the problem, frequency, previous evaluation, and treatment. Additional important information needed includes the partner's response, a family history, early development, sexual information, sexual abuse including molestation and rape, early sexual experiences, current relationship, schooling and occupations, religious beliefs, medical and psychiatric histories, use of alcohol and drugs, and goals of treatment.

D. **Contraceptive history** is also imperative. This includes current method used (if any) and satisfaction with it, as well as methods used in the past and their success or failure. If the patient is not currently sexually active, it is still useful to ask her if she would like to discuss contraception to ensure that she is aware of the different methods available. In addition, heterosexual women who are using only barrier methods should be educated about the availability of emergency contraception in the event of failure of the primary method (see Chapter 22).

II. **Physical examination** is part of a continuum that includes a careful history and a focused physical examination.

A. **General examination**

1. **Vital signs. Blood pressure, pulse, and weight** should be obtained routinely.

2. **Neck.** The **thyroid and lymph nodes** (especially the supraclavicular) should be examined. The presence of webbing should be noted.

3. **Cardiopulmonary.**

a. **Auscultation of lungs** should be done to detect rales, rhonchi, or decreased breath sounds.

b. **Cardiac auscultation** is also essential.

4. **Breast.** A careful breast examination is particularly important and, at this time, the **patient should be taught how to do BSE.** It is often helpful to have the patient repeat or demonstrate a portion of the breast examination at this time to facilitate her comfort with doing her BSE.

a. The breasts should be carefully inspected, noting **size, symmetry, and contour** (i.e., masses, dimpling, and flattening).

b. The **skin should be observed for edema and venous pattern.**

c. The **nipples should be checked for inversion, rashes, ulcerations, or discharge.**

d. **Palpation** should then be done systematically, examining the entire breast including the periphery, tail, and areola. The pads of three fingers should be used in a rotary motion to compress the breast tissue gently against the chest wall.

5. **Axillae** should be **palpated for possible nodes.**

6. **Abdomen.** An abdominal examination is performed to check for **organomegaly, masses, ascites, or tenderness.** Note the presence or absence of any incisions that should correlate with the patient's surgical history.

B. **Pelvic examination**

1. The pelvic examination is usually **performed in the lithotomy position,** with the patient's thighs flexed and abducted, her feet in stirrups, and her buttocks extended slightly beyond the edge of the examining table. The woman should **empty her bladder prior** to the examination.

2. The patient's **external genitalia are first examined.**

a. **Pubic hair distribution** is noted.

b. The **labia minora, clitoris, urethral orifice, and introitus** are examined, looking for any inflammation, ulceration, swelling, or nodules.

          c. Any lesions are palpated. In the event that a lesion is identified and not previously discussed, a detailed history must be elicited.

    3. The **labia are then separated and the patient is asked to strain.** Any loss of urine or protrusion (i.e., anterior vaginal wall, cervix, or posterior vaginal wall) is noted.

    4. The **vagina** and **cervix** are examined by inserting a warm speculum into the vagina. The vagina is inspected for **inflammation, ulcers, atrophy, discharge,** and **masses.** This evaluation might be more thorough when performed at the end of the examination while **slowly withdrawing the speculum.** The cervix is inspected for **ulcerations, nodules, masses, bleeding,** or **discharge.** At this time, a Pap smear and, if needed, an endometrial biopsy should be obtained (see Chapter 19).

          a. Speculums are available in both **plastic** (disposable) and **metal.**

          b. Types of speculums include **Pedersens** and **Graves. Both** types **are** available in small, medium, and large sizes.

          c. A small-sized speculum should be used for most women.

          d. Some **menopausal women** may require a **small Pedersen** speculum.

          e. Children may require a **nasal speculum** for adequate examination.

    5. **The bimanual examination** is performed while the clinician is in the standing position. The index and middle fingers of a gloved, lubricated hand are inserted into the vagina.

          a. The vaginal wall is palpated for nodularity and tenderness.

          b. The **cervix is then identified and palpated,** noting its position if significantly deviated from the midline, shape, and consistency and checking for cervical motion tenderness.

          c. The uterus is palpated by placing the other hand on the abdomen about midway between the umbilicus and symphysis pubis and pressing down toward the pelvic hand. The uterus is identified and its position (e.g., anteversion, retroversion, anteflexion, retroflexion, midposition) is noted. It is examined for **size, shape, consistency, mobility, tenderness,** and **masses.**

          d. The adnexa are examined by placing the abdominal hand on one side of the lower abdomen and the pelvic hand in the same lateral fornix and palpating the adnexal area (now between the two hands). The **size, shape, consistency, and mobility** of the adnexa and **any palpable masses** should be noted. Ovaries should not be palpable 3 to 5 years after menopause. **If an ovary is palpated, a tumor must be suspected.** The uterus also involutes with time.

    6. Recent evidence indicates that the **rectovaginal examination** is **no longer** necessary to be **routinely performed.** In the event that this examination is indicated, place the index finger into the vagina, while the middle finger is placed into the rectum. The maneuvers of the bimanual examination are repeated, with special attention to the region behind the cervix and the posterior uterine wall. If the patient is older than 50 years of age, the stool may be tested for blood (guaiac). Due to dietary influences on the results and the rates of false-positive and false-negative results, the routine use of this test has become controversial.

III. Screening procedures. As the primary health care provider for women, it is important that the provider employ screening procedures as part of health care maintenance.

    A. Risk factors for gynecologic cancers

        1. **Endometrium:** unopposed estrogen exposure (i.e., estrogen therapy without progestin, tamoxifen, late menopause, polycystic ovary disease, estrogen-secreting ovarian tumors); nulliparity; obesity; family history; long history of menstrual irregularities; endometrial hyperplasia; or other malignancy such as ovary, breast, and colon.

        2. **Ovary:** low or no parity, decreased fertility, delayed childbearing, family history of ovarian cancer, and no history of oral contraceptive use.

3. **Cervix:** initial sexual intercourse during the adolescent years, multiple sexual partners, or cigarette smoking. HPV appears to be an important factor, although its exact role has yet to be determined (see Chapter 4).
4. **Vulva:** chronic vulvar irritation, previously uncontrolled chronic vulvar dystrophy, condyloma acuminatum, granulomatous vulvar lesions, immunosuppression, vulvar intraepithelial neoplasia, or smoking.

B. **Warning signs for various gynecologic cancers**
   1. **Endometrium.** Postmenopausal uterine bleeding, prolonged heavy menstrual flow especially if preceded by periods of amenorrhea, and intermenstrual spotting are indications for **further investigation.**
   2. **Ovary. There are no early warning signs.**
      a. Most symptoms are related to the increasing tumor mass such as abdominal discomfort or upper abdominal fullness.
      b. Related pleural effusions may cause fatigue, increasing abdominal girth, urinary frequency, or shortness of breath.
   3. **Cervix.** The initial symptom can be a thin, watery, blood-tinged vaginal discharge. A classic symptom is intermittent, painless metrorrhagia, which is often only postcoital spotting or spotting after douching. As the tumor grows, bleeding becomes heavier, more frequent, and of longer duration. Late symptoms include pain referred to the flank or leg. Dysuria, hematuria, rectal bleeding, or obstipation commonly occur.
   4. **Vulva.** The most common symptom is pruritus. A lump, sore, pain or bleeding may also be the first symptom.

C. **Cancer screening procedures.** The American College of Obstetricians and Gynecologists (ACOG) and the U.S. Preventive Services Task Force recommend a cancer-related health checkup for **all women who have been sexually active or who have reached age 18.**
   1. After a woman has had three or more consecutive, satisfactory, normal cervical Pap tests, the Pap test may be performed less frequently, for example, every 2 to 3 years, depending on risk factors and the discretion of the clinician.
   2. **All sexually active women** should have **annual** breast and pelvic examinations and Pap smears depending upon risk factors.
   3. **Perimenopausal and postmenopausal women with** a history or evidence of **abnormal vaginal bleeding** are at high risk for endometrial cancer and should have an **endometrial biopsy or curettage** without delay.
      a. Some clinicians use age 35 as a cutoff for performing an endometrial biopsy for abnormal bleeding. However, in **younger women with risk factors** for endometrial cancer such as obesity and amenorrhea, it is reasonable to **perform** an **endometrial biopsy.**
      b. **Dilation and curettage** (D & C) is recommended when endometrial hyperplasia or questionable endometrial carcinoma are present and when there is insufficient tissue for diagnosis by endometrial biopsy.
      c. **Hysteroscopy** has been increasingly used in association with endometrial biopsy or D & C to identify polyps or fibroids.
      d. **Ultrasonography** can also be used in the evaluation of postmenopausal bleeding.
         (1) An **endometrial stripe** <5-mm thick usually indicates a benign lesion and no biopsy is needed unless bleeding persists.
         (2) An endometrial stripe >10-mm thick indicates that a biopsy **should** be done.
   4. Most guidelines agree that **screening mammograms** should be done every 1 to 2 years for women who are 50 to 75 years.
      Routine screening, except in high-risk patients, should not be done prior to age 40. However, recommendations for routine screening of women 40 to 49 range from never to every 1 to 2 years (see Chapter 9 and Appendix A).

5. **Breast examination guidelines.**
   a. **Women ages 20 to 40** should have a breast examination every 3 years.
   b. **Women older than age 40** should have a breast examination every year.
   c. **All women older than age 20** should perform a BSE monthly.
   d. **Women with personal or family histories of breast cancer** may need more frequent physical examinations or periodic mammography prior to age 50.
6. **Colorectal screening** guidelines may vary among organizational recommendations (see Appendix, Table 3 and section II.B.7.).
   a. **Women older than 40** should have a digital rectal examination every year.
   b. **Women older than age 50** should have a sigmoidoscopic examination every 3 to 10 years depending on risk factors (see Appendix, Table 3).
7. **Ovarian cancer screening** guidelines. No techniques that have proved to be effective in reducing the disease-specific mortality of ovarian cancer are currently available.
   a. The American College of Preventive Medicine currently does **not** recommend routine pelvic examinations for the detection of ovarian cancer.
   b. However, pelvic examinations may be performed for diagnostic purposes, or CA 125 or ultrasound may be used to screen asymptomatic women depending upon risk factors.
      (1) These same recommendations apply to women with either none or one first-degree relative with ovarian cancer.
      (2) Screening of women with familial cancer syndrome may be appropriate due to their elevated risk of cancer; however, direct **evidence** of effectiveness is **lacking**.

D. **Laboratory tests**
1. **A rubella titer for women of childbearing age on first gynecologic visit. A varicella titer should also be drawn if there is an uncertain or no history of chickenpox.**
2. **A wet-mount smear of vaginal discharge** as indicated.
3. **A Veneral Disease Research Laboratory (VDRL) test** at first visit **and** as indicated.
4. **Chemistry screening** including cholesterol is done as indicated by the medical and family history.
5. **Gonococcal and chlamydial cultures** if indicated by history or symptoms.
6. **HIV testing should be offered.**
7. **Hepatitis B surface antigen and hepatitis C antibody** test should be offered.

E. **Immunizations**
1. **Measles, mumps,** and **rubella booster** should be given to anyone born after 1956 unless they have previously had two doses. It is recommended that women abstain from becoming pregnant for 12 weeks after receiving this vaccine.
2. **Tetanus-diptheria booster** should be offered as indicated.
3. **Hepatitis A series** is recommended for high-risk adult groups (following the hepatitis B recommendations).
4. **Hepatitis B vaccine** series is recommended for anyone with risk factors including sexual activity, occupation, and needle use.
5. **Varicella vaccine** is recommended for anyone who has not had varicella (chickenpox) previously. It is recommended that women abstain from becoming pregnant for 12 weeks after receiving this vaccine.
6. **Influenza vaccine** is recommended yearly in patients 65 years or older and for those of any age with significant chronic disease (see Appendix, Table 3).

7. **Pneumovax vaccine** is recommended for anyone 65 years or older or for those with any medical problem that increases the risk of developing pneumococcal pneumonia (see Appendix, Table 3).

IV. **Education and counseling** are essential parts of health care maintenance. The function of health care education is to equip people intellectually and emotionally to make sound decisions on matters affecting their health, safety, and welfare. Subjects that frequently need to be addressed include the following: **nutrition** (e.g., general obesity; iron, vitamins, and calcium intake), **exercise, substance abuse** (e.g., tobacco, alcohol, street drugs, prescription and over-the-counter medications including herbal remedies, and caffeine), and **stress reduction.**

In addition, the **primary care provider should be familiar with postmenopausal hormonal therapy** (see Chapter 25) and **contraception** (see Chapter 22).

A. **Tampons.** Toxic shock syndrome (TSS) has led to many inquiries about the safety of tampons. TSS is a **multisystem illness with a wide range of signs and symptoms.** A prodromal illness consisting of malaise, myalgias, low-grade fever, vomiting, or diarrhea has been reported in some patients. These symptoms later progress to the acute systemic illness. Onset of the acute illness generally occurs precipitously with the appearance of fever ($\geq 38.8°C$; $102°F$), chills, severe hypotension, myalgias, pharyngitis, conjunctivitis, leukocytosis, and a generalized desquamative rash.

1. **The causes of TSS are not yet thoroughly understood** but it has been hypothesized that a **staphylococcal toxin,** either alone or in conjunction with other as yet unidentified factors, causes the widespread systemic illness.
2. Currently, fewer than 300 cases are reported annually to the Centers for Disease Control.
3. **The greatest risk is with high-absorbency tampons and with continuous use of tampons during menses.** There is up to a 30% recurrence rate, and multiple recurrences have been observed. There is a 2.6% to 13.0% case fatality.
4. **Women can significantly decrease their risk of developing TSS** by avoiding the use of tampons during menses and using other products, such as napkins or minipads. It has also been suggested that the intermittent use of tampons, such as alternating them with napkins, may reduce the risk of TSS.
5. Studies have suggested that **women who use oral contraceptives may have a decreased risk** of developing TSS.
6. **Women who have had an episode of TSS should be advised to discontinue tampon use altogether.**

B. **Feminine hygiene products. Vaginal discharge and bad odor** cause concern in many women, and some find even normal odor and discharge unpleasant. Common causes of bad odors include intertrigo; smegma; accumulation of sebum and sweat; the smell associated with a copper intrauterine device (IUD); infection caused by Monilia, bacterial vaginosis, or *Trichomonas* species; semen; old blood; a retained tampon; or, less commonly, a cervical carcinoma. **Once a specific lesion has been excluded and if no pathogenic organism is found** in routine laboratory tests, then **explanation and reassurance** may be all that is needed. In some patients, **improved local hygiene** may be all that is necessary (i.e., a daily bath).

1. **Deodorant sprays, douches, and wipes should be discouraged** as they are likely to cause soreness of the vulvar skin, contact dermatitis, or allergy.
2. **Douches can cause the vagina to become dry and can cause vaginitis** since the natural secretions are washed away.
3. **If no pathogenic organism** is found in routine laboratory tests **but the discharge is excessive and smelly,** an **infection with unusual microorganisms should be suspected.** Treatments should aim either

to bolster the natural defenses by reducing the vaginal pH or to kill all microorganisms using an antiseptic preparation [e.g., povidone-iodine (Betadine)].

References

1. American Cancer Society. *Cancer facts and figures.* Atlanta, GA: American Cancer Society, 1998.
2. The American College of Obstetricians and Gynecologists. *Report of task force on routine cancer screening.* ACOG opinion No. 128, October 1993.
3. American Cancer Society. Summary of American Cancer Society recommendations for the early detection of cancer in asymptomatic people. *CA Cancer J Clin* 1993;43:42.
4. American College of Obstetricians and Gynecologists. *Cervical cytology: evaluation and management of abnormalities.* Washington, DC: American College of Obstetricians and Gynecologists, 1993. ACOG Technical Bulletin, no. 183.
5. American College of Physicians Task Force on Adult Immunization/Infectious Diseases Society of America. *Guide for adult immunization,* 3rd ed. Philadelphia: American College of Physicians, 1994.
6. American College of Preventive Medicine Practice policy statement. Screening asymptomatic women for ovarian cancer. *Am J Preventive Med* 1997;13:444–446.
7. *Am J Preventative Med* 1998;14(2):156–158.
8. Breast cancer screening for women ages 40–49. *NIH Consensus Statement* January 1997;15(1):1–35.
9. *Guide to clinical preventive services,* 2nd ed. Report of the U.S. Preventive Services Task Force. Baltimore: Williams & Wilkins, 1996.
10. Precis IV. Washington, DC: American College of Obstetricians and Gynecologists.
11. Wagner G. Toxic shock syndrome: a review. *Am J Obstet Gynecol* 1983;46:93.
12. *Women's health consensus program handbook.* Little Falls, NJ: Health Learning Systems, 1990.
13. U.S. Department of Health and Human Services/Public Health Service. Adults/older adults screening: Papanicolaou smear. In: *Clinician's handbook of preventive services.* Washington, DC: U.S. Government Printing Office, 1994.

33. COMPLEMENTARY AND ALTERNATIVE MEDICINE

Harley Goldberg

I. **Introduction.** Complementary and alternative medicine (CAM) constitutes approaches to health and health care, treatments for disease, and cultural health care systems that lie outside conventional Western medical practice. These varied treatments are often grouped into categories by either treatment or condition. Since they arose before or outside the sphere of scientific method, they often lack a scientific evidence base; although this is beginning to change. Like early Western medicine, these traditions grew upon the clinical observations of respected clinicians. How these therapies or practices are integrated with conventional care is dependent upon how the individual person balances their life, preventive care, and health care. Most often, patients do not tell their provider about the alternative care they use. It is very important to ask specific questions about the patient's use of other treatments and clinicians.

Overall, the evidence base in CAM is weak. Dosages, interactions, adverse effects, and other more subtle aspects of care are poorly understood. Patients often have **misconceptions** such as **"because it's natural, it must be safe."** The most important aspect of patient care in regard to CAM is no different than patient care in any arena: open, honest, nonjudgmental discussion focused on the patient's values and health care choices.

It is not surprising that the majority of users of CAM **are** women. The majority of health care users and decision makers are women. This is not a new phenomenon, women for ages have been carriers of the healing traditions now categorized as CAM. Although there are claims for many treatments, in this overview we focus on the treatments most commonly used for women's health, and those for which some evidence exists to evaluate safety or effectiveness. They are often used for varying conditions. The use of specific vitamins or minerals for prevention or treatment of various diseases is discussed in the appropriate chapters in this manual (such as the use of calcium and vitamin D in osteoporosis) and is not addressed here.

II. **Alternative and complementary therapies for menopausal symptoms**
   A. **Dietary soy and phytoestrogens.** There are three main categories of phytoestrogens: isoflavones, lignins, and resorcylic acid lactones. Isoflavones are found in soy and other legumes. Lignins are found in flax seed oil, whole grains, fruits, and vegetables. Resorcylic acid lactones are found in fungi and are less common in normal diets.
      1. Women using soy proteins and other phytoestrogens **have** demonstrated a modest decline in the frequency and/or severity of vasomotor symptoms associated with menopause (1,2). The minimum dose required for effect is not known.
      2. Evidence of the effect of phytoestrogens on **lipid profiles is conflicting** (3,4), and the effect on the clinically relevant end point, cardiovascular events, is unknown. However, soy does have a beneficial effect on cardiovascular risk factors.
         a. In a meta-analysis of 38 controlled trials (5) an average of 47 g of soy protein daily was associated with reduced cholesterol (23.2 mg/dL or 9.3%), **reduced low-density lipoprotein (LDL) cholesterol** (21.7 mg/dL or 12.9%), and **reduced triglycerides** (13.3 mg/dL or 10.5%). **High-density lipoprotein (HDL) was unaffected.**
         b. There is physiologic evidence that soy competitively inhibits hormone replacement therapy (HRT) or endogenous hormones. It is possible that concomitant use of soy with HRT **may decrease** total effect.
      3. The effect of phytoestrogens on bone mineral density (BMD) and the clinically relevant end point of fractures is not known (6).

4. The incidence of adverse effects from soy proteins was not different from placebo. The most common adverse reaction was mild gastrointestinal (GI) complaints.

5. Epidemiologic studies associate a diet high in phytoestrogens with a reduction in breast cancer rates and improved breast cancer survival and decreased osteoporotic fractures especially in women of Asian descent (7–10). There are several other confounding variables, such as a low-fat, high-fiber diet, and other cultural and lifestyle issues.

6. A case control study of 332 multiethnic Hawaiian women with endometrial cancer matched with 511 controls showed that high consumption of phytoestrogens was associated with a decreased risk of endometrial cancer (11).

B. Ipriflavone is a nonsteroidal synthetic isoflavone. It maintains BMD in the perimenopausal period, and is associated with a modest improvement in BMD in postmenopausal women (12–15).

1. There may be some benefit in vasomotor symptoms as well (12).

2. The dose of ipriflavone in these trials was 200 mg tid.

3. There may be reduced effectiveness when combining ipriflavone with HRT, possibly resulting from competition for estrogen receptor sites (15).

C. Progesterone cream. There is very limited evidence that progesterone cream may decrease vasomotor symptoms (16). There is insufficient evidence for any other effects. There is evidence that progesterone cream does not preserve or improve bone density or lipid levels.

1. Patients using over-the-counter progesterone cream in conjunction with traditional estrogen replacement therapy should be counseled and treated as if they were on unopposed estrogen (17).

2. There is the indirect risk that use of "natural hormones" will decrease the use of effective therapy.

D. Dehydroepiandrosterone (DHEA). DHEA is a steroid hormone related to testosterone and estrogen. It was classified as a supplement by the Dietary Supplement Health and Education Act of 1994. Endogenous DHEA is made from cholesterol in the adrenal glands. Levels decrease with aging, and by the seventh decade, may be as low as 10% to 20% of their peak values. There is inadequate evidence to support the use of DHEA for menopausal symptoms, and the potential for adverse effects is high (18–22).

III. Botanicals. Many herbal remedies are recommended in lay press for menopause and other gynecologic uses. They are classified as food or dietary supplements, not as drugs. Yet they have biologically active components, physiologic effects, adverse effects, and herb-drug effects. They should be considered pharmacologically active compounds, although as a rule they are relatively weak. In addition, the manufacturing of these products is not regulated by the Food and Drug Administration, and therefore there is inconsistency in the quality of products on the market.

A. Black cohosh *(Cimicifuga racemosa).* One of the most commonly recommended herbs for women is black cohosh. Although there are physiologic studies, there are no randomized controlled trials (RCTs) evaluating its effectiveness (23,24). Several open trials supported by the manufacturer of Remifemin (an alcohol extract of black cohosh) showed reduction in hot flashes and improved mood.

1. **Traditional use.** Menopausal symptoms, premenstrual syndrome (PMS), dysmenorrhea.

2. **Dose.** For menopause and PMS, the clinical studies that exist have been sponsored by and use a single product that is a specific black cohosh extract (Remifemin) standardized to contain 1 mg triterpene glycosides per 20 mg tablet. Most studies used doses of **40 to 80 mg twice daily,** providing 4 to 8 mg triterpene glycosides. (The manufacturer now claims that improvement in the extraction process permits using their currently recommended lower dose of **20 mg twice daily,** providing 2 mg triterpene glycosides.)

3. **Physiologic effect.** Competitively inhibits estradiol binding to estrogen receptors.
4. **Mechanism of action unknown.**
5. **Adverse effects.** Most commonly GI symptoms, headaches, and dizziness.
6. **Contraindications.** Pregnancy, lactation, estrogen dependent tumors. May potentiate antiproliferative effect of tamoxifen.
7. **Safety.** Although adverse event reporting is extremely limited, at present it is thought to be likely safe for the indications discussed here at the discussed doses. Effect on osteoporosis and cardiovascular disease unknown. Theoretical risk of use with estrogen positive tumors.
8. **Effectiveness.** Based on limited number and quality of studies, possibly effective for menopausal symptoms.

B. **Dong quai** *(Angelica polymorpha).* A single clinical trial shows no significant difference between dong quai and placebo for vasomotor symptoms and vaginal and epithelial effects (25). Although it is usually used in a mixture in Chinese formulas, as an isolated herb it cannot be recommended for menopause symptoms.
1. **Traditional use.** Menopause, PMS, dysmenorrhea.
2. **Dose.** Dosage is 1 to 3 g per day in divided doses.
3. **Physiologic effect.** Animal studies demonstrate both uterine stimulation (water and alcohol-soluble components) and uterine inhibition (volatile oil component).
4. **The mechanism of action is unknown.** Several coumarin constituents are present, and it may have an antiplatelet effect.
5. **Adverse effects.** Possible bleeding, diarrhea, fever, and known photosensitivity.
6. **Contraindications.** Pregnancy, lactation, and bleeding dyscrasias. Interaction with warfarin anticoagulants. Unknown effect on estrogen dependent tumors.
7. **Safety.** It is possibly unsafe with large doses and there is the potential for drug-herb interaction as described previously.
8. **Effectiveness.** One RCT shows no effect as an isolated agent on menopausal symptoms.

C. **Chastetree** *(Vitex angus-castus)*
1. **Traditional use.** Menopause, PMS, dysmenorrhea.
2. **Dose.** The dosage is 20 mg per day.
3. **Physiologic effect.** Claimed to have antiinflammatory, antiandrogenic, and progesterone effects.
4. **Adverse effects.** Abdominal pain, cramping, diarrhea, headache, and rash.
5. **Contraindications.** Pregnancy and lactation.
6. **Safety.** Foreign studies show possibly safe.
7. **Effectiveness.** Possibly effective in PMS, insufficient information in other clinical conditions.

D. **Ginger** *(Zingiber officinale)*
1. **Traditional use.** Nausea, vomiting, dyspepsia, GI complaints, and motion sickness.
2. **Dose:** The dosage is 1 to 2 g powdered extract tid.
3. **Physiologic effect.** Antiemetic, promotes secretion of saliva and gastric juices, and cholagogue (promotes the flow of bile into the intestine). Physiologic studies indicate there may be hypoglycemic, hypotensive or hypertensive, and positive cardiac inotropic activities. It also may inhibit platelets and prostaglandins.
4. **Adverse effects.** Heartburn, diarrhea, and abdominal discomfort.
5. **Contraindications.** Theoretical risk of teratogenicity in pregnancy and lactation.
6. **Safety.** Likely safe in usual doses.

7. **Effectiveness.** A systematic review of clinical trials for nausea and vomiting concluded it is possibly effective and low risk.
E. **Ginkgo *(Ginkgo biloba)***
1. **Traditional use.** Asthma, memory loss, headache, tinnitus, vertigo, dizziness, difficulty concentrating, mood disturbances, and hearing disorders.
2. **Indication.** Dementia and peripheral arterial occlusive disease.
3. **Dose.** The dosage is 120 to 240 mg dry leaf extract in 2 to 3 divided doses.
4. **Physiologic effect.** Inhibition of platelet aggregating factor and thrombus formation, arterial vasodilatation, and reduced capillary fragility.
5. **Adverse effects.** Bleeding and contact dermatitis.
6. **Contraindications.** Concomitant use of anticoagulants, antiplatelet agents.
7. **Safety.** Likely safe.
8. **Effectiveness.** Small but significantly positive effect in patients with dementia, no clear benefit in patients without cognitive impairment.
F. **St. John's wort *(Hypericum perforatum)***
1. **Traditional use.** Depression, gastritis, insomnia, enuresis, PMS, and menopause.
2. **Indication.** Mild to moderate depression.
3. **Dose.** The dosage is 300 mg extract (standardized to 0.3% hypericin) tid.
4. **Physiologic effect.** Mechanism of action unknown. Inhibits reuptake of GABA, serotonin, dopamine, and norepinephrine *in vitro*.
5. **Adverse effects.** GI, allergic reactions, constipation, dizziness, dry mouth, and fatigue.
6. **Contraindications.** Pregnancy and lactation and in children.
7. **Interactions.** Induces hepatic cytochrome P450 system, thereby potentially interacting with any drug cleared by this system including protease inhibitors, nonnucleoside reverse transcriptase inhibitors, cyclosporin, calcium channel blockers, beta-blockers, digoxin, phenytoin, phenobarbital, tamoxifen, or oral contraceptives. In addition, potentiation of selective serotonin reuptake inhibitors (SSRIs) has been reported, creating serotonism (headache, sweating, dizziness, agitation).
8. **Safety.** When used without any other drugs, it is likely safe. The interactions noted previously are important limitations to the safe use of this herb.
9. **Effectiveness.** Multiple RCTs and meta-analysis has demonstrated the effectiveness of St. John's wort in mild to moderate depression. It has been shown to be as effective as tricyclic antidepressants, and a comparison to SSRIs is currently underway at the National Institutes of Health.

References

1. Albertazzi P, et al. The effect of dietary soy supplementation on hot flushes. *Obstet Gynecol* 1998;91:6–11.
2. Washburn S, et al. Effect of soy protein supplementation on serum lipoproteins, blood pressure, and menopausal symptoms in perimenopausal women. *Menopause* 1999;6(1):7–13.
3. Baird DD, et al. Dietary intervention study to assess estrogenicity of dietary soy among postmenopausal women. *J Clin Endocrinol Metab* 1995;80:1685–1690.
4. Baum J, et al. Long-term intake of soy protein improves blood lipid profiles and increases mononuclear cell low-density-lipoprotein receptor messenger RNA in hypercholesterolemic, post-menopausal women. *Am J Clin Nutr* 1998;68:545–551.
5. Anderson JW, et al. Meta-analysis of the effects of soy protein rich intake on serum lipids. *N Engl J Med* 1995;33:276–282.
6. Potter SM, et al. Soy protein and isoflavones: their effect on blood lipids and bone density in postmenopausal women. *Am J Clin Nutr* 1998;68[Suppl]:1375S–1379S.
7. Knight DC, Eden JA. A review of the clinical effects of phytoestrogens. *Obstet Gynecol* 1996;87:897–904.

8. Ingram D, Sanders K, Kolybaba M, et al. Case-control study of phytoestrogens and breast cancer. *Lancet* 1997;350:990–994.
9. Rose DP, Boyar AP, Wynder EL. International comparisons of mortality rates for cancer of the breast, ovary, prostate, and colon, and per capita food consumption. *Cancer* 1986;58:2363–2371.
10. Ziegler RG, Hoover RN, Pike MC, et al. Migration patterns and breast cancer risk in Asian-American women. *J Natl Cancer Inst* 1993;85:1819–1827.
11. Goodman M, Wilkens LR, Hankin JN, et al. The association of dietary phytoestrogens with the risk for endometrial cancer. *Am J Epidemiol* 1997;146:294–306.
12. Agnusdei D, et al. Prevention of early postmenopausal bone loss using low doses of conjugated estrogens and the non-hormonal, bone-active drug ipriflavone. *Osteopososis Int* 1995;5:462–466.
13. Agnusdei D, et al. A double blind, placebo-controlled trial of ipriflavone for prevention of postmenopausal spinal bone loss. *Calcif Tissue Int* 1997;61:142–147.
14. Agnusdei D, Bufalino L. Efficacy of ipriflavone in established osteoporosis and long-term safety. *Calcif Tissue Int* 1997;61:S23–S27.
15. de Aloysio D, et al. Bone density changes in postmenopausal women with the administration of ipriflavone alone or in association with low-dose ERT. *Gynecol Endocrinol* 1997;121:289–293.
16. Leonetti HB, Longo S, Anasti J. Transdermal progesterone cream for vasomotor symptoms and postmenopausal bone loss. *Obstet Gynecol* 1999;94(2):225–228.
17. Cooper A, et al. Systemic absorption of progesterone from Progest cream in postmenopausal women. *Lancet* 1998;351:1255–1256.
18. Casson PR, Santoro N, Elkind-Hirsch K, et al. Postmenopausal dehydroepiandrosterone administration increases free insulin-like growth factor-I and decreases high-density lipoprotein: a six-month trial. *Fertil Steril* 1998;70(1):107–110.
19. Casson PR, Faquin LC, Stentz FB, et al. Replacement of dehydroepiandrosterone enhances T-lymphocyte insulin binding in postmenopausal women. *Fertil Steril* 1995;63:1027–1031.
20. Labrie F, Diamond P, Cusan L, et al. Effect of 12-month dehydroepiandrosterone replacement therapy on bone, vagina, and endometrium in postmenopausal women. *J Clin Endocrinol Metab* 1997;82:3498–3505.
21. Morales AJ, Nolan J, Nelson JC, et al. Effects of replacement dose of dehydroepiandrosterone in men and women of advancing age. *J Clin Endocrinol Metab* 1994;78:1360–1367.
22. Mortola JF, Yen SSC. The effects of oral dehydroepiandrosterone on endocrine-metabolic parameters in postmenopausal women. *J Clin Endocrinol Metab* 1990;71:696–704.
23. Düker E-M, Kopanski L, Jarry H, et al. Effects of extracts from *Cimicifuga racemosa* on gonadotropin release in menopausal women and ovariectomized rats. *Planta Med* 1991;57:420–424.
24. Foster S. Black cohosh: cimicifuga racemosa—a literature review. *Herbal Gram* 1999(Winter):35–49.
25. Hirata JD, Swiersz LM, Zell B, et al. Does dong quai have estrogenic effects in postmenopausal women? A double-blind, placebo-controlled trial. *Fertil Steril* 1997;68:981–986.

Appendix. **THE PERIODIC HEALTH EXAMINATION: AGE-SPECIFIC CHARTS**

Table 1. Birth to 10 years

Interventions Considered and Recommended for the Periodic Health Examination	Leading Causes of Death Conditions originating in perinatal period Congenital anomalies Sudden infant death syndrome (SIDS) Unintentional injuries (non-motor vehicle) Motor vehicle injuries

INTERVENTIONS FOR THE GENERAL POPULATION

SCREENING
Height and weight
Blood pressure
Vision screen (age 3–4 yr)
Hemoglobinopathy screen (birth)[1]
Phenylalanine level (birth)[2]
T_4 and/or TSH (birth)[3]

COUNSELING
Injury Prevention
Child safety car seats (age <5 yr)
Lap-shoulder belts (age ≥5 yr)
Bicycle helmet; avoid bicycling
   near traffic
Smoke detector, flame retardant
   sleepwear
Hot water heater temperature
   <120–130°F
Window/stair guards, pool fence
Safe storage of drugs, toxic
   substances, firearms & matches
Syrup of ipecac, poison control
   phone number
CPR training for parents/caretakers

Diet and Exercise
Breast-feeding, iron-enriched
   formula and foods
   (infants & toddlers)
Limit fat & cholesterol; maintain caloric
   balance; emphasize grains, fruits,
   vegetables (age ≥2 yr)
Regular physical activity*

Substance Use
Effects of passive smoking*
Anti-tobacco message*

Dental Health
Regular visits to dental care provider*
Floss, brush with fluoride toothpaste daily*
Advice about baby bottle tooth decay*

IMMUNIZATIONS
Diphtheria-tetanus-pertussis (DTP)[4]
Oral poliovirus (OPV)[5]
Measles-mumps-rubella (MMR)[6]
H. influenzae type b (Hib) conjugate[7]
Hepatitis B[8]
Varicella[9]

CHEMOPROPHYLAXIS
Ocular prophylaxis (birth)

INTERVENTIONS FOR HIGH-RISK POPULATIONS

POPULATION	POTENTIAL INTERVENTIONS (See detailed high-risk definitions)
Preterm or low birth weight	Hemoglobin/hematocrit (HR1)
Infants of mothers at risk for HIV	HIV testing (HR2)
Low income; immigrants	Hemoglobin/hematocrit (HR1); PPD (HR3)
TB contacts	PPD (HR3)
Native American/Alaska Native	Hemoglobin/hematocrit (HR1); PPD (HR3); hepatitis A vaccine (HR4); pneumococcal vaccine (HR5)
Travelers to developing countries	Hepatitis A vaccine (HR4)
Residents of long-term care facilities	PPD (HR3); hepatitis A vaccine (HR4); influenza vaccine (HR6)
Certain chronic medical conditions	PPD (HR3); pneumococcal vaccine (HR5); influenza vaccine (HR6)
Increased individual or community lead exposure	Blood lead level (HR7)
Inadequate water fluoridation	Daily fluoride supplement (HR8)
Family h/o skin cancer; nevi; fair skin, eyes, hair	Avoid excess/midday sun, use protective clothing* (HR9)

[1]Whether screening should be universal or targeted to high-risk groups will depend on the proportion of high-risk individuals in the screening area, and other considerations. [2]If done during first 24 hr of life, repeat by age 2 wk. [3]Optimally between day 2 and 6, but in all cases before newborn nursery discharge. [4]2, 4, 6, and 12–18 mo; once between ages 4–6 yr (DTaP may be used at 15 mo and older). [5]2, 4, 6–18 mo; once between ages 4–6 yr. [6]12–15 mo and 4–6 yr. [7]2, 4, 6 and 12–15 mo; no dose needed at 6 mo if PRP-OMP vaccine is used for first 2 doses. [8]Birth, 1 mo, 5 mo; or, 0–2 mo, 1–2 mo later, and 6–18 mo. If not done in infancy: current visit, and 1 and 6 mo later. [9]12–18 mo; or older child without hx of chickenpox or previous immunization. Include information on risk in adulthood, duration of immunity, and potential need for booster doses.

*The ability of clinician counseling to influence this behavior is unproven.

OVERVIEW

HR1 = Infants age 6–12 mo who are: living in poverty, Black, Native American or Alaska Native, immigrants from developing countries, preterm or low birth weight infants, or infants whose principal dietary intake is unfortified cow's milk.

HR2 = Infants born to high-risk mothers whose HIV status is unknown. Women at high risk include: past or present injection drug use; persons who exchange sex for money or drugs, and their sex partners; injection drug-using, bisexual, or HIV-positive sex partners currently or in past; persons seeking treatment for STDs; blood transfusion during 1978–1985.

HR3 = Persons infected with HIV, close contacts of persons with known or suspected TB, persons with medical risk factors associated with TB, immigrants from countries with high TB prevalence, medically underserved low-income populations (including homeless), residents of long-term care facilities.

HR4 = Persons ≥2 yr living in or traveling to areas where the disease is endemic and where periodic outbreaks occur (e.g., countries with high or intermediate endemicity; certain Alaska Native, Pacific Island, Native American, and religious communities). Consider for institutionalized children aged ≥2 yr. Clinicians should also consider local epidemiology.

HR5 = Immunocompetent persons ≥2 yr with certain medical conditions, including chronic cardiac or pulmonary disease, diabetes mellitus, and anatomic asplenia. Immunocompetent persons ≥2 yr living in high-risk environments or social settings (e.g., certain Native American and Alaska Native populations).

HR6 = Annual vaccination of children ≥6 mo who are residents of chronic care facilities or who have chronic cardiopulmonary disorders, metabolic diseases (including diabetes mellitus), hemoglobinopathies, immunosuppression, or renal dysfunction.

HR7 = Children about age 12 mo who: 1) live in communities in which the prevalence of lead levels requiring individual intervention, including residential lead hazard control or chelation, is high or undefined; 2) live in or frequently visit a home built before 1950 with dilapidated paint or with recent or ongoing renovation or remodeling; 3) have close contact with a person who has an elevated lead level; 4) live near lead industry or heavy traffic; 5) live with someone whose job or hobby involves lead exposure; 6) use lead-based pottery; or 7) take traditional ethnic remedies that contain lead.

HR8 = Children living in areas with inadequate water fluoridation (<0.6 ppm).

HR9 = Persons with a family history of skin cancer; a large number of moles; atypical moles; poor tanning ability; or light skin, hair, and eye color.

Table 2. Ages 11–24 years

Interventions Considered and Recommended for the Periodic Health Examination	Leading Causes of Death Motor vehicle/other unintentional injuries Homicide/Suicide Malignant neoplasms Heart diseases

INTERVENTIONS FOR THE GENERAL POPULATION

SCREENING
Height & weight
Blood pressure[1]
Papanicolaou (Pap) test[2] (females)
Chlamydia screen[3] (females <20 yr)
Rubella serology or vaccination hx[4]
    (females > 12 yr)
Assess for problem drinking

COUNSELING
Injury Prevention
Lap/shoulder belts
Bicycle/motorcycle/ATV helmets*
Smoke detector*
Safe storage/removal of firearms*

Substance Use
Avoid tobacco use
Avoid underage drinking & illicit
    drug use*
Avoid alcohol/drug use while
    driving, swimming, boating, etc.*

Sexual Behavior
STD prevention: abstinence*; avoid high-risk behavior*; condoms/female barrier with spermicide*
Unintended pregnancy: contraception

Diet and Exercise
Limit fat & cholesterol; maintain caloric balance;
    emphasize grains, fruits, vegetables
Adequate calcium intake (females)
Regular physical activity*

Dental Health
Regular visits to dental care provider*
Floss, brush with fluoride toothpaste daily*

IMMUNIZATIONS
Tetanus-diphtheria (Td) boosters (11–16 yr)
Hepatitis B[5]
MMR (11–12 yr)[6]
Varicella (11–12 yr)[7]
Rubella[4] (females > 12 yr)

CHEMOPROPHYLAXIS
Multivitamin with folic acid (females
    planning/capable of pregnancy)

INTERVENTIONS FOR HIGH-RISK POPULATIONS

POPULATION	POTENTIAL INTERVENTIONS (See detailed high-risk definitions)
High-risk sexual behavior	RPR/VDRL (HR1); screen for gonorrhea (female) (HR2), HIV (HR3), chlamydia (female) (HR4); hepatitis A vaccine (HR5)
Injection or street drug use	RPR/VDRL (HR1); HIV screen (HR3); hepatitis A vaccine (HR5); PPD (HR6); advice to reduce infection risk (HR7)
TB contacts; immigrants; low income	PPD (HR6)
Native Americans/Alaska Natives	Hepatitis A vaccine (HR5); PPD (HR6); pneumococcal vaccine (HR8)
Travelers to developing countries	Hepatitis A vaccine (HR5)
Certain chronic medical conditions	PPD (HR6); pneumococcal vaccine (HR8); influenza vaccine (HR9)
Settings where adolescents and young adults congregate	Second MMR (HR10)
Susceptible to varicella, measles, mumps	Varicella vaccine (HR11); MMR (HR12)
Blood transfusion between 1978–1985	HIV screen (HR3)
Institutionalized persons; health care/lab workers	Hepatitis A vaccine (HR5); PPD (HR6); influenza vaccine (HR9)
Family h/o skin cancer; nevi; fair skin, eyes, hair	Avoid excess/midday sun, use protective clothing* (HR13)
Prior pregnancy with neural tube defect	Folic acid 4.0 mg (HR14)
Inadequate water fluoridation	Daily fluoride supplement (HR15)

[1]Periodic BP for persons aged ≥21 yr. [2]If sexually active at present or in the past: q ≤ 3 yr. If sexual history is unreliable, begin Pap tests at age 18 yr. [3]If sexually active. [4]Serologic testing, documented vaccination history, and routine vaccination against rubella (preferably with MMR) are equally acceptable alternatives. [5]If not previously immunized: current visit, 1 and 6 mo later. [6]If no previous second dose of MMR. [7]If susceptible to chickenpox.

* The ability of clinician counseling to influence this behavior is unproven.

OVERVIEW

HR1 = Persons who exchange sex for money or drugs, and their sex partners; persons with other STDs (including HIV); and sexual contacts of persons with active syphilis. Clinicians should also consider local epidemiology.

HR2 = Females who have two or more sex partners in the last year; a sex partner with multiple sexual contacts; exchanged sex for money or drugs; or a history of repeated episodes of gonorrhea. Clinicians should also consider local epidemiology.

HR3 = Males who had sex with males after 1975; past or present injection drug use; persons who exchange sex for money or drugs, and their sex partners; injection drug-using, bisexual, or HIV-positive sex partner currently or in the past; blood transfusion during 1978–1985; persons seeking treatment for STDs. Clinicians should also consider local epidemiology.

HR4 = Sexually active females with multiple risk factors including: history of prior STD; new or multiple sex partners; age under 25; nonuse or inconsistent use of barrier contraceptives; cervical ectopy. Clinicians should consider local epidemiology of the disease in identifying other high-risk groups.

HR5 = Persons living in, traveling to, or working in areas where the disease is endemic and where periodic outbreaks occur (e.g., countries with high or intermediate endemicity; certain Alaska Native, Pacific Island, Native American, and religious communities); men who have sex with men; injection or street drug users. Vaccine may be considered for institutionalized persons and workers in these institutions, military personnel, and day-care, hospital, and laboratory workers. Clinicians should also consider local epidemiology.

HR6 = HIV positive, close contacts of persons with known or suspected TB, health care workers, persons with medical risk factors associated with TB, immigrants from countries with high TB prevalence, medically underserved low-income populations (including homeless), alcoholics, injection drug users, and residents of long-term care facilities.

HR7 = Persons who continue to inject drugs.

HR8 = Immunocompetent persons with certain medical conditions, including chronic cardiac or pulmonary disease, diabetes mellitus, and anatomic asplenia. Immunocompetent persons who live in high-risk environments or social settings (e.g., certain Native American and Alaska Native populations).

HR9 = Annual vaccination of residents of chronic care facilities; persons with chronic cardiopulmonary disorders, metabolic diseases (including diabetes mellitus), hemoglobinopathies, immunosuppression, or renal dysfunction; and health care providers for high-risk patients.

HR10 = Adolescents and young adults in settings where such individuals congregate (e.g., high schools and colleges), if they have not previously received a second dose.

HR11 = Healthy persons aged ≥13 yr without a history of chickenpox or previous immunization. Consider serologic testing for presumed susceptible persons aged ≥13 yr.

HR12 = Persons born after 1956 who lack evidence of immunity to measles or mumps (e.g., documented receipt of live vaccine on or after the first birthday, laboratory evidence of immunity, or a history of physician-diagnosed measles or mumps).

HR13 = Persons with a family or personal history of skin cancer; a large number of moles; atypical moles; poor tanning ability; or light skin, hair, and eye color.

HR14 = Women with prior pregnancy affected by neural tube defect who are planning pregnancy.

HR15 = Persons aged <17 yr living in areas with inadequate water fluoridation (<0.6 ppm).

Table 3. Ages 25–64 years

Interventions Considered and Recommended for the Periodic Health Examination	Leading Causes of Death Malignant neoplasms Heart diseases Motor vehicle and other unintentional injuries HIV infection Suicide and homicide

INTERVENTIONS FOR THE GENERAL POPULATION

SCREENING
Blood pressure
Height and weight
Total blood cholesterol
   (men age 35–65, women
   age 45–65)
Papanicolaou (Pap) test (women)[1]
Fecal occult blood test[2] and/or
   sigmoidoscopy (≥50 yr)
Mammogram ± clinical breast
   exam[3] (women 50–69 yr)
Assess for problem drinking
Rubella serology or vaccination hx[4]
   (women of childbearing age)

COUNSELING
Substance Use
Tobacco cessation
Avoid alcohol/drug use while
   driving, swimming, boating, etc.

Diet and Exercise
Limit fat & cholesterol; maintain
   caloric balance; emphasize
   grains, fruits, vegetables
Adequate calcium intake (women)
Regular physical activity*

Injury Prevention
Lap/shoulder belts
Motorcycle/bicycle/ATV helmets*
Smoke detector
Safe storage/removal of firearms*

Sexual Behavior
STD prevention: avoid high-risk behavior*; con-
   doms/female barrier with spermicide
Unintended pregnancy: contraception

Dental Health
Regular visits to dental care provider*
Floss, brush with fluoride toothpaste daily*

IMMUNIZATIONS
Tetanus-diphtheria (Td) boosters
Rubella[4] (women of childbearing age)

CHEMOPROPHYLAXIS
Multivitamin with folic acid (women planning or capable of pregnancy)
Discuss hormone prophylaxis (peri- and postmenopausal women)

INTERVENTIONS FOR HIGH-RISK POPULATIONS

POPULATION	POTENTIAL INTERVENTIONS (See detailed high-risk definitions)
High-risk sexual behavior	RPR/VDRL (HR1); screen for gonorrhea (female) (HR2), HIV (HR3), chlamydia (female) (HR4); hepatitis B vaccine (HR5); hepatitis A vaccine (HR6)
Injection or street drug use	RPR/VDRL (HR1); HIV screen (HR3); hepatitis B vaccine (HR5); hepatitis A vaccine (HR6); PPD (HR7); advice to reduce infection risk (HR8)
Low income; TB contacts; immigrants; alcoholics	PPD (HR7)
Native Americans/Alaska Natives	Hepatitis A vaccine (HR6); PPD (HR7); pneumococcal vaccine (HR9)
Travelers to developing countries	Hepatitis B vaccine (HR5); hepatitis A vaccine (HR6)
Certain chronic medical conditions	PPD (HR7); pneumococcal vaccine (HR9); influenza vaccine (HR10)
Blood product recipients	HIV screen (HR3); hepatitis B vaccine (HR5)
Susceptible to measles, mumps, or varicella	MMR (HR11); varicella vaccine (HR12)
Institutionalized persons	Hepatitis A vaccine (HR6); PPD (HR7); pneumococcal vaccine (HR9); influenza vaccine (HR10)
Health care/lab workers	Hepatitis B vaccine (HR5); hepatitis A vaccine (HR6); PPD (HR7); influenza vaccine (HR10)
Family h/o skin cancer; fair skin, eyes, hair	Avoid excess/midday sun, use protective clothing* (HR13)
Previous pregnancy with neural tube defect	Folic acid 4.0 mg (HR14)

[1]Women who are or have been sexually active and who have a cervix; q ≤ 3 yr. [2]Annually. [3]Mammogram q1–2 yr, or mammogram q1–2 yr with annual clinical breast examination. [4]Serologic testing, documented vaccination history, and routine vaccination (preferably with MMR) are equally acceptable alternatives.

*The ability of clinician counseling to influence this behavior is unproven.

OVERVIEW

HR1 = Persons who exchange sex for money or drugs, and their sex partners; persons with other STDs (including HIV); and sexual contacts of persons with active syphilis. Clinicians should also consider local epidemiology.

HR2 = Women who exchange sex for money or drugs, or who have had repeated episodes of gonorrhea. Clinicians should also consider local epidemiology.

HR3 = Men who had sex with men after 1975; past or present injection drug use; persons who exchange sex for money or drugs, and their sex partners; injection drug-using, bisexual, or HIV-positive sex partner currently or in the past; blood transfusion during 1978–1985; persons seeking treatment for STDs. Clinicians should also consider local epidemiology.

HR4 = Sexually active women with multiple risk factors including: history of STD; new or multiple sex partners; nonuse or inconsistent use of barrier contraceptives; cervical ectopy. Clinicians should also consider local epidemiology.

HR5 = Blood product recipients (including hemodialysis patients), persons with frequent occupational exposure to blood or blood products, men who have sex with men, injection drug users and their sex partners, persons with multiple recent sex partners, persons with other STDs (including HIV), travelers to countries with endemic hepatitis B.

HR6 = Persons living in, traveling to, or working in areas where the disease is endemic and where periodic outbreaks occur (e.g., countries with high or intermediate endemicity; certain Alaska Native, Pacific Island, Native American, and religious communities); men who have sex with men; injection or street drug users. Consider for institutionalized persons and workers in these institutions, military personnel, and day-care, hospital, and laboratory workers. Clinicians should also consider local epidemiology.

HR7 = HIV positive, close contacts of persons with known or suspected TB, health care workers, persons with medical risk factors associated with TB, immigrants from countries with high TB prevalence, medically underserved low-income populations (including homeless), alcoholics, injection drug users, and residents of long-term care facilities.

HR8 = Persons who continue to inject drugs.

HR9 = Immunocompetent institutionalized persons aged ≥50 yr and immunocompetent persons with certain medical conditions, including chronic cardiac or pulmonary disease, diabetes mellitus, and anatomic asplenia. Immunocompetent persons who live in high-risk environments or social settings (e.g., certain Native American and Alaska Native populations).

HR10 = Annual vaccination of residents of chronic care facilities; persons with chronic cardiopulmonary disorders, metabolic diseases (including diabetes mellitus), hemoglobinopathies, immunosuppression, or renal dysfunction; and health care providers for high-risk patients.

HR11 = Persons born after 1956 who lack evidence of immunity to measles or mumps (e.g., documented receipt of live vaccine on or after the first birthday, laboratory evidence of immunity, or a history of physician-diagnosed measles or mumps).

HR12 = Healthy adults without a history of chickenpox or previous immunization. Consider serologic testing for presumed susceptible adults.

HR13 = Persons with a family or personal history of skin cancer; a large number of moles; atypical moles; poor tanning ability; or light skin, hair, and eye color.

HR14 = Women with previous pregnancy affected by neural tube defect who are planning pregnancy.

Table 4. Age 65 and older

Interventions Considered and Recommended for the Periodic Health Examination	Leading Causes of Death
	Heart diseases
	Malignant neoplasms (lung, colorectal, breast)
	Cerebrovascular disease
	Chronic obstructive pulmonary disease
	Pneumonia and influenza

INTERVENTIONS FOR THE GENERAL POPULATION

SCREENING
Blood pressure
Height and weight
Fecal occult blood test[1] and/or
  sigmoidoscopy
Mammogram ± clinical breast
  exam[2] (women ≤69 yr)
Papanicolaou (Pap) test (women)[3]
Vision screening
Assess for hearing impairment
Assess for problem drinking

COUNSELING
Substance Use
Tobacco cessation
Avoid alcohol/drug use while
  driving, swimming, boating, etc.*

Diet and Exercise
Limit fat & cholesterol; maintain
  caloric balance; emphasize
  grains, fruits, vegetables
Adequate calcium intake (women)
Regular physical activity*

Injury Prevention
Lap/shoulder belts
Motorcycle and bicycle helmets*
Fall prevention*
Safe storage/removal of firearms*
Smoke detector*
Set hot water heater to <120–130°F*
CPR training for household members

Dental Health
Regular visits to dental care provider*
Floss, brush with fluoride toothpaste daily*

Sexual Behavior
STD prevention: avoid high-risk sexual
  behavior; use condoms

IMMUNIZATIONS
Pneumococcal vaccine
Influenza[1]
Tetanus-diphtheria (Td) boosters

CHEMOPROPHYLAXIS
Discuss hormone prophylaxis (women)

INTERVENTIONS FOR HIGH-RISK POPULATIONS

POPULATION	POTENTIAL INTERVENTIONS (See detailed high-risk definitions)
Institutionalized persons	PPD (HR1); hepatitis A vaccine (HR2); amantadine/rimantadine (HR4)
Chronic medical conditions; TB contacts; low income; immigrants; alcoholics	PPD (HR1)
Persons ≥75 yr; or ≥70 yr with risk factors for falls	Fall prevention intervention (HR5)
Cardiovascular disease risk factors	Consider cholesterol screening (HR6)
Family h/o skin cancer; nevi; fair skin, eyes, hair	Avoid excess/midday sun, use protective clothing* (HR7)
Native Americans/Alaska Natives	PPD (HR1); hepatitis A vaccine (HR2)
Travelers to developing countries	Hepatitis A vaccine (HR2); hepatitis B vaccine (HR8)
Blood product recipients	HIV screen (HR3); hepatitis B vaccine (HR8)
High-risk sexual behavior	Hepatitis A vaccine (HR2); HIV screen (HR3); hepatitis B vaccine (HR8); RPR/VDRL (HR9)
Injection or street drug use	PPD (HR1); hepatitis A vaccine (HR2); HIV screen (HR3); hepatitis B vaccine (HR8); RPR/VDRL (HR9); advice to reduce infection risk (HR10)
Health care/lab workers	PPD (HR1); hepatitis A vaccine (HR2); amantadine/rimantadine (HR4); hepatitis B vaccine (HR8)
Persons susceptible to varicella	Varicella vaccine (HR11)

[1]Annually. [2]Mammogram q1–2 yr, or mammogram q1–2 yr with annual clinical breast exam. [3]All women who are or have been sexually active and who have a cervix: q ≤ 3 yr. Consider discontinuation of testing after age 65 yr if previous regular screening with consistently normal results.

*The ability of clinician counseling to influence this behavior is unproven.

OVERVIEW

HR1 = HIV positive, close contacts of persons with known or suspected TB, health care workers, persons with medical risk factors associated with TB, immigrants from countries with high TB prevalence, medically underserved low-income populations (including homeless), alcoholics, injection drug users, and residents of long-term care facilities.

HR2 = Persons living in, traveling to, or working in areas where the disease is endemic and where periodic outbreaks occur (e.g., countries with high or intermediate endemicity; certain Alaska Native, Pacific Island, Native American, and religious communities); men who have sex with men; injection or street drug users. Consider for institutionalized persons and workers in these institutions, and day-care, hospital, and laboratory workers. Clinicians should also consider local epidemiology.

HR3 = Men who had sex with men after 1975; past or present injection drug use; persons who exchange sex for money or drugs, and their sex partners; injection drug-using, bisexual, or HIV-positive sex partner currently or in the past; blood transfusion during 1978–1985; persons seeking treatment for STDs. Clinicians should also consider local epidemiology.

HR4 = Consider for persons who have not received influenza vaccine or are vaccinated late; when the vaccine may be ineffective due to major antigenic changes in the virus; for unvaccinated persons who provide home care for high-risk persons; to supplement protection provided by vaccine in persons who are expected to have a poor antibody response; and for high-risk persons in whom the vaccine is contraindicated.

HR5 = Persons aged 75 years and older; or aged 70–74 with one or more additional risk factors including; use of certain psychoactive and cardiac medications (e.g., benzodiazepines, antihypertensives); use of ≥ 4 prescription medications; impaired cognition, strength, balance, or gait. Intensive individualized home-based multifactorial fall prevention intervention is recommended in settings where adequate resources are available to deliver such services.

HR6 = Although evidence is insufficient to recommend routine screening in elderly persons, clinicians should consider cholesterol screening on a case-by-case basis for persons ages 65–75 with additional risk factors (e.g., smoking, diabetes, or hypertension).

HR7 = Persons with a family or personal history of skin cancer; a large number of moles; atypical moles; poor tanning ability; or light skin, hair, and eye color.

HR8 = Blood product recipients (including hemodialysis patients), persons with frequent occupational exposure to blood or blood products, men who have sex with men, injection drug users and their sex partners, persons with multiple recent sex partners, persons with other STDs (including HIV), travelers to countries with endemic hepatitis B.

HP9 = Persons who exchange sex for money or drugs and their sex partners; persons with other STDs (including HIV); and sexual contacts of persons with active syphilis. Clinicians should also consider local epidemiology.

HR10 = Persons who continue to inject drugs.

HR11 = Healthy adults without a history of chickenpox or previous immunization. Consider serologic testing for presumed susceptible adults.

Table 5. Pregnant women**

Interventions Considered and Recommended for the Periodic Health Examination

INTERVENTIONS FOR THE GENERAL POPULATION

SCREENING
First visit
Blood pressure
Hemoglobin/hematocrit
Hepatitis B surface antigen (HBsAg)
RPR/VDRL
Chlamydia screen (<25 yr)
Rubella serology or vaccination history
D(Rh) typing, antibody screen
Offer CVS (<13 wk)[1] or amniocentesis
  (15–18 wk)[1] (age ≥35 yr)
Offer hemoglobinopathy screening
Assess for problem or risk drinking
Offer HIV screening[2]

Follow-up visits
Blood pressure
Urine culture (12–16 wk)

Offer amniocentesis (15–18 wk)[1]
  (age ≥35 yr)
Offer multiple marker testing[1] (15–18 wk)
Offer serum a-fetoprotein[1] (16–18 wk)

COUNSELING
Tobacco cessation; effects of passive
  smoking
Alcohol/other drug use
Nutrition, including adequate calcium
  intake
Encourage breastfeeding
Lap/shoulder belts
Infant safety car seats
STD prevention: avoid high-risk sexual
  behavior*; use condoms*

CHEMOPROPHYLAXIS
Multivitamin with folic acid[3]

INTERVENTIONS FOR HIGH-RISK POPULATIONS

POPULATION	POTENTIAL INTERVENTIONS (See detailed high-risk definitions)
High-risk sexual behavior	Screen for chlamydia (1st visit) (HR1), gonorrhea (1st visit) (HR2), HIV (1st visit) (HR3); HBsAg (3rd trimester) (HR4); RPR/VDRL (3rd trimester) (HR5)
Blood transfusion 1978–1985	HIV screen (1st visit) (HR3)
Injection drug use	HIV screen (HR3); HBsAg (3rd trimester) (HR4); advice to reduce infection risk (HR6)
Unsensitized D-negative women	D(Rh) antibody testing (24–28 wk) (HR7)
Risk factors for Down syndrome	Offer CVS[1] (1st trimester), amniocentesis[1] (15–18 wk) (HR8)
Prior pregnancy with neural tube defect	Offer amniocentesis[1] (15–18 wk), folic acid 4.0 mg[3] (HR9)

[1]Women with access to counseling and follow-up services, reliable standardized laboratories, skilled high-resolution ultrasound, and, for those receiving serum marker tasting, amniocentesis capabilities. [2]Universal screening is recommended for areas (states, counties, or cities) with an increased prevalence of HIV infection among pregnant women. In low-prevalence areas, the choice between universal and targeted screening may depend on other considerations. [3]Beginning at least 1 mo before conception and continuing through the first trimester.

*The ability of clinician counseling to influence this behavior is unproven.
**See Tables 2 and 3 for other preventive services recommended for women of childbearing age.

OVERVIEW

HR1 = Women with history of STD or new or multiple sex partners. Clinicians should also consider local epidemiology. Chlamydia screen should be repeated in 3rd trimester if at continued risk.

HR2 = Women under age 25 with two or more sex partners in the last year, or whose sex partner has multiple sexual contacts; women who exchange sex for money or drugs; and women with a history of repeated episodes of gonorrhea. Clinicians should also consider local epidemiology. Gonorrhea screen should be repeated in the 3rd trimester if at continued risk.

HR3 = In areas where universal screening is not performed due to low prevalence of HIV infection, pregnant women with the following individual risk factors should be screened; past or present injection drug use; women who exchange sex for money or drugs; injection drug-using, bisexual, or HIV-positive sex partner currently or in the past; blood transfusion during 1978–1985; persons seeking treatment for STDs.

HR4 = Women who are initially HBsAg-negative who are at high risk due to injection drug use, suspected exposure to hepatitis B during pregnancy, multiple sex partners.

HR5 = Women who exchange sex for money or drugs, women with other STDs (including HIV), and sexual contacts of persons with active syphilis. Clinicians should also consider local epidemiology.

HR6 = Women who continue to inject drugs.

HR7 = Unsensitized D-negative women.

HR8 = Prior pregnancy affected by Down syndrome, advanced maternal age (≥35 yr), known carriage of chromosome rearrangement.

HR9 = Women with previous pregnancy affected by neural tube defect.

SUBJECT INDEX

Page numbers in italics indicate figures; those followed by t indicate tabular material.